Life Support Systems Design

Diving and Hyperbaric Applications

M. L. Nuckols, Ph.D., PE
U. S. Naval Academy
Annapolis, MD

Ace J. Sarich, MSc, PE
Marine Acoustics, Inc.
Arlington, VA

Wayne C. Tucker, Ph.D.
Naval Undersea Warfare Center
Newport, RI

PEARSON CUSTOM PUBLISHING

Cover art: Daniel Frolich

Printed in the United States of America

10 9 8 7 6 5 4 3 2

ISBN 0-536-59616-6
BA 96161

 PEARSON CUSTOM PUBLISHING
75 Arlington Street, Boston, MA 02116
A Pearson Education Company

Table of Contents

Acknowledgments

The authors would like to express their sincere appreciation to the Production and Editorial staff at Simon & Schuster Publishing Company for their cooperation in the preparation for publication of this manuscript. They would also like to thank the many research organizations, industrial manufacturers and all those who are actively involved in the development of systems to enhance our ability to do work underwater. Many of these organizations contributed valuable illustrations and technical information for this book. The authors also wish to particularly thank Hilbert Schenck for generously providing his assistance in the preparation of the chapter on humidity control.

To the target audience of this book, the students pursuing a career of ocean exploration and research, the authors gratefully acknowledge their valuable inputs during past courses in which the notes making up this manuscript where used. Their helpful suggestions for clarifying this material are appreciated. These students continue to provide the enthusiasm and motivation to us all to keep apace of this rapidly advancing technology.

Preface

Welcome to my 1-atmosphere diving bell in which we will be making a hypothetical observation dive to 300 feet beneath the ocean's surface to survey the wreckage of the *Andrea Doria*. You will notice that this capsule, although only eight feet in diameter, contains most of the comforts of home. The atmosphere inside this capsule is indistinguishable from the air in which we breath on the surface, thanks to an environmental control system which continually monitors and adjusts the temperature and humidity to satisfy our needs.

We have just reached our destination when for some unexplained reason we have apparently suffered a complete shutdown of our main power supply and primary life support systems! It appears that we have become entangled in some type of obstacle on the bottom and severed our power cable which connects us to the surface. Please don't Panic!!

Auxiliary battery power is presently supplying the eerie, low intensity lighting in our sealed compartment. These batteries should last for at least 48 hours. It is at least some consolation to know that our capsule having ½-inch thick walls, constructed of high-yield strength steel, will keep us from being crushed by the outside pressures which are over 10 times those inside.

Our immediate concern shifts to our supply of oxygen. Presently, our bodies are consuming approximately 0.3-0.5 liters per minute to support our resting metabolic functions. This oxygen is being taken from the capsule atmosphere, which if not replenished, will slowly reduce the oxygen content in this atmosphere from its initial value of approximately 21% by volume. If the oxygen content is allowed to drop to 16%, we will begin experiencing labored breathing, confusion, and finally unconsciousness. Even if we didn't replenish this atmosphere with fresh oxygen, at the rate at which we are consuming oxygen we should have nearly 6 hours before these symptoms become noticeable, and up to 13 hours before we are unconscious. We fortunately brought along an additional supply to extend these times by 12 hours. But by all means, please stay calm as increased anxiety will only increase our oxygen consumption rates and
thus, reduce these times considerably.

But wait; even of more concern is the buildup of carbon dioxide which our environmental sensors are detecting. Since we no longer have power to operate the ventilation fans in our capsule, the air from our atmosphere is no longer being forced through the carbon dioxide absorption system which we have on board. The carbon dioxide which our bodies are generating through normal metabolism is now being dumped into our capsule environment. As in the case of oxygen, our bodies are tolerant of only a slight variation in the carbon dioxide content in the air which we breathe. Even though we can tolerate short exposures at carbon dioxide levels of up to 3%-4%, we will begin experiencing respiratory discomfort, a feeling of air hunger, and perhaps dizziness and nausea when breathing only 1%-2% carbon dioxide for extended durations; at 6%, we will most assuredly be on the brink of unconscious. Based on our present rates of carbon dioxide generation, our capsule environment is predicted to reach 2% levels of CO_2 in approximately 2-3/4 hours and 6% in slightly over 6 hours. Don't be surprised though if you experience a headache and reduced sensory perceptions (hearing, seeing, etc) before these times are reached. Again, steady yourself; further anxiety will only speed up the timetable.

You say that it is getting cold? Unfortunately, the capsule is not insulated, and without the electrical heating system which was more than adequate when power was available, the temperature inside the capsule quickly reaches the surrounding water temperature of about 40° F. We need to try to stay as warm as possible, since any shivering will only increase our oxygen consumption and carbon dioxide generation rates.

One way that we can rewarm the cabin atmosphere and ward off the extremely uncomfortable consequences of being cold is to pressurize the bell with our emergency gas banks. By increasing the cabin pressure, we can immediately feel a renewed warmth, not unlike the rise in temperature that we see when inflating an automobile tire. If done in stages, we may have a chance to offset the continual heat loss from the bell to the surrounding water, and maintain a tolerable cabin temperature until rescue is made.

But, alas, the increase in cabin pressure is seen to offer only momentary relief from the extreme cold. The lack of insulation and immense heat sink provided by the ocean quickly dissipates all temperature excesses above the ambient water temperature. In addition, the increased cabin pressure has caused even further problems. The physiological responses of our bodies to the levels of carbon dioxide in the cabin are increased proportionately to increases in pressure. An environment having only 0.5% carbon dioxide will be as toxic to our bodies at a pressure of 10 atmospheres as when we breathe 5% carbon dioxide at surface pressure. The horrible consequences of breathing these toxic levels will only occur sooner!

Finally, the unwise, albeit desperate, act of pressurizing our cabin may have eliminated our last safe means of escape. By exposing our bodies to an ever increasing atmospheric pressure, we are in fact building up a decompression debt, just as the deep sea diver. The inert gases in our atmosphere are slowly being dissolved into our bodies. If allowed to continue, once our capsule is rescued and brought back to the surface, catastrophic results will await our bodies when the hatch is opened unless we are permitted a slow decompression. Otherwise, these dissolved gases will come out of solution too rapidly, causing bubbles to form in our body tissues and blood. Not unlike the diver experiencing decompression sickness, our symptoms will be pain in the joints, nausea, dizziness, possibly paralysis or even death. But of course slow decompression will be impossible since our oxygen supply is being depleted and our atmosphere is being contaminated with carbon dioxide. A resupply of electrical power appears to be our only hope!

Abrupt Environmental Changes vs Adaptation

The rather dramatic demonstration given above is intended to show what can happen when our bodies are rapidly put in a foreign environment without adequate life support. Our bodies can not tolerate abrupt changes in the environment in which we have grown to be accustomed. Through the ages living organisms have been able to make evolutionary changes in reaction to some environmental stress. For example, inhabitants of cold, arctic regions are reported to have adopted an increased resting metabolic rate (Brown et al, 1954) as a defense against the cold. Similarly, the famous Korean diving women (Ama), who are exposed daily to severe hypothermia (reduction of body temperature due to cold stress) have been reported to have increased resting metabolic rates in winter (Kang et al, 1963). Desert rodents have apparently developed an amazing water conservation mechanism in their airways to reduce the moisture leaving their bodies during respiration (Jackson ,Schmidt-Neilsen, 1964). In so doing, they are reported to sustain life in dry, arid climates without a source of drinking water. I would dare to say that our bodies could adapt to an environment containing 10% oxygen, rather than the 21% which we are presently accustomed, if that change occurred over the time span of many generations. After all, we were able to descend from liquid breathing animals, so say the evolutionists.

However, the abrupt changes that a diver sees as he descends into the deep; the astronaut sees in his space capsule or as he walks in space; the fireman sees as he fights a blazing inferno; or the crew of a submersible or hyperbaric chamber sees; demand adequate life support to sustain life.

As noted in the scenario above, in each case the oxygen supply and carbon dioxide removal requirements must be satisfied. Adequate thermal protection must be provided. Pressure equilibriums must be maintained. Sufficient food and water, and depending on the length of the mission, certain human comforts must be provided. Such is the mission of the life support systems engineer.

Book Objectives

An interdisciplinary field of study, underwater life support systems design requires the application of engineering principles with a knowledge of human physiology. Specifically, the study of life support systems design should have a strong background in the following areas:

a) human physiology related to respiration and the thermo-regulatory system
b) underwater physics including the interrelationship of pressure and temperature to gas volumes, their properties, and their solution in other materials
c) the chemistry involved in the absorption of gas constituents including carbon dioxide and other toxic contaminants
d) decompression theory required to predict the safe exposures to elevated pressure environments
e) pressure vessel design including design methods for exposures to both external and internal pressures
f) heat transfer including conduction, convection, and radiation modes
g) fluid dynamics involved in hydrostatic pressures and pipe flow
h) psychrometry at elevated pressures required to maintain adequate moisture levels in cabin environments

In addition to these basic fundamentals, the student should be exposed to the practical technological areas in the field of life support engineering including;

a) conventional options and designs in breathing apparatus design
b) environmental control systems (ECS) design
c) optional methods and the current state-of-the-art in thermal protection
d) gas storage and delivery systems

In this book, underwater physics, including the transport of light, heat, and gases in and about the diver are explored with particular emphasis on the effects of hyperbaric exposures to the diver's ability to function. An understanding of the uptake of inert gases in the human body at elevated pressures, and decompression theory and its practice are covered. Carbon dioxide absorption processes are reviewed and a systemic procedure for CO_2 scrubber design are studied. Hardware design methods for both conventional and saturation diving systems are presented, including the design of pressure vessels and environmental control systems for deep diving applications, and the design of shallow-water, open-circuit breathing apparatus.

Upon completion of this textbook, the student is intended to have a working knowledge of the engineering principles and special vocabulary of the life support systems engineer. Once equipped with this knowledge, the student should be prepared to apply these fundamentals and conventional technologies to an exercise in creative design. This is best accomplished by requiring the student, either acting alone or as a member of a design team, to conceptually design a life support system for some specified application. The student should be encouraged to not be constrained by current technologies, but rather, he/she should be rewarded for applying his/her own creative abilities to the mission at hand. In so doing, the student can explore the potential of new methods or designs, while obtaining a fuller appreciation for the demands of a life support engineer.

Life Support Considerations

A Delicate Balance

Oxygen Consumption
0.25 - 3.6 SLPM
(0.05 - 0.7 lbm/hr)

Metabolic Heat Output
280 - 4800 Btu/hr
(82 - 1406 watts)

Thermal Constraints
Tcore = 36 - 38 C
Avg Skin Temp > 25 C
Net heat loss < 3 kcal/kg

Carbon Dioxide Output
0.2 - 2.9 SLPM
(0.05 - 0.75 lbm/hr)

Water Intake:
Drink 3.3 lb/day
Foods 1.5 lb/day
Metabolic   0.7 lb/day
    Total   5.5 lb/day

Water Output:
Urine   3.3 lb/day
Feces   0.2 lb/day
Resp/Sweat 2.0 lb/day
    Total   5.5 lb/day

1

Introduction to Diving and Hyperbaric Systems

Objectives

The objectives of this chapter are to:
- present a brief history of man's attempts to conduct useful work beneath the oceans
- introduce the student to the development of dive systems, emphasizing the interdisciplinary nature of the technologies involved in these developments
- discuss alternative options to do work underwater.

1.1   History of Diving

It is unknown when man first discovered he could hold his breath and go underwater, but the origins of diving can be traced back more than 5000 years. Early breathhold divers worked in water less than 100 feet deep and were harvesters of materials for use as food and trade such as shellfish, sponges, coral and mother-of-pearl.

Throughout the history of military conflicts, divers were used. Early breathhold skin divers cut anchor lines to set enemy ships adrift. They were also effective in punching holes in the bottoms of these ships and in building harbor defenses at home as well as destroying those of the enemy abroad. In 332 B.C. Alexander the Great not only sent divers to remove obstacles in the harbor of Tyre (Lebanon) but also

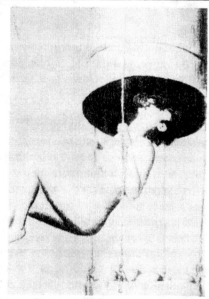

Figure 1-1: Early divers' air supply was simply an inverted, weighted barrel. (Courtesy of U.S. Navy)

went underwater himself to view the progress.

With the advent of commercial and military activities at sea came the inevitable need for salvage divers. Early salvage focused around the major shipping ports of the eastern Mediterranean. By the first century B.C., the first depth pay scale was established which recognized that effort and risk increased with depth. Divers working in 24 feet of water could claim one-half share of everything they recovered; while in 12 feet they kept one-third; and in 3 feet one-tenth. The incremental rewards with increasing depth motivated the development of operational capabilities at depth.

Early advances in diving focused on providing an air supply that would permit the diver to stay underwater longer than one or two minutes. The first such efforts attempted to use hollow tubes extending to the surface. Little was accomplished by the breathing tubes except as a tactic in military operations where they permitted an undetected approach to a military stronghold. It soon became apparent that it is impossible to breath from a tube to the surface from any depth below a few inches because of the force the water exerts on a diver's chest. This force increases with depth and is a major factor in diving. Any successful diving operation must overcome the pressure. Many imaginative devices were designed throughout history. However, since the problem of pressure underwater was not fully understood, most of the early designs were impractical.

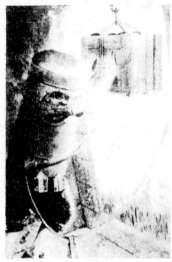

Figure 1-2: Later diver's dress was still an inverted barrel that the diver could walk in, but fresh air could be pumped from the surface. (Courtesy of U.S. Navy)

Possibly the earliest designs which foreshadowed later successful developments occurred in the 16th and 17th centuries. However, as well conceived as they might have been, these designs did not have the necessary supporting technology to be successful.

The earliest successful device which allowed divers to remain underwater for durations of hours rather than minutes was the diving bell. Early bells were literally bell-shaped wooden barrels with the bottom open to the sea.

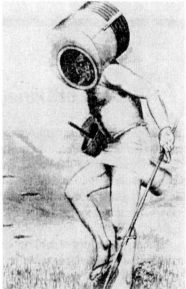

Figure 1-3: Some early concepts foreshadowed later developments but lacked the necessary supporting technology. (Courtesy of U.S. Navy)

The first reference to a practical diving bell was made in 1531. These tubs were large, strong inverted tubs weighted to sink in a vertical position. The air trapped inside would allow the diver to breath without returning to the surface. If the bell were positioned over the work, the diver could sometimes remain in the bell. More often, however, the diver would leave the bell holding his breath to work, and return to the bell to breathe. As CO_2 levels increased and oxygen percentage dropped, divers soon recognized that the "fouled" air in the bell would be unfit to breathe after a certain amount of time. Although they did not fully understand why, they knew the air must be replaced with fresh air to extend their time on the bottom.

In the 1680's a Massachusetts adventurer named William Phipps modified the diving bell by replenishing the diver's air supply with weighted inverted buckets. In 1690 Edmund Halley, for whom the comet is named also used a diving bell replenished with barrels in which he and four others remained at 60 feet for 1.5 hours. Later, Halley improved the bell and spent more than four hours at 65 feet.

In 1715 John Lethbridge developed a one-man enclosed "diving engine". The leather-coated barrel had a glass viewport and arm holes with water-tight sleeves. The Lethbridge suit was slung from a ship. Lethbridge achieved success with his invention while salvaging wrecks in Europe. He reported that he could dive to a maximum of 72 feet and remain underwater for 34 minutes.

The next significant advance in diving occurred at the turn of the 19th century with the development of a pump capable of delivering air under pressure. Credit is given to Augustus Siebe for developing the first practical diving dress. He was actually one of several who produced a successful apparatus at the same time. However, Siebe's modification of John and Charles Deane's patent diving dress sealed the helmet to the dress and collar by using a short waist-length suit which permitted exhaust air to escape under the hem. By 1840 Siebe had adopted a full-length waterproof suit and added an exhaust valve to the system. This is the direct ancestor of the standard deep sea diving dress which was used for more than 100 years for heavy work underwater.

With the ability for men to dive routinely to 60 or 70 feet and work for 6 or 7 hours a day, a new problem was noted that "of the seasoned divers, not a man escaped the repeated attacks of rheumatism and cold". Actually, what appeared to be rheumatism was, in fact, a symptom of a far more serious diver's disease -- decompression sickness.

At the same time improvements to a practical diving dress were being made, other inventors were improving the diving bell by adding high capacity air pumps. This eventually led to the construction of chambers large enough to permit several men to engage in dry work on the bottom and was a big advantage to the excavation of bridge footings or construction of tunnel sections. These so-called "caissons" (big box) were accessed through an air lock at the surface so that men, debris, or materials could be passed in and out while maintaining pressure inside.

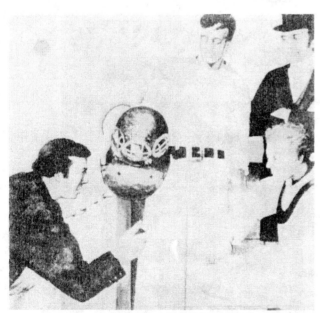

Figure 1-4: Augustus Siebe is credited with the first successful deep-sea diving dress. (Courtesy of U.S. Navy)

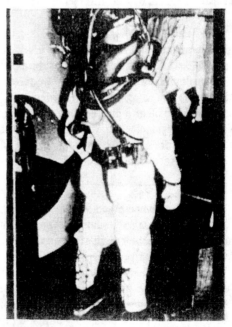

Figure 1-5: The introduction of helium to divers' breathing gases allowed deeper dives. (Courtesy of U.S. Navy)

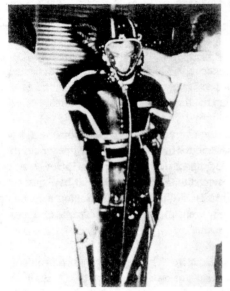

Figure 1-6: Lighter rigs for shallow water allowed somewhat more mobility. (Courtesy of U.S. Navy)

As caisson work was extended to greater operating pressures workers experienced more and more physiological problems which became so severe that fatalities were occurring with alarming frequency. The malady was originally named "caissons disease" but workers on the Brooklyn Bridge project in New York gave the sickness its most recognized name, "the bends", based on the contorted posture of the suffering worker.

The actual cause of the bends was first described in 1878 by French physiologist Paul Bert. Bert determined that breathing air under pressure forced quantities of nitrogen into solution in the blood and tissues. He determined that if pressure was reduced too quickly, the nitrogen could not be eliminated from the blood and tissues of the body in a natural manner, and bubbles would then form in the blood and tissues as the nitrogen came out of solution. The bubbles formed throughout the body caused the wide range of symptoms associated with the disease, including paralysis and death.

Bert recommended that the caisson workers return to the surface slowly while the atmospheric pressure was gradually reduced to surface conditions. His study led to an immediate improvement for the workers since they also discovered that pain could be relieved by returning to the pressure of the caisson. Within a few years, specifically designed "re-compression" chambers were used at job sites to control and treat the bends. Bert's recommendation that divers use a gradual but steady ascent was not a complete success. Some divers continued to suffer from the bends. Dives deeper than 120 feet repeatedly resulted in the bends and it was also noted that beyond 120 feet divers became markedly inefficient and often lost consciousness.

An English physiologist, J. S. Haldane, conducted experiments with Royal Navy divers from 1905 to 1907 and determined that part of the problem was simply due to the fact that divers were not ventilating their helmets properly. This poor ventilation resulted in the build up of high levels of carbon dioxide. Establishing a standard flow rate measured at the pressure of the diver and by providing pumps of sufficient capacity to maintain the flow solved this problem.

Haldane also composed a set of diving tables using stage decompression. Although they have been refined over the years, these tables remain the foundation of accepted practice in bringing a diver safely to the surface. Haldane's work extended the practical operating depth for air divers to slightly more than 200 feet. This limit was imposed by the ability of the hand pumps to provide the air supply at that time. Before long, more powerful pumps became available and divers experienced another malady at greater depths. In the 1920's the "rapture of the deep" was identified as

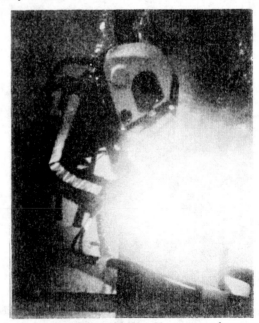

Figure 1-7: During World War II many underwater techniques such as welding were developed, and are still in use today. (Courtesy of U.S. Navy)

nitrogen narcosis where the diver becomes more and more intoxicated breathing nitrogen at higher and higher pressures. Special breathing mixtures were developed using helium and oxygen for breathing gases in deep diving.

While Siebe and others gave man the ability to remain underwater for extended periods with enough flexibility to do a significant amount of work, other inventors searched for methods to release the diver from the surface hose. The solution sought after was to provide the diver with his own portable air supply. The concept remained theoretical until technology was able to provide high pressure compressors and tanks of adequate strength to handle the high pressure needed to provide a practical air supply.

Historically, the development of self-contained breathing apparatus (SCUBA) has involved many significant inventions which, for the lack of supporting technology, could not be exploited. Two main paths were followed: open-circuit SCUBA; and closed-circuit SCUBA.

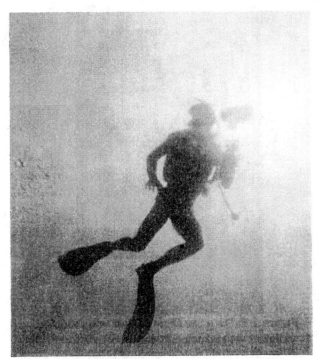

Figure 1-8: After World War II, open circuit SCUBA became available commercially. (Courtesy of U.S. Navy)

The first major component of open-circuit apparatus was designed by Benoist Rouquayrol in 1866. The demand regulator adjusted the flow of air from the tank to meet the breathing and pressure requirements of the diver. Since tanks of sufficient strength could not be built at the time, Rouquayrol adapted his regulator to surface-supplied equipment. However, Jules Verne saw the potential of Rouquayrol's invention when he wrote Twenty Thousand Leagues under the Sea in 1869:

> Captain Nemo: You know as well as I do, Professor, that man can live underwater, providing he carries with him a sufficient supply of breathable air. In submarine works, the workman, clad in an impervious dress, with his head in a metal helmet, receives air from above by means of forcing pumps and regulators.
>
> Professor Aronnax: That is a diving apparatus.
>
> Nemo: Just so; but under these conditions the man is not a liberty; he is attached to the pump which sends him air through an India rubber tube, an if we were obliged to be thus held to the Nautilus, we could not go far.
>
> Aronnax: And the means of getting free?
>
> Nemo: It is to use the Rouquayrol apparatus invented by two of your own countrymen, which I have brought to perfection for my own use. It consists of a reservoir of thick iron plates in which I store the air under a pressure of 50 atmospheres.

In reality, Rouquayrol's concept of a demand regulator to a successful open-circuit SCUBA was to wait more than 60 years.

In 1878, the first commercially practical self-contained breathing apparatus was developed by H.A. Fleuss. Closed-circuit SCUBA using 100% oxygen did not require the large quantity of gas needed for compressed air (21% oxygen). Thus the need for high-strength tanks was set aside. Fleuss was not aware of the limitation caused by the problem of oxygen poisoning when breathing 100% oxygen under pressure. Many years later researchers determined that the maximum safe depth for breathing 100% oxygen was about 25 feet. Two years after its invention, the Fleuss SCUBA received wide recognition when Alexander Lambert walked 1000 feet into a flooded tunnel under the Severn River in England. In complete darkness he found and closed crucial valves so the tunnel could be drained.

By World War I the Fleuss SCUBA was improved with a demand regulator and tanks capable of holding oxygen at more than 2000 psi. This became the basis for submarine escape equipment used in the Royal Navy.

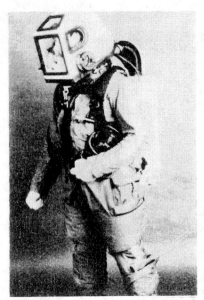

Figure 1-9: Deep Sea Diving Dress was modified to lighter weight materials during oil platform diving in the 1960's. (Courtesy of U.S. Navy)

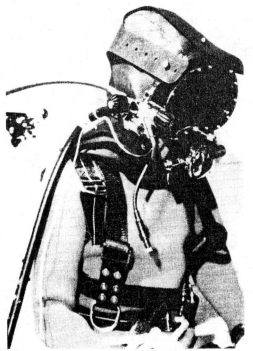

Figure 1-10: Demand regulators combined with surface-supplied air allowed better communications and efficient gas consumption. (Courtesy of U.S. Navy)

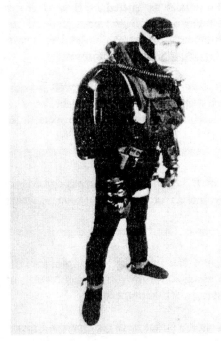

Figure 1-11: Closed-circuit, mixed-gas SCUBA allowed extended durations for free diving, especially for combat swimmers. (Courtesy of U.S. Navy)

In 1933, a French Naval Officer, Commander LePrieur constructed an open-circuit SCUBA using compressed air. However, LePrieur did not include a demand-regulator in his design, and the diver's main focus was diverted to manual control of his air supply. This, coupled with the short duration of dives due to inefficiency, limited the practical use of LePrieur's apparatus and the focus remained on closed-circuit SCUBA.

Although closed-circuit was restricted to shallow water, its design soon reached high efficiency. By World War II Navy swimmers on both sides were using closed-circuit SCUBA in combat. British divers, working out of midget submarines placed explosive charges under the keel of the German Battleship TIRPITZ. Italian divers rode "chariot torpedoes" fitted with seats and manual controls in repeated attacks against British shipping. In the final stages of the war, Japanese divers employed the underwater equivalent of kamikaze pilots - the Kaiten diver-guided torpedo.

Open-circuit SCUBA made a significant breakthrough during the war. Working in a small Mediterranean village in German-occupied France, Captain Jacques-Yves Cousteau, a French Naval Officer and Emil Gagnan, an engineer, combined an improved demand regulator with high-pressure air tanks. Cousteau and his companions brought their "Aqua Lung" to a high state of development as they explored and photographed underwater. Cousteau used his gear successfully to a depth of 180 feet. At the end of the war, the Aqua Lung became commercially available opening diving to anyone with suitable training. The freedom SCUBA brought to the world led to a rapid growth of diving as a sport. Science and commerce also benefitted since biologists, geologists, zoologists, archaeologists, and other scientists had direct access to the underwater world. An entire industry, centered on commercial diving, flourished during offshore oil petroleum production.

As divers continued to dive deeper and develop saturation techniques, technology was taking another turn towards the use of submersibles and remotely operated vehicles (ROVs). Much of the expense of using divers is eliminated if ROVs can do the job. Also, safety (and litigation due to accidents) is less important with ROVs.

1.2 The Application of Diving Systems to Underwater Intervention

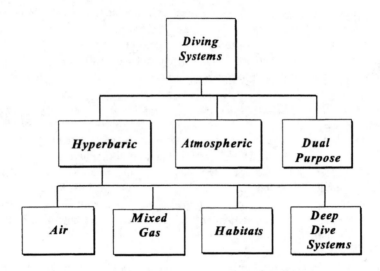

Figure 1-12: Underwater intervention methods using diving systems.

The debate continues concerning the use of divers instead of submersibles or remote vehicles to complete certain underwater missions. However, there is simply no better manipulator on the market today that can compare with the fine dexterity and motor skills achievable with the human hand. Additionally, the most sophisticated computer systems on the market today can not come close to the analysis and immediate problem solving capabilities of the human brain. Having the human "on site" is still the most efficient and cost-effective means of completing many underwater missions, particularly in relatively shallow depths. These are some of the primary reasons that developments in systems to support the diver will continue to be important for the foreseeable future.

Options for human intervention in undersea missions covers a wide spectrum, with final selection usually based on mission depth and complexity. It is generally convenient to characterize these options as either hyperbaric, atmospheric, or a combination of both as depicted in Figure 1-12.

1.2.1 Hyperbaric Dive Systems

With hyperbaric dive systems the diver's body is exposed to the ambient conditions that exist at the mission depth. Under these conditions the diver must contend with numerous physical and physiological concerns associated with breathing high pressure gases, often in cold, dark surroundings. There are a number of different types of hyperbaric dive systems including:

1.2.1.1   Air Diving Systems

Air diving systems are perhaps the most commonly used systems for relatively shallow operations due to their lack of complexity and inexpensive gas supply. Such air systems may be:

Self-contained, such as the familiar open-circuit *SCUBA* (**S**elf **C**ontained **U**nderwater **B**reathing **A**pparatus) used by most sport divers, shown in Figure 1-8. With these systems divers have freedom of movement around the dive site but have a limited breathing gas supply which they must carry in high pressure flasks. Because of this limited gas supply, open-circuit SCUBA systems are usually limited to depths of less than 130 feet.

Surface-supplied, such as those systems depicted in Figures 1-9 and 1-10. Unlike SCUBA, surface-supplied air diving systems usually have an unlimited air source supplied through an umbilical from the surface, giving the diver prolonged bottom time. However, due to the surface connection, the diver's excursion distance and mobility around the dive site is limited. These systems are limited to depths less that 190 feet due to the excessive narcotic effect of breathing nitrogen in air at high pressures.

1.2.1.2   Mixed-Gas Diving Systems

When the physiological effects of breathing high pressure gases make breathing air unsafe, mixed-gas systems are used. These systems typically use a mixture of nitrogen and oxygen (nitrox) or helium and oxygen (heliox) as the breathing medium. Some mixed- gas systems may be characterized as *bounce diving systems* (sometimes referred to as conventional dive systems) in which the diver will initiate each dive from the surface and then return to surface conditions, often incurring lengthy decompression obligations with each dive. These systems can be either surface-supplied, such as the semi-closed system shown in Figure 1-5, or self-contained, such as the system shown in Figure 1-11. Because of the umbilical connection between the diver and the surface, the surface-supplied, mixed-gas systems suffer many of the same limitations seen with surface-supplied air systems discussed above, but are capable of operational depths of up to 350 feet (heliox mixtures) when the proper percentages of oxygen and inert gases are utilized.

1.2.1.3   Underwater Habitats

Underwater habitats, similar to that shown in Figure 1-13, provide a means for divers to remain under pressure, often for days or even weeks, until the mission is completed. The feasibility of using habitats to support *saturation diving* was first demonstrated operationally in the early 1960's through several parallel efforts including, Edwin Link's *Man-In-The-Sea Program*, Jacques Cousteau's *Conshelf* experiments, and the U.S. Navy's *Sealab Program* (Penzias and Goodman, 1973). During these missions divers live in dry shelters, located on the sea floor, from which they are able to make dive excursions away from the habitat without the need to decompress after each excursion dive. This ability to delay decompression obligations is possible since the divers return to the high pressure atmosphere within the habitat instead of returning to the surface after each dive excursion. The divers' bodies become completely "saturated" with the inert gases within the habitat during these missions, necessitating a lengthy decompression at the end of the mission. However, the duration of this single, delayed decompression period is generally far less than the accumulative decompression times that would be required to complete the same mission with a series of bounce dives.

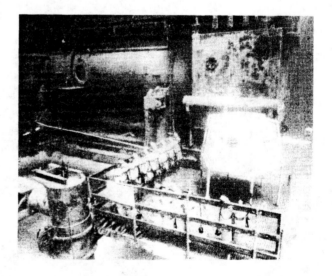

Figure 1-13: "Aquarius" underwater habitat operated by the NOAA's National Undersea Research Program (courtesy of the National Oceanic and Atmospheric Administration).

Underwater habitats are continuing to find

applications in many scientific missions where researchers are required to be at a particular worksite for long periods. NOAA's *Aquarius* habitat continues to provide a safe underwater haven for missions of up to 30 days at a maximum depth of 120 feet.

1.2.1.4 Deep Diving Systems

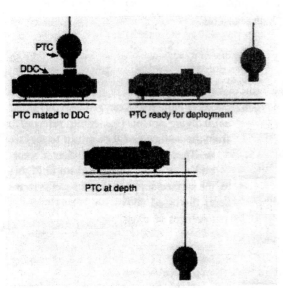

Figure 1-14: Saturation dive system. (U.S. Navy Dive Manual, Vol 2, 1991)

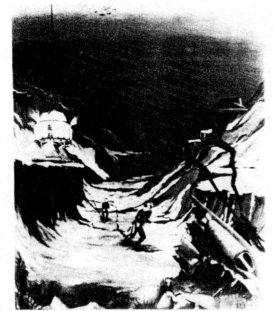

Figure 1-15: Divers being lowered to the work site via a personnel transfer capsule (PTC). Saturation diving techniques have greatly extended working depths and durations. (Courtesy of U.S. Navy)

Another method used to support divers during saturation missions involves the use of *deep diving systems* (otherwise referred to as saturation diving systems), shown in Figures 1-14 and 1-15. As with habitat missions, the diver(s) remains under pressure, often for days or even weeks, until the mission is completed. However, unlike habitat diving, the diver lives in a pressurized *deck decompression chamber (DDC)* on board a surface platform. Periodically he will be lowered to the worksite in a pressurized *personnel transfer capsule (PTC)* to conduct work and then return to the surface chamber. This transfer to the worksite is repeated until the mission is completed, at which time the diver will decompress inside the DDC under the watch of surface support personnel. When the DDC is aboard a surface vessel, the decompression proceeds as the ship is returning to its port, minimizing onsite manpower requirements resulting in a more cost-effective operation. This saturation technique has become the most widely used method for deep military and commercial diving today with open water depth capabilities in excess of 1000 feet.

1.2.2 Atmospheric Dive Systems

Atmospheric dive systems, like those shown in Figure 1-16, maintain the same pressure inside the suit as a dive sees at the surface, thereby isolating the diver from high ambient pressures. These systems allow the diver to descend to depths in excess of 1500 feet and return to the surface without the need to undergo any decompression, as well as provide a fair amount of thermal protection from cold water temperatures at depth. They additionally eliminate most of the operational and physiological problems that plague divers when using many of the hyperbaric dive systems discussed above. While extremely heavy and bulky on the surface, these systems are remarkably mobile underwater and have the ability to do gross motor tasks such as shackling and threading nuts. Atmospheric dive systems allow long bottom times at depth, greater repetitive dive capability, and added diver security.

1.2.3 Lockout Submersibles

Lockout submersibles offer the same features as any other research submersible, as well as, provide an alternate method for divers to gain access to an underwater worksite. These dual-purpose vehicles, such as the *Johnson Sea-Link* shown in Figure 1-17, have at least two separate compartments--one allows the vehicle operator to remain at one atmosphere pressure during a dive, while a diver can be pressurized in a second

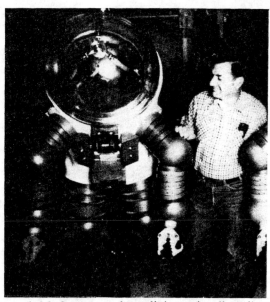

Figure 1-16: One-atmosphere diving suits allow divers to descend to over 1000 feet and return to the surface without decompression stops. (Courtesy of U.S. Navy)

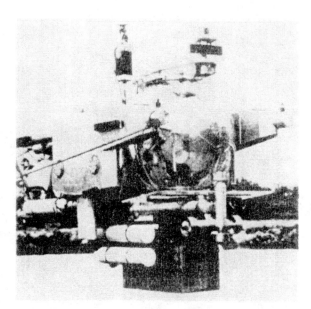

Figure 1-17: Lockout submersible "Johnson Sea-Link" (courtesy of Harbor Branch Oceanographic Institute)

compartment to the surrounding seawater pressure. This allows the diver to exit the submersible at the worksite and begin decompressing on the way to the surface. By delaying compression of the diver's compartment until reaching the worksite at the bottom, the diver's bottom time and decompression obligation can be minimized. Although highly effective in the past for placing divers at the worksite, the improvements in manipulators and other work systems has eliminated the need for diver lockout from the Johnson Sea-Link, as well as many other, dual-purpose submersibles.

1.3   Closure

The primary aim of this chapter has been to introduce the student to the development of dive systems and to classify the different diving and hyperbaric system options. It should be apparent that the design of such systems can be complex, requiring many interdisciplinary and integrative factors to be taken into account.

This book has been written in such a manner as to provide a basic understanding of the physiological and technical aspects which must be considered in the design of diving and hyperbaric systems. With this understanding, we can continue to advance diving capabilities from the early successes of breathhold skin divers more than 5000 years ago.

2

Diving Physics

Objectives

The objectives of this chapter are to
- review fundamental units of measurement in both the English and SI systems
- give an overview of gas laws and their applications to life support systems design
- understand the concept of residual volumes with regards to storage containers, and give methods for calculating these residual volumes
- understand the relationships of gas partial pressures with gas mixtures at varying pressures
- understand the variables which affect the solubility of gases in liquids
- review methods for determining the properties of gases, including the relationships of real and ideal gas behaviors
- give a brief overview of the transmission of light and sound in water.

2.1 Units of Measurement

2.1.1 English System

In the English system there are 5 primary dimensions, as follows

Dimensions	Symbol	Increments
Length	L	foot (ft)
Time	t	second (sec)
Force	F	pound force (lbf)
Mass	M	pound mass (lbm)
Temperature	T	degrees (°F, °R)

A major source of confusion is the relationship between force and mass. This relationship is explained by Newton's 2nd Law; i.e.

$$F = M \cdot a \tag{2-1}$$

where a is the acceleration of gravity, having units of L/t^2.

Dimensionally, Newton's Law can be stated as

$$F \sim \frac{M \cdot L}{t^2} \tag{2-2}$$

We can make this relationship an equality by introducing a constant, K, such that

$$F = K \frac{M \cdot L}{t^2} = K \cdot M \cdot a \tag{2-3}$$

Dimensionally, K must have the units

$$K = \frac{F \cdot t^2}{M \cdot L} \tag{2-4}$$

which in the English system, K would have the units $\frac{lbf \cdot sec^2}{lbm \cdot ft}$.

Generally, we define a dimensional constant, $g_c = \frac{1}{K}$ such that

$$F = \frac{M \cdot a}{g_c} \tag{2-5}$$

The magnitude of g_c can readily be found from a fundamental definition of physics, which says

"1 lbf is defined as the force acting upon a mass of 1 lbm to cause that mass to accelerate at 32.174 ft/sec²".

Therefore, by applying this definition we find the magnitude of g_c as

$$g_c = \frac{M \cdot a}{F} = \frac{1\ lbm \cdot 32.174\ ft/sec^2}{1\ lbf} \tag{2-6}$$

or

$$g_c = 32.174\ \frac{lbm - ft}{lbf - sec^2} \qquad [\ English\ System\ ] \tag{2-7}$$

2.1.2 International System (SI)

The International System (SI) has only 4 primary dimensions, including

Dimensions	Symbol	Increments
Length	L	meter (m)
Time	t	second (sec)
Mass	M	kilogram (kg)
Temperature	T	degrees (°C, °K)

Note that force is not a primary dimension in the SI system. Rather, it is a derived secondary dimension with units of *Newtons (N)* defined as

"A newton is the force acting upon a 1 kg mass to cause an acceleration of 1 meter per sec²".

Therefore, in the SI system we can show that the units and magnitude of g_c will be as follows

$$g_c = \frac{M \cdot a}{F} = \frac{1 \; kg \cdot 1 \; \frac{m}{sec^2}}{1 \; N} = \frac{1 \; kg \cdot m}{N \cdot sec^2}$$

However, since the newton is defined as

$$1 \; N = 1 \; \frac{kg \cdot m}{sec^2}$$

then

$$g_c = 1.0 \qquad [\; SI \; System \;]$$

i.e., g_c is dimensionless in the SI System with a magnitude of 1.0.

2.1.3 Weight: A Special Case of Newton's 2nd Law

Weight is defined as the force originating from the effect of gravity on a body. Therefore, weight, W, can be determined by

$$W = \frac{m \cdot g}{g_c} \qquad\qquad (2\text{-}8)$$

where g is the acceleration due to gravity.

Note that g will vary as we move further away from the earth's surface, and even at different locations along the earth's crust. In the vacuum of outer space where g approaches zero

$$W = \frac{m \cdot 0}{g_c} = 0$$

I.e., weightlessness results. On the earth's surface, however, an object having a mass of 1 pound mass (lbm) will weigh 1 pound force (lbf) when the local acceleration of gravity equals 32.174 ft/sec^2.

Example: An air column having a cross-sectional area of 1 square inch, projecting from the surface of the earth to the limits of the earth's atmosphere, has an air mass of 14.69 lbm. What is the weight of this air column when the local acceleration of gravity at the earth's surface is 32.174 ft/sec^2?

Solution: Since

$$W = m\,\frac{g}{g_c} = 14.69\ lbm\ \frac{32.174\ ft/sec^2}{32.174\ \dfrac{lbm-ft}{lbf-sec^2}} = 14.69\ lbf$$

Note: A gravitational force (weight) of 14.69 lbf per square inch is referred to as 1 standard atmosphere, and represents the weight of air pressing on the earth's surface.

2.1.4 Derived Units of Measurement

Density, ρ: mass per unit volume

$$\rho \sim \frac{M}{L^3} \sim \frac{lbm}{ft^3} \quad [\ English\ ]; \qquad\qquad \rho \sim \frac{kg}{m^3} \quad [\ SI\ ] \qquad\qquad (2\text{-}9)$$

Specific Volume, v: volume per unit mass

$$v = \frac{1}{\rho} \sim \frac{L^3}{M} \sim \frac{ft^3}{lbm} \quad [\ English\ ]; \qquad v \sim \frac{m^3}{kg} \quad [\ SI\ ] \qquad\qquad (2\text{-}10)$$

Specific Weight, γ: weight per unit volume

$$\gamma \sim \frac{W}{L^3} \sim \frac{lbf}{ft^3} \quad [\ English\ ]; \qquad \gamma = \rho\,\frac{g}{g_c} = \frac{1}{v}\,\frac{g}{g_c} \qquad\qquad (2\text{-}11)$$

Note: If the local acceleration of gravity is 32.174 ft/sec^2, then the magnitudes of density and specific weight are identical.

Example: Air at a temperature of 70°F at an atmospheric pressure of 1 standard atmosphere has a density of 0.075 lbm/ft^3.

a) What is the specific volume of the air?

$$v = \frac{1}{\rho} = \frac{1}{0.075 \, \frac{lbm}{ft^3}} = 13.33 \, \frac{ft^3}{lbm}$$

b) What is the specific weight of the air if the local acceleration of gravity is 30.5 ft/sec²?

$$\gamma = \rho \cdot \frac{g}{g_c} = 0.075 \, \frac{lbm}{ft^3} \cdot \frac{30.5 \, \frac{ft}{sec^2}}{32.174 \, \frac{lbm-ft}{lbf-suc^2}} = 0.071 \, \frac{lbf}{ft^3}$$

c) What is the density of the air in SI units?

$$\rho = 0.075 \, \frac{lbm}{ft^3} \, x \, 0.4536 \, \frac{kg}{lbm} \, x \, \frac{1 \, ft^3}{0.02832 \, m^3} = 1.201 \, \frac{kg}{m^3}$$

Pressure, *P*:   force per unit area

$$P \sim \frac{F}{L^2} \sim \frac{lbf}{ft^2} \quad (psf) \tag{2-12}$$

or

$$P \sim \frac{lbf}{in^2} \quad (psi) \qquad [\, English \,] \tag{2-13}$$

and

$$P \sim \frac{N}{m^2} \quad (Pascal) \qquad [\, SI \,] \quad \textbf{(2-14)}$$

Pressure can also be expressed as the equivalent height of a column of liquid that can be supported by that pressure. If, for example, we fill a test tube with mercury, as shown in the figure, and then invert that test tube with its open end submerged in an open dish filled with mercury, the weight of the earth's atmosphere (at sea level) pressing on the exposed mercury surface in the dish will support a column of mercury in the tube of 760 millimeters (29.92 inches). Likewise, a column of freshwater 33.9 feet high, or a column of seawater 33.0

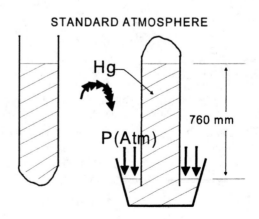

STANDARD ATMOSPHERE

feet high, would be supported by this atmospheric pressure.

These liquid columns represent the equivalent heights supported by a "standard atmosphere". Thus, the pressure of a standard atmosphere can be given as

1 standard atmosphere (Atm)	=	760 mm Hg
	=	33.9 feet of fresh water
	=	33.0 feet of seawater (FSW)
	=	14.69 lbf/in² (psi)

2.1.5 Absolute vs. Gage Pressure

A pressure reading referenced to a perfect vacuum is referred to as *absolute* pressure. To signify that a reading is in absolute terms, units such as *psia* (meaning psi, absolute) or *Ata* (atmospheres, absolute) will be used. Barometers are used to obtain absolute pressure readings. A pressure reading referenced to the local atmospheric pressure is called *gage* pressure. Units such as *psig* (meaning psi, gage) or *Atm* (atmospheres, gage) will be used. Bourdon tube pressure gauges give pressure referenced to the local atmosphere. Since local atmospheric pressure varies from one site to another, it is important to record this local value when specifying pressure as gage pressure. Absolute pressure can then be found from gage readings as

$$P_{Absolute} = P_{Gage} + P_{Atmospheric} \qquad (2\text{-}15)$$

Example: A Bourdon-type pressure gauge indicates a pressure reading of 32.0 psig in an enclosed container. The local atmospheric pressure of 28 in Hg is recorded from a barometer. What is the absolute pressure in this container?

$$P_{Atmospheric} = 28 \ in \ Hg \ x \ 0.491 \ \frac{psi}{in \ Hg} = 13.75 \ psia$$

and

$$P_{Absolute} = P_{Gage} + P_{Atmospheric}$$

$$P_{Absolute} = 32.0 \ psig + 13.75 \ psia = 45.75 \ psia$$

Example: A scuba bottle is placed inside a pressure capsule (diving bell) where the atmospheric pressure inside the bell was initially measured at 15 psia at sealevel. Under these conditions, a Bourdon tube gauge attached to the scuba bottle shows a pressure of 3000 psig. If the diving bell is now pressurized until the atmospheric pressure inside the bell is 460 psia, what pressure will the Bourdon tube gauge show for the scuba bottle?

Solution: At the surface

$$P_{Absolute} = P_{Gage} + P_{Atmospheric}$$

$$P_{Absolute} = 3000 + 15 = 3015 \ psia$$

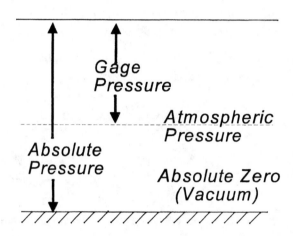

Note that absolute pressure in the bottle is unaffected by the local atmospheric pressure; such that, even though the pressure inside the bell is elevated to 460 psia, the absolute pressure inside the bottle is still 3015 psia. Therefore, when the pressure in the bell is raised to 460 psia, the gauge attached to the bottle will show

$$P_{Gage} = P_{Absolute} - P_{Atmospheric}$$

$$P_{Gage} = 3015 - 460 = 2555 \ psig$$

Indeed, the bottle gage pressure will continue to drop as the surrounding atmospheric pressure inside the bell increases. This drop in gage pressure, as the surrounding pressure rises, is indicative of the reduction of gas that would be available from this bottle when used in high pressure environments. The stored gas that could be supplied from this bottle would be limited to the gas supplied until the pressure inside the bottle dropped to bell atmospheric pressure. The remainder of the gas left in the bottle when the bottle gage pressure comes to equilibrium with the bell atmospheric pressure would be unavailable (see Residual Volume).

2.1.6 Hydrostatic Pressure

The absolute pressure exerted on a diver beneath sealevel consists of the weight of the atmosphere pressing on the ocean surface (14.69 psia) plus the

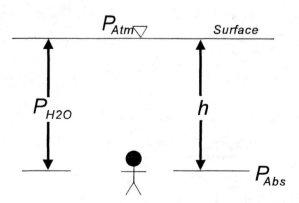

weight of the water column above the diver. The pressure due to this water column, called the hydrostatic pressure can be found as

$$P_{H_2O} = \gamma_{liq} \cdot h \qquad (2\text{-}16)$$

where h is the water depth (or height of the water column), ft; γ_{liq} is the specific weight of water, lbf/ft³. Note: for freshwater, $\gamma_{FW} = 62.4$ lbf/ft³; for seawater, $\gamma_{SW} = 64.0$ lbf/ft³.

It is easy to confirm that an additional pressure equivalent to 1 standard atmosphere (14.7 psi) will be exerted on the diver for every 33 feet of increasing depth in seawater, since

$$P_{H_2O} = \gamma_{liq} \cdot h = \frac{64 \frac{lbf}{ft^3} \cdot 33\ ft}{144 \frac{in^2}{ft^2}} = 14.7\ psi \quad (\ 1\ std\ atm\ )$$

Thus, as the diver's depth increases, the pressures on the diver will increase as follows:

Depth-Pressure Relationship in Seawater				
Depth, FSW	**ATM**	**Psig**	**Ata**	**Psia**
0	0	0	1	14.7
33	1	14.7	2	29.4
66	2	29.4	3	44.1
99	3	44.1	4	58.8
132	4	58.8	5	73.5
Etc				

This relationship between depth and the corresponding pressure can be quantified as follows:

Gage Pressure

$$P\ (Atm) = \frac{D\ (ft)}{33} \qquad or \qquad P\ (psig) = \frac{D\ (ft)}{33}\ (14.7) = 0.445 \cdot D\ (ft) \qquad (2\text{-}17)$$

Absolute Pressure

$$P\ (Ata) = \frac{D\ (ft) + 33}{33} \qquad or \qquad P\ (psia) = \frac{D\ (ft) + 33}{33}\ (14.7) \qquad (2\text{-}18)$$

Example: You are going to dive to 50 meters. What will be the absolute pressure in atmospheres? What will the gage pressure be in kg/cm² ?

Solution:

$$50 \ meters \ x \ 3.28 \ \frac{ft}{meter} = 164 \ feet$$

$$P \ (Ata) = \frac{D \ (ft) \ + \ 33}{33} = \frac{164 \ + \ 33}{33} = 5.97 \ Ata$$

$$P_{Gage} = P_{Absolute} - P_{Atmospheric} = 5.97 \ Ata \ - \ 1.0 \ Atm \ = \ 4.97 \ Atm$$

$$4.97 \ Atm \ x \ 1.0333 \ \frac{kg/cm^2}{Atm} = 5.13 \ \frac{kg}{cm^2}$$

2.2   Buoyancy

When any object is placed in a liquid medium, the net force on that object in the direction of the earth's gravity is equal to the difference between the force due to gravity (weight) and the buoyant force acting on that body. I.e.,

$$F_{net} = m \left(\frac{g}{g_c} \right) - F_B \qquad (2\text{-}19)$$

where F_{net} is the net force acting on the body, lbf; m is the mass of the object, lbm; g is the acceleration of gravity, ft/sec²; and, F_B is the buoyant force acting on the body, lbf.

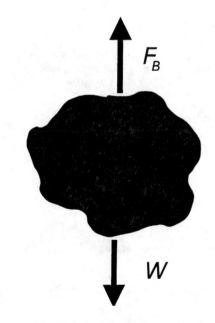

The buoyant force is dictated by *Archimedes Principle* which says:

"*A body immersed in a liquid, either wholly or partially, is buoyed up by a force equal to the weight of the liquid that is displaced by that body.*" I.e.,

$$F_B = \gamma_{liq} \cdot V \qquad (2\text{-}20)$$

where γ_{liq} is the specific weight of the liquid, lbf/ft³; and V is the displaced liquid volume or volume of the object, ft³.

By noting that the mass of the object can be found as the product of its density and volume, and recalling the relationship for specific weight to density, Equation (2-11), we can calculate the net force acting on a totally submerged object as

$$F_{net} = V \cdot (\gamma_o - \gamma_{liq}) \qquad (2\text{-}21)$$

where γ_o is the specific weight of the object, lbf/ft³.

This expression emphasizes that the net force on the object will be positive (meaning that the buoyancy force is negative) if the specific weight of the object is greater than that of the liquid, causing the object to sink (negative buoyancy). On the other hand, the object will float if the specific weight of the object is less than that of the liquid (positive buoyancy). The object will have neutral buoyancy if $\gamma_o = \gamma_{liq}$, simulating a weightless environment.

Example: What will weigh more, 10 lbm of lead or 10 lbm of concrete?

Solution: Both objects will weigh the same on the surface since $W = m \cdot g/g_c$. However, the lead will weigh more submerged due to its higher specific weight when compared to concrete.

Example: What is the net downward force that would be measured on a block of concrete with dimensions 18" x 12" x 9" in air? In seawater? Assume that the specific weight of concrete is 150 lbf/ft³, the specific weight of air is 0.075 lbf/ft³, and the specific weight of seawater is 64 lbf/ft³.

Solution: First, we calculate the volume of the concrete block as

$$V = \frac{18 \ in \ x \ 12 \ in \ x \ 9 \ in}{1728 \ \frac{in^3}{ft^3}} = 1.125 \ ft^3$$

In air, the net force on the block will be

$$F_{net} = V \cdot (\gamma_o - \gamma_{liq}) = 1.125 \ ft^3 \left(150 \ \frac{lbf}{ft^3} - 0.075 \ \frac{lbf}{ft^3} \right) = 168.8 \ lbf$$

Note the insignificance of the air to this net force due to the relative magnitude of the specific weight of the air to that of concrete.   However, when submerged in seawater the net force on the block will be

$$F_{net} = V \cdot (\gamma_o - \gamma_{liq}) = 1.125 \ ft^3 \left(150 \ \frac{lbf}{ft^3} - 64 \ \frac{lbf}{ft^3} \right) = 96.8 \ lbf$$

or 72 lbf less than in air.

2.3   Temperature

Temperature is normally measured in degrees Fahrenheit (°F) or degrees Celsius (°C). However, temperatures are converted for most thermodynamic calculations to degrees Rankine (°R) in the English system, or degrees Kelvin (°K) in the SI system. The Rankine and Kelvin temperature scales are called *absolute temperature* scales. Zero degrees on the absolute temperature scale marks absolute zero; where theoretically, all molecular motion of matter would stop.

The single most common error when calculating gas properties, as we will discuss in the next section, is neglecting to convert temperatures to the absolute temperature scale. These conversions can be easily made as follows:

Fahrenheit to Rankine:

$$°R = °F + 459.67 \tag{2-22}$$

Celsius to Kelvin:

$$°K = °C + 273 \tag{2-23}$$

Fahrenheit to Celsius:

$$°C = \frac{5}{9} \cdot (°F - 32) \tag{2-24}$$

Celsius to Fahrenheit:

$$°F = \frac{9}{5} \cdot °C + 32 \tag{2-25}$$

2.4   Gas Laws

Gases are affected by three interrelated factors, including
- temperature
- pressure
- volume

At low pressures, this interrelationship can be approximated by any form of the *Ideal Gas Law*

$$P \cdot V = m \cdot R \cdot T \qquad\qquad P \cdot v = R \cdot T \qquad\qquad (2\text{-}26)$$

$$P \cdot V = N \cdot R_u \cdot T \qquad\qquad \frac{P}{\rho} = R \cdot T \qquad\qquad (2\text{-}27)$$

where

P	=	absolute pressure, lbf/ft^2
V	=	gas volume, ft^3
m	=	mass of gas, lbm
R	=	gas constant, ft-lbf/lbm-°R
T	=	absolute temperature, °R
N	=	moles of gas
R_u	=	Universal gas constant = 1544 ft-lbf/mol-°R
		= 0.0821 L-atm/mol-°K
v	=	specific volume, ft^3/lbm

For a fixed container where the gas mass will remain constant, we can write the *general gas law* for an ideal gas as

$$\frac{P \cdot V}{T} = constant \qquad\qquad [\; General\ Gas\ Law\ ] \qquad\qquad (2\text{-}28)$$

This expression dictates that as a diver's depth increases (with a corresponding increase in absolute pressure), the volume of that fixed volume of gas must decrease if the temperature remains constant. Likewise, if the absolute temperature increases while the pressure remains constant, the volume of a fixed container of gas must increase.

2.5   Standard Conditions

2.5.1   Engineering Units

The routine variations in pressure and temperature that occur beneath the sea makes it essential that we specify these conditions when referring to any volume measurement. A short-hand method of specifying these conditions is through the definition of standard conditions; i.e., *STPD* (standard temperature and pressure, dry gas). In engineering units STPD is defined as 70°F, 14.7 psia, dry. A volumetric measurement of 1 *standard cubic foot*, indicated by the letters *SCF*, contains the volume of dry gas in a 1 cubic foot container at conditions of 70°F and 14.7 psia. As the temperature and pressure vary away from these standard conditions, the actual gas volume, designated as *actual cubic feet (ACF)*, will change according to the general gas law above. However, even though the actual volume will vary as the environmental conditions change, the volume of the gas will remain constant when specified in SCF.

It is often necessary to convert between standard and actual volumetric conditions during engineering calculations. This is easily accomplished using the following expression which has been derived from the general gas law:

$$V\ (SCF)\ =\ V\ (ACF)\ \cdot\ P\ (Ata)\ \cdot\ \frac{530^{\circ}R}{T\ (^{\circ}F)\ +\ 460} \tag{2-29}$$

where T and P are the actual environmental temperature and pressure.

2.5.2 Scientific Units

In scientific units *STPD* is defined as 0°C, [handwritten: 70°F] 14.7 psia, dry. The volumetric measurement of 1 *standard liter (SL)* contains the dry gas in a 1 liter container at 0°C (32°F) and 14.7 psia. Again, the actual volume (actual liters, AL) of the container will change with changes in pressure and temperature; however, we can still designate this volume as a constant when we refer to standard conditions.

We can likewise convert between standard and actual volumetric conditions during scientific calculations using the following expression derived from the general gas law:

$$V\ (SL)\ =\ V\ (AL)\ \cdot\ P\ (Ata)\ \cdot\ \frac{273^{\circ}K}{T\ (^{\circ}C)\ +\ 273} \tag{2-30}$$

where T and P are the actual environmental temperature and pressure.

Example: It is often necessary to convert between engineering and scientific units when dealing with underwater life support systems design. For instance, a diver's level of metabolic oxygen consumption is generally given in standard liters, while gas storage capacities are generally given in standard cubic feet. Assuming a diver's oxygen consumption rate is specified as 1.5 standard liters per minute (designated as SLPM), what would be the corresponding consumption rate expressed in standard cubic feet per minute (designated SCFM)? There are 28.32 liters in a cubic foot.

Solution: The general gas law states that the quantity PV/T is a constant for ideal gases. Thus, we can equate gas volumes that are expressed at different conditions by applying these conditions to the general gas law as follows:

$$\left[\frac{P\cdot V}{T}\right]_{SCFM}\ =\ \left[\frac{P\cdot\left(\dfrac{V,\ lit}{28.32\ \dfrac{lit}{ft^{3}}}\right)}{T}\right]_{SLPM}$$

Rearranging, and solving for the gas volume in SCFM, we have

$$V\ (SCFM) = V\ (SLPM)\ x\ \frac{1\ ft^3}{28.32\ liters}\ x\ \frac{530°R}{492°R}\ x\ \frac{1\ Ata}{1\ Ata}$$

$$V\ (SCFM) = \frac{V\ (SLPM)}{26.3} = \frac{1.5}{26.3} = 0.057\ SCFM$$

2.6 Residual Volumes in Storage Containers

When consuming gas from a pressurized container the amount of gas available from this container for consumption is dependent on the surrounding ambient conditions. For instance, at a depth of 1000 FSW, where the surrounding water pressure is approximately 460 psia, gas can be removed from a storage container until the pressure in that container reaches pressure equilibrium with the surrounding seawater. The gas remaining in the flask following equilibrium is called the bottle *residual volume*, a volume which is generally unavailable to the diver. Further removal of this residual gas can only be accomplished by pulling a vacuum on the interior of the container relative to the surrounding water pressure, or by reducing the surrounding water pressure. Both of these options are usually impractical during deep sea operations.

The *rated capacity* of a gas storage container, generally expressed in standard cubic feet (SCF), is the volume that the gas contained in the flask would occupy if it was expanded to an atmospheric pressure of 14.7 psia and 70°F (i.e., standard conditions). The rated capacity should not be confused with the gas that is available, since the available gas volume will be variable and depend on the surrounding pressure that the gas will be utilized.

Typical Bottle Sizes and Capacities						
Nominal Capacity	Service Pressure Psi	Capacity SCF	Outside Dia Inches	Length Inches	Weight Lbs	Buoy-ancy Lbs
Steel 120	3500	120.0	7.25	27.9	38.0	+1.0
Steel 100	3500	100.1	7.25	23.9	33.0	0.0
Steel 80	3500	80.6	7.25	19.7	27.0	-1.0
Alum 80	3000	77.4	7.25	26.0	31.7	+3.9
Alum 63	3000	63.0	7.25	21.8	26.9	+2.3
Alum 50	3000	48.5	6.9	19.0	15.3	+4.4
Alum 30	3000	30.0	4.87	21.8	11.8	+1.1
Alum 15	2015	13.7	4.4	16.5	5.4	+1.7
Alum 13	3000	13.3	4.4	12.9	5.8	+0.7

Example: The rated capacity of an aluminum storage container used with a SCUBA apparatus is 80 SCF when pressurized to 3000 psig at 70°F. What is the actual volume (referred to as the "water volume") of this container in actual cubic feet, ACF?

Solution: The general gas law can be used to find the actual container volume as follows:

$$\left[\frac{P \cdot V}{T}\right]_{SCF} = \left[\frac{P \cdot V}{T}\right]_{ACF}$$

or

$$V_{ACF} = V_{SCF} \left[\frac{P_{SCF}}{P_{ACF}}\right]\left[\frac{T_{ACF}}{T_{SCF}}\right] = 80 \ ft^3 \left[\frac{14.7 \ psia}{3014.7 \ psia}\right]\left[\frac{530°R}{530°R}\right]$$

$$V_{ACF} = 0.39 \ ft^3$$

Note that the residual volume, equal to this actual container volume, will remain in the SCUBA bottle if the shutoff valve is opened and the stored gas is allowed to escape to the surrounding atmosphere. This unavailable gas volume remaining in the bottle is relatively minor when the gas is expanded to 1 Ata, or surface conditions (0.39 ft³ unavailable out of 80 ft³ total volume--less than 0.5%). However, the unavailable gas volume can become significant as the atmospheric pressure at which the stored gas is being used increases.

For example, if the same storage container is used at 1000 FSW at an ambient temperature of 40°F, the expanded volume of this gas when in equilibrium with the working conditions will be as follows:

$$V_{1000'} = V_{STD} \left[\frac{P_{STD}}{P_{1000'}}\right]\left[\frac{T_{1000'}}{T_{STD}}\right] = 80 \ ft^3 \left[\frac{14.7 \ psia}{460.2 \ psia}\right]\left[\frac{500°R}{530°R}\right]$$

$$V_{1000'} = 2.41 \ ft^3 \ @ \ 460.2 \ psia \ and \ 40°F$$

After the gas comes into equilibrium with the working conditions at 1000 FSW, the storage container will still have a residual volume of 0.39 ACF (also at a pressure of 460.2 psia and a temperature of 40°F) which will be unavailable to the diver. Unlike surface conditions, where the unavailable gas was less than 0.5% of the stored volume, the unavailable gas at 1000 FSW is greater than 16% of the rated capacity (0.39 ft³ unavailable out of 2.41 ft³ total volume). The available gas to the diver at 1000 FSW and 40°F will now be only

$$V_{Available} = V_{1000'} - V_{Residual}$$

$$V_{Available} = 2.41 - 0.39 = 2.02 \ ft^3 \ @ \ 1000 \ FSW \ and \ 40°F$$

The unavailable volume will continue to increase as the depth at which the gas is to be used increases.

2.7 Special Gas Laws

2.7.1 Boyles Law

A special application of the general gas law says:

If temperature is constant, the volume of a gas will vary inversely with absolute pressure, while density will vary directly with absolute pressure. I.e.,

$$P \cdot V = constant \qquad [\ For \ constant \ temperature \ ] \qquad \text{(2-31)}$$

Example: At the surface a diver inflates his life vest to an internal volume of 140 in^3 to compensate for the added weight of tools that he will be carrying to a submerged seawater work site. What will be the internal volume of his life vest, and the resulting change in buoyancy, after the diver reaches a depth of 150 FSW if we ignore any temperature change?

Solution: First, we will label the conditions at the surface as condition #1, and those at 150 FSW as condition #2. At the surface, P_1 is 1 Ata. At 150 FSW,

$$P_2 = \frac{D + 33}{33} = \frac{150 + 33}{33} = 5.54 \ Ata$$

Rearranging Boyle's Law, we can solve for the gas volume inside the vest at 150 FSW as

$$V_2 = V_1 \left(\frac{P_1}{P_2} \right) = 140 \ in^3 \left(\frac{1 \ Ata}{5.54 \ Ata} \right) = 25.3 \ in^3$$

From Archimedes Principle, we know that the buoyant force from the vest at the surface would be the following:

$$F_{B_1} = \gamma_{SW} \cdot V_1 = 64 \ \frac{lbf}{ft^3} \cdot \frac{140 \ in^3}{1728 \ \frac{in^3}{ft^3}} = 5.2 \ lbf$$

At 150 FSW, the buoyant force will be reduced to

$$F_{B_2} = \gamma_{SW} \cdot V_2 = 64 \ \frac{lbf}{ft^3} \cdot \frac{25.3 \ in^3}{1728 \ \frac{in^3}{ft^3}} = 0.94 \ lbf$$

The reduction in volume of the life vest due to the increased pressure results in a loss of 4.3 lbf of buoyancy. If the diver does not correct for this lost buoyancy, he will find it difficult to remain at the work site, and run the risk of plunging at an ever increasing rate of descent.

Example: What will be the change in the gas volume in a lift bag if an ascent is made from 30 meters to 10 meters?

Solution: Labeling condition #1 as those conditions at 30 meters, and condition #2 as the conditions at 10 meters, we find

$$P_1 = \frac{D, ft + 33}{33} = \frac{\left(30 \ m \cdot 3.28 \ \frac{ft}{m} \right) + 33}{33} = 3.98 \ Ata$$

And

$$P_2 = \frac{\left(10\ m\ \cdot\ 3.28\ \frac{ft}{m}\right)\ +\ 33}{33} = 1.99\ Ata$$

If we assume no change in temperature, then

$$P_1\ V_1\ =\ P_2\ V_2$$

and thus

$$\frac{V_2}{V_1}\ =\ \frac{P_1}{P_2}\ =\ \frac{3.98\ Ata}{1.99\ Ata}\ =\ 2$$

The gas volume will double unless the gas is allowed to vent from the bag. If unchecked, this volume expansion will cause a continuing increase in buoyancy, resulting in an ever-increasing rate of ascent. This uncontrolled ascent is commonly referred to as "blowup".

Example: A diver takes a full breath of air from his breathing apparatus at a depth of 33 FSW ($P_1 = 2$ Ata). Suddenly, he panics after sighting a shark and begins a rapid ascent, forgetting to exhale as he rises. What will be the volume change in the diver's lungs after reaching the surface ($P_2 = 1$ Ata)?

Solution: Again, since

$$P_1\ V_1\ =\ P_2\ V_2$$

then

$$V_2\ =\ V_1\ \frac{P_1}{P_2}\ =\ 2\ V_1 \qquad \textit{(twice the original volume)}$$

Under these conditions, the lungs would suffer severe damage as a result of this excessive over-inflation, leading to fatality if the diver is not recompressed immediately (see *gas embolism* Chapter 3).

2.7.2 Charles' Law

Another special case of the general gas law says:

The amount of change in either volume or pressure is directly related to the change in absolute temperature. I. e.,

$$\frac{P}{T} = constant \qquad\qquad [\ For\ constant\ volume\ ]$$

$$\frac{V}{T} = constant \qquad\qquad [\ For\ constant\ pressure\ ]$$

(2-32)

Example: A gas container for SCUBA is rapidly filled to 2500 psig, resulting in the gas temperature inside the container rising to 180°F. What will be the gas pressure if the container is lowered in 45°F water and allowed to come to temperature equilibrium with the surrounding water?

Solution: Setting condition #1 as the state of the initial filled container and condition #2 as the condition of the container after coming to temperature equilibrium, we have

$$P_2 = P_1 \frac{T_2}{T_1} = (\ 2500 + 14.7 psia\ ) \cdot \frac{(\ 45° + 460°R\ )}{(\ 180° + 460°R\ )} = 1984.3\ psia$$

A pressure gauge attached to the container at sealevel would measure the following:

$$P_{2_{Gage}} = P_{2_{Absolute}} - P_{Atmospheric}$$

$$P_2 = 1984.3\ psia - 14.7\ psia = 1969.6\ psig$$

Example: A lift bag is inflated underwater to a volume of 3 ft³ with air at 90° F. If this bag travels through a thermocline such that the surrounding water temperature drops to 50°F, how much lifting capability will be lost?

Solution: The volume of the lift bag initially (condition #1) will be reduced after it comes to equilibrium with the cold water (condition #2), found as

$$V_2 = V_1 \frac{T_2}{T_1} = 3\ ft^3 \cdot \frac{(\ 50° + 460°R\ )}{(\ 90° + 460°R\ )} = 2.78\ ft^3$$

The resulting change in buoyant force from the lift bag can be calculated (we will assume that the temperature change has a negligible effect on the specific weight for the seawater):

$$F_B = \gamma \cdot V$$

thus

$$\Delta F_B = \Delta(\gamma_{SW} \cdot V) \approx \gamma_{SW} \cdot \Delta V = 64 \; \frac{lbf}{ft^3} \cdot (\; 2.78 \; - \; 3.0 \;) \; ft^3 = -14.1 \; lbf$$

More air would have to be added to this lift bag to continue its ascent to the surface.

2.8   Dalton's Law (Law of Partial Pressures)

Dalton's Law*: The total pressure exerted by a mixture of gases is equal to the sum of the pressures of each component of that mixture if it alone were present and occupied the total volume.*

A one cubic foot container of air at a pressure of 1 Ata (14.7 psia) contains approximately 79%, by volume, nitrogen and 21% oxygen. If we could physically remove all of the oxygen molecules in this container, and thus allow the nitrogen molecules to occupy the entire volume, the pressure in this container would be 79% of the original pressure, or 0.79 Ata. This pressure is referred to as the *partial pressure*, P_{N2}, of the nitrogen in that container.

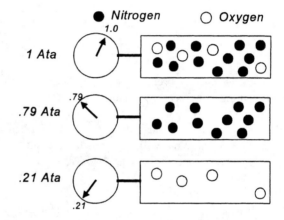

Likewise, if we removed only the nitrogen molecules, and allowed the oxygen to occupy the entire volume, the pressure in this container would be 21% of the original pressure, or 0.21 Ata. This is the partial pressure of oxygen, P_{O2}, in the container.

Thus, we can say that partial pressure for any gas is the pressure that would be exerted by that gas if it alone occupied the total container volume. Dalton's Law says that the sum of these partial pressures will equal the total system pressure. That is,

$$P_T = P_{N2} + P_{O2} \qquad\qquad\qquad (2\text{-}33)$$

where P_{N2} is the partial pressure of nitrogen, Ata or psia; P_{O2} is the partial pressure of oxygen, Ata or psia; and P_T is the total system pressure, Ata or psia.

In the above example,

$$P_T = 0.79 \; Ata \; + \; 0.21 \; Ata \; = \; 1.0 \; Ata$$

Or in general, for multiple gas mixtures we can say

$$P_T = \sum_{i=1}^{n} P_i \qquad\qquad\qquad (2\text{-}34)$$

where *n* is the number of gas components; P_i is the partial pressure of the ith component of the gas mixture; and

$$P_i = X_i \cdot P_T \qquad\qquad (2\text{-}35)$$

where X_i is the volume fraction of the ith component.

Example: What are the partial pressures of oxygen and nitrogen in air if the total pressure is 5 Ata?

Solution: Using the above definition for partial pressures, we can find that

$$P_{O2} = 0.21 \cdot (5\ Ata) = 1.05\ Ata$$

$$P_{N2} = 0.79 \cdot (5\ Ata) = 3.95\ Ata$$

$$P_T = \sum_{i=1}^{2} P_i = 1.05 + 3.95 = 5.00\ Ata$$

Note: A diver breathing air at 5 Ata would experience a higher P_{O2} (1.05 Ata) than if that diver was breathing pure oxygen at sealevel (1.0 Ata).

Example: A gas mixture contains 80% helium, 5% oxygen, 4% carbon dioxide, 10% nitrogen, and 1% water vapor. What will be the partial pressures of each component when the mixture is pressurized to an ambient environment seen at 200 FSW?

Solution: At 200 FSW, the ambient pressure will be

$$P_T = \frac{200 + 33}{33} = 7.06\ Ata$$

At this total pressure the partial pressures of each gas component can be found as

$$P_{He} = 0.80 \cdot (7.06\ Ata) = 5.65\ Ata$$

$$P_{O2} = 0.05 \cdot (7.06\ Ata) = 0.35\ Ata$$

$$P_{CO2} = 0.04 \cdot (7.06\ Ata) = 0.28\ Ata$$

$$P_{N2} = 0.10 \cdot (7.06\ Ata) = 0.70\ Ata$$

$$P_{H2O} = 0.01 \cdot (7.06\ Ata) = 0.07\ Ata$$

Summing the partial pressures of these gases, we can see that Dalton's Law is satisfied since

$$P_T = \sum_{i=1}^{5} P_i = 5.65 + 0.35 + 0.28 + 0.70 + 0.07 = 7.06\ Ata$$

2.8.1 Percent Surface Equivalent (%SEV)

Often we are dealing with extremely small volume fractions of gas components (such as carbon dioxide, carbon monoxide, water vapor, etc), particularly when working at large depths beneath the ocean's surface. To avoid the need to express these trace gas constituents as small volume fractions, we can use another unit of measurement for partial pressures referred to as *percent surface equivalent, or %SEV*. %SEV is defined as the volume percentage of a gas at surface conditions (i.e., 1 Ata) which would have the same partial pressure as the actual gas being breathed at elevated pressures.

For example, a gas mixture containing 1% carbon dioxide at an atmospheric pressure of 4 Ata will have the same partial pressure for carbon dioxide as a gas mixture containing 4% CO_2 at the surface. In both cases the P_{CO_2} is said to be 4 %SEV, equivalent to a partial pressure of 0.04 Ata. This unit can be calculated from the actual gas volume fraction using the relationship

$$\%SEV = X \cdot P_T \cdot 100\% \qquad or \qquad X = \frac{\%SEV}{P_T \cdot 100\%} \qquad (2\text{-}36)$$

where X is the actual volume fraction of the gas, and P_T is the total pressure at which the gas is being used, Ata.

Example: Air at sealevel has a trace of carbon dioxide, approximately 0.035% by volume. At what depth would air need to be compressed to reach a partial pressure of carbon dioxide equal to 0.5 %SEV (P_{CO_2} = 0.005 Ata)?

Solution: A gas containing 0.035% carbon dioxide has a volume fraction for CO_2 of

$$X_{CO_2} = \frac{\% \ CO_2}{100}$$

We saw previously that we can find the partial pressure of any gas component, knowing the volume fraction and the total pressure as

$$P_i = X_i \cdot P_T$$

This expression can also be used to find the total pressure at which this carbon dioxide partial pressure will occur

$$P_T = \frac{P_i}{X_i} = \frac{0.005 Ata}{0.00035} = 14.29 \ Ata$$

However, since we also know that the depth is related to seawater pressure as

$$P_T = \frac{D + 33}{33} \qquad \therefore \qquad D = 438 \ FSW$$

We will see later that if a diver could breathe air at a depth of 438 FSW, with a 0.035% carbon dioxide content, that diver would experience the same physiological effects from the carbon dioxide as if he was breathing 0.5% carbon dioxide at sealevel (see carbon dioxide toxicity).

Example: A SCUBA bottle is charged with a gas containing 2% carbon dioxide. What will be the exposure in %SEV for carbon dioxide if a diver breathed that gas at a depth of 132 FSW (5 Ata)?

Solution: The volume fraction of carbon dioxide in this gas mixture is

$$X_{CO2} = \frac{\%\ CO_2}{100} = \frac{2}{100} = 0.02$$

giving a partial pressure of carbon dioxide at 132 FSW of

$$P_{CO2} = X_{CO2} \cdot P_T = 0.02 \cdot 5\ Ata = 0.10\ Ata$$

This partial pressure is equivalent to that which we would experience by breathing 10% carbon dioxide at 1 Ata, or 10 %SEV. We will see in the next chapter that this concentration of carbon dioxide will result in diver unconsciousness in a short period of time.

2.9   Henry's Law

The solubility of gases in liquids at any temperature is proportional to the partial pressure of the gas that is in contact with that liquid.

This simple statement, referred to as Henry's Law, has its primary applications to human physiology in the absorption and off-gassing of inert gases to and from human tissues (see decompression theory), and the gas exchange processes occurring in our lungs and blood capillaries (see diving physiology).

Mathematically, we can express Henry's Law as

$$c_b = k_H \cdot P_i \tag{2-37}$$

where c_b is the molar concentration of the dissolved gas in the liquid, mol/L; P_i is the partial pressure of the gas in contact with the liquid, Ata; and k_H is a constant that depends only on temperature, mol/L-Ata (see Table 2-1).

Table 2-1: Solubility Constants For Selected Gases

kₕ, mol/L-Ata			
Temp, °C	**Nitrogen** Mw = 28.01	**Helium** Mw = 4.003	**Hydrogen** Mw = 2.016
15	7.699×10^{-4}	3.957×10^{-4}	8.388×10^{-4}
20	7.077×10^{-4}	3.913×10^{-4}	8.083×10^{-4}
25	6.572×10^{-4}	3.887×10^{-4}	7.838×10^{-4}
30	6.155×10^{-4}	3.876×10^{-4}	7.650×10^{-4}
35	5.816×10^{-4}	3.881×10^{-4}	7.500×10^{-4}

If we assume that our bodies consist of mostly water, we can uses Henry's Law to determine the equilibrium concentration of nitrogen that is dissolved in our bodies as a result of breathing air (assume that air contains approximately 79% nitrogen) at sealevel (1 Ata). For instance at 25°C, k_{N2} is given in Table 2-1 as 6.572×10^{-4} mol/L-Ata, and the amount of dissolved nitrogen in our blood at sealevel could be approximated as

$$c_{N2} = k_{N2} \cdot P_{N2} = 6.572 \times 10^{-4} \frac{mol}{L - Ata} \cdot 0.79 \; Ata$$

$$c_{N2} = 5.192 \times 10^{-4} \frac{mol}{L} \quad [\;called \; Molarity, \; M]$$

We can convert this Molarity concentration into a mass concentration by multiplying the molarity concentration by the molecular weight of nitrogen to obtain

$$c_{N2} = 5.192 \times 10^{-4} \left(\frac{mol}{L}\right) \cdot 28.01 \left(\frac{gm}{mol}\right) = 1.45 \times 10^{-2} \frac{gm}{L}$$

However, if we dive to 190 FSW (6.76 Ata) and breathe air (P_{N2} = 5.34 Ata) until our bodies absorb enough nitrogen to reach a new equilibrium, the concentration of nitrogen in our blood would increase to approximately

$$c_{N2} = k_{N2} \cdot P_{N2} = 6.572 \times 10^{-4} \frac{mol}{L - Ata} \cdot 5.34 \; Ata$$

$$c_{N2} = 3.510 \times 10^{-3} \frac{mol}{L}$$

or at 190 FSW

$$c_{N2} = 3.510 \times 10^{-3} \; \frac{mol}{L} \cdot 28.01 \; \frac{gm}{mol} = 9.83 \times 10^{-2} \; \frac{gm}{L}$$

or over 5 times as much dissolved nitrogen as compared to sealevel conditions. If not brought out of solution slowly during the diver's ascent back to the surface (i.e., decompress), this increase in dissolved nitrogen in a diver's blood and his other body tissues can lead to a dangerous condition commonly referred to as the "bends". A further discussion of the consequences of dissolved gases at elevated pressures will be given in Chapter 4 when we examine a common theory of decompression and derive ways to predict decompression schedules.

2.10 Gas Properties

At pressures other than sealevel, diver's are forced to breathe gas mixtures other than air to avoid dangerous physiological factors (these will be discussed later). Conventionally, these respiratory mixtures have contained varying percentages of nitrogen and oxygen (referred to as *nitrox*), helium and oxygen (referred to as *heliox*), or some combination of these three gases (*trimix*). However, some research, particularly in European and Asian countries, has been directed to the use of gas mixtures containing high percentages of hydrogen and oxygen (*hydrox*).

In many engineering calculations, it is important to have methods to derive the properties of any combination of gases at temperatures and pressures which covers the limits of divers' capabilities. The following relationships can be used to calculate the physical and thermal properties of an infinite number of gas mixtures.

2.10.1   Molecular Weight, M_{mix}

$$M_{mix} = \sum_{i=1}^{n} M_i \cdot X_i \qquad (2\text{-}38)$$

where M_{mix} is the molecular weight of the gas mixture; n is the number of gas components in the mixture; M_i is the molecular weight of the ith component (see Table 2-2); and X_i is the volume fraction of the ith component.

Table 2-2: Properties of Gases Commonly Found in Breathing Mixtures
(Properties taken from U.S. Navy Diving-Gas Manual at 70°F)

Gas	Molecular Weight	Specific Heat c_p, Btu/lbm- °F	Thermal Conductivity Btu/ft-hr-°F
Oxygen	32.0	0.22	0.0150
Nitrogen	28.01	0.25	0.0148
Helium	4.003	1.24	0.086
Hydrogen	2.016	3.43	0.101
Carbon Dioxide	44.01	0.20	0.0093
Carbon Monoxide	28.01	0.25	0.0132
Water Vapor	18.02	1.00	0.0140

Example: What is the molecular weight of a gas mixture containing 10% oxygen and 90 % helium?

Solution:

$$M_{mix} = \sum_{i=1}^{n} M_i \cdot X_i = 32\,(0.1) + 4.003\,(0.9) = 6.803$$

2.10.2 Specific Heat, c_{pmix}

$$c_{p_{mix}} = \frac{\sum_{i=1}^{n} M_i \cdot X_i \cdot c_{p_i}}{M_{mix}} \qquad (2\text{-}39)$$

where c_{pmix} is the specific heat of the gas mixture, Btu/lbm-°F; and c_{pi} is the specific heat of the ith component (see Table 2-2).

Example: What is the specific heat of the same gas mixture containing 10% oxygen and 90% helium?

Solution:

$$c_{p_{mix}} = \frac{\sum_{i=1}^{n} M_i \cdot X_i \cdot c_{p_i}}{M_{mix}} = \frac{32\,(0.1)\,(0.22) + 4.003\,(0.9)\,(1.24)}{6.803}$$

$$c_{p_{mix}} = 0.76\ \frac{Btu}{lbm - °F}$$

2.10.3 Gas Constant, R_{mix}

$$R_{mix} = \frac{R_u}{M_{mix}} \qquad (2\text{-}40)$$

where R_{mix} is the gas constant for the gas mixture, ft-lbf/lbm-°R; and R_u is the Universal Gas Constant, 1544 ft-lbf/mol-°R.

Example: What is the gas constant for the mixture in the above example?

Solution: Using the molecular weight calculated earlier, we get

$$R_{mix} = \frac{R_u}{M_{mix}} = \frac{1544\ \frac{ft-lbf}{mol-°R}}{6.803\ \frac{lbm}{mol}} = 227.1\ \frac{ft-lbf}{lbm-°R}$$

2.10.4   Gas Density, ρ_{mix}

Gases at relatively low pressures behave as *ideal gases*, which we saw previously can be described using one form of the Ideal Gas Law (a discussion of non-ideal gas behavior will follow later). With ideal gas behavior, we can write:

$$\frac{P}{\rho} = R \cdot T$$

Rearranging to solve for the density of a gas mixture, we get

$$\rho_{mix} = \frac{P}{R_{mix} \cdot T} \qquad\qquad (2\text{-}41)$$

where ρ_{mix} is the density of the gas mixture, P is the *absolute pressure*, R_{mix} is the gas constant (calculated above), and T is *absolute temperature*. We must be careful when calculating density to insure that proper dimensions are used; otherwise severe errors will result in our design analyses. If we wish to calculate density in units of lbm/ft³ using pressure in psia, a conversion of 144 in²/ft² will be necessary in the above equation.

    Example: What is the density of a gas mixture containing 10% oxygen and 90% helium at a pressure of 1.0 Ata (14.7 psia) and 70°F?

    Solution: Using the stated conditions and the gas constant found above, we have

$$\rho_{mix} = \frac{P}{R_{mix} \cdot T} = \frac{14.7 \, \frac{lbf}{in^2} \cdot 144 \, \frac{in^2}{ft^2}}{227.1 \, \frac{ft\text{-}lbf}{lbm\text{-}°R} \cdot (70° + 460°R)} = 0.0176 \, \frac{lbm}{ft^3}$$

2.10.5   Gas Viscosity, μ_{mix}

The viscosity of most gases is little affected by pressure, but shows a strong dependency on temperature. To obtain the viscosity of a gas mixture, we first need to find the viscosities of each gas component at the desired temperature. The temperature dependencies for viscosities of individual gas components can be approximated using the following:

$$\mu_i = A \left[\frac{459.67 + T}{529.67} \right]^b \qquad\qquad (2\text{-}42)$$

where μ_i is the viscosity of the ith gas component, lbm/ft-sec; T is the gas temperature, °F; and A and b are constants given in Table 2-3 below.

Table 2-3: Constants Used to Calculate Gas Viscosities

Gas	A	b
Oxygen	1.364 x 10^{-5}	0.810
Helium	1.323 x 10^{-5}	0.6694
Nitrogen	1.184 x 10^{-5}	0.7704
Carbon Dioxide	0.991 x 10^{-5}	0.999
Air	1.212 x 10^{-5}	0.710

Example: What are the viscosities of oxygen and helium at 70°F?

Solution: Using the constants A and b given in the above table, we obtain for oxygen at 70°F

$$\mu_{O_2} = 1.364 \ x \ 10^{-5} \cdot \left[\frac{459.67 + 70°}{529.67°} \right]^{0.81} = 1.364 \ x \ 10^{-5} \ \frac{lbm}{ft-sec}$$

and for helium

$$\mu_{He} = 1.323 \ x \ 10^{-5} \cdot \left[\frac{459.67 + 70°}{529.67°} \right]^{0.6694} = 1.323 \ x \ 10^{-5} \ \frac{lbm}{ft-sec}$$

We can confirm in the above equations that the value of the constant A is actually the viscosity of each gas component at 70°F. Variations in these gas viscosities away from 70°F can be found using the above temperature relationships.

Once the viscosity of each gas component is known at the desired temperature, the viscosity of the gas mixture can be found using the following expression:

$$\mu_{mix} = \sum_{i=1}^{n} \left[\frac{X_i \cdot \mu_i}{\sum_{j=1}^{n} X_j \cdot \Phi_{ij}} \right] \tag{2-43}$$

where μ_{mix} is the viscosity of the gas mixture, lbm/ft-sec; n is the number of gas components; μ_i is the viscosity of the ith component; X_i is the volume fraction of the ith component; and Φ_{ij} is a dummy variable defined as

$$\Phi_{ij} = \frac{1}{\sqrt{8}} \cdot \left[1 + \frac{M_i}{M_j} \right]^{-0.5} \cdot \left[1 + \sqrt{\frac{\mu_i}{\mu_j}} \left(\frac{M_j}{M_i} \right)^{\frac{1}{4}} \right]^2 \tag{2-44}$$

where M_i and M_j are molecular weights of the ith and jth components.

Example: What is the viscosity of the 10% oxygen/90% helium gas mixture at 70°F?

Solution: First, the equation which allows us to calculate the viscosity of the gas mixture is expanded for a 2 component mixture ($n = 2$). We will designate component #1 as helium, and oxygen as component #2 in this example. This expansion looks like the following:

$$\mu_{mix} = \frac{X_{He} \cdot \mu_{He}}{X_{He} \cdot \Phi_{He\,He} + X_{O_2} \cdot \Phi_{He\,O_2}} + \frac{X_{O_2} \cdot \mu_{O_2}}{X_{He} \cdot \Phi_{O_2\,He} + X_{O_2} \cdot \Phi_{O_2\,O_2}}$$

where

$$\Phi_{He\,O_2} = \frac{1}{\sqrt{8}} \cdot \left[1 + \frac{M_{He}}{M_{O_2}} \right]^{-0.5} \cdot \left[1 + \sqrt{\frac{\mu_{He}}{\mu_{O_2}}} \left(\frac{M_{O_2}}{M_{He}} \right)^{\frac{1}{4}} \right]^2$$

Recalling the molecular weights and viscosities that we obtained above for each of the gas components, we obtain

$$\Phi_{He\,O_2} = \frac{1}{\sqrt{8}} \cdot \left[1 + \frac{4.003}{32} \right]^{-0.5} \cdot \left[1 + \sqrt{\frac{1.323 \times 10^{-5}}{1.364 \times 10^{-5}} \left(\frac{32}{4.003} \right)^{\frac{1}{4}}} \right]^2$$

$$\Phi_{He\,O_2} = 2.3514$$

It is left to the reader to show that

$$\Phi_{O_2\,He} = 0.3033$$

$$\Phi_{He\,He} = 1.0000$$

$$\Phi_{O_2\,O_2} = 1.0000$$

Note: We can confirm that for all identical subscript pairs, such as Φ_{11}, Φ_{22}, Φ_{33}, etc, the value of the dummy variable will always be equal to 1.0000.

Now that we have found the viscosities of each component, and the values of all dummy variables, we can calculate the viscosity of this 2-component heliox gas mixture as

$$\mu_{mix} = \left[\frac{0.9\,(1.323)}{0.9\,(1) + 0.1\,(2.3514)} + \frac{0.1\,(1.364)}{0.9\,(0.3033) + 0.1\,(1)} \right] \times 10^{-5}$$

$$\mu_{mix} = 1.4147 \times 10^{-5} \; \frac{lbm}{ft\text{-}sec}$$

Note: Observe that the viscosity of the mixture is greater than the viscosities of either of the two components.

Viscosities of other gas mixtures can be similarly found using the method described above. While more laborious than the calculations shown for a 2-component mixture, the viscosities for 3-, 4-, and greater components can likewise be found.

2.10.6   Thermal Conductivity, *K*

An identical method as used above to find the viscosities of gas mixtures can be used to calculate the thermal conductivities of gases, by replacing values of μ_i in Equations 2-43 and 2-44 with values of the gas thermal conductivities given in Table 2-2. It is left to the reader to find the thermal conductivity of the 10% oxygen/90% helium mixture used in the above examples.

2.11 Non-ideal Gas Behavior

A gas is said to behave as an *ideal gas* if (a) the molecules in the gaseous state do not exert any force, either attractive or repulsive, on one another, and (b) the volumes of the molecules are negligibly small when compared to that of the container. At low atmospheric pressures and normal temperatures, these two assumptions would seem reasonable for most real gases. Under these conditions, the molecules of real gases are relatively far apart, and attractive forces between their molecules are negligible.

Under these conditions, we say previously that the behavior of the ideal gas can be described with the expression

$$P \cdot V = n \cdot R_u \cdot T$$

where P is gas absolute pressure, Ata; V is the gas volume, liters; n is the number of moles contained in the volume; T is the absolute temperature, °K; and R_u is a proportionality constant, referred to as the universal gas constant, 0.0821 L-Ata/°K-mol. Note that 1 mol of an ideal gas will always satisfy

$$\frac{P\ V}{R_u\ T} = 1 \qquad\qquad (2\text{-}45)$$

no matter what the temperature or pressure.

However, we can not assume that this ideal gas behavior will hold under all conditions. For example, without intermolecular forces, real gases could not condense to form liquids at higher pressures and/or lower temperatures. At high pressures, the density of the gas increases; the molecules are much closer to one another. The intermolecular forces can become significant enough to affect the motion of the molecules resulting in significant deviations from ideal gas behavior. Similarly, at low temperatures, the kinetic energy of the gas molecules decreases, depriving them of the drive they need to break away from their mutual attractive influences.

In 1873, the Dutch physicist J. D. van der Waals first dealt with deviations from Eq (2-45) which result at high pressures and low temperatures by mathematically accounting for the intermolecular forces and finite molecular volumes for real gases. According to kinetic molecular theory, gas pressure is the result of collisions between the molecules and the walls of the container, and its magnitude will depend on how "hard" the molecules strike the wall. Van der Waal rationalized that the impact of a molecule against the wall of the vessel in which it was contained would be softened due to the intermolecular attractions of its neighboring molecules. He stated that this "softening" effect would be proportional to the square of the number of molecules per unit volume in the container, or $(n/V)^2$. Thus, van der Waal suggested that the pressure that would be exerted by an ideal gas, P_{ideal}, could be related to the experimentally measured pressure, P_{real}, by the expression

$$P_{ideal} = P_{real} + \frac{a\,n^2}{V^2}$$

where *a* is simply a proportionality constant in this pressure correction. He also corrected for the finite, although small, volume of the gas molecules by noting that the effective container volume used in Eq (2-45) should be

$$V_{corrected} = V - n\,b$$

where *b* is a constant which attempts to account for the volume of the gas molecules. Taking into account the above corrections for pressure and volume, Eq (2-45) can now be written as

$$\left(P + \frac{a\,n^2}{V^2} \right)(V - n\,b) = n\,R\,T \qquad (2\text{-}46)$$

which is known as the *van der Waal's equation*. Constants *a* and *b*, given in Table 2-4 have been experimentally determined for common gases to give the best possible agreement between van der Waal's equation and actual gas behavior.

Table 2-4: Van der Waals Constants of Some Common Gases

Gas	a (atm-L²/mol²)	b (L/mol)
He	0.034	0.0237
Ne	0.211	0.0171
Ar	1.34	0.0322
H_2	0.244	0.0266
N_2	1.39	0.0391
O_2	1.36	0.0318
CO_2	3.59	0.0427
CH_4	2.25	0.0428
H_2O	5.46	0.0305

Note that the magnitude of *a* indicates how strongly a given type of gas molecule attracts one another. Also, *b* roughly correlates with the molecular size. The closer that *a* and *b* approach zero, the more closely that a gas can be approximated as an ideal gas. Helium molecules have the weakest attraction for one another as indicated by *a*.

Figure 2-1 compares the behaviors of several gases with that of an ideal gas ($PV/R_uT = 1$ for an ideal gas) over a range of pressures from zero to 400 Ata. Observe that for pressures up to 50 Ata (1617 FSW), oxygen, helium and hydrogen are within 5% of ideal gas behavior.

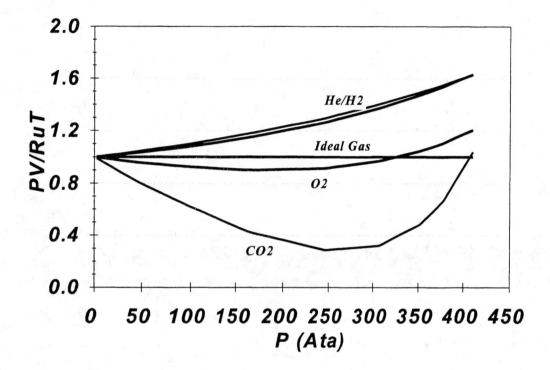

Figure 2-1: Comparison of real gas behavior with that of an ideal gas at various pressures. All pressures were calculated based on 1 mole of gas at 27 C.

2.12 Light Transmission in Water

Visible light consists of a narrow band of electromagnetic radiation waves having wavelengths between 4 x 10^{-7} and 7 x 10^7 meters, see Figure 2-2. Daylight is comprised of a color spectrum including red (6.5 - 7.0 x 10^{-7} meters), orange (6.0 - 6.5 x 10^{-7} meters), yellow (5.5 - 6.0 x 10^{-7} meters), green (5.0 - 5.5 x 10^{-7} meters), blue (4.5 - 5.0 x 10^{-7} meters), and violet (4.0 - 4.5 x 10^{-7} meters).

A fundamental principle of physics states that all forms of electromagnetic waves which fall on a transparent body will be either absorbed, reflected, or transmitted through that body. As sunlight falls on a body of water, that portion of the light which is absorbed will vary with wavelength; colors having the longest wavelengths are absorbed quickest, while the shorter wavelengths are found at greater depths beneath the surface. Thus, colors underwater are continually modified with depth as the wavelengths of the visible spectrum are progressively absorbed by the water, or effectively filtered out. Just two inches beneath the surface, all the infra-red rays of the color spectrum are absorbed by the water. Within 20 to 30 feet, all reds have been filtered out. Orange, yellow, and one by one, the other colors vanish as depth increases. Beyond approximately one hundred feet, only blue and violet remain. This creates the blue-green cast characteristic of most deep water.

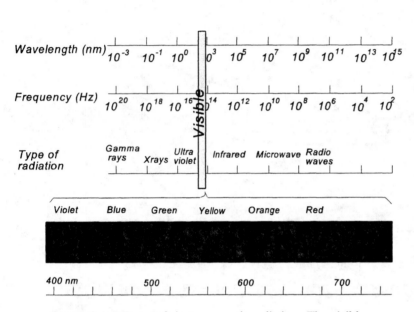

Figure 2-2: Types of electromagnetic radiation. The visible region ranges from 400 nm (violet) to 700 nm (red).

A second physical phenomenon which pertains to the portion of light which is transmitted into water has a direct effect on the apparent size and location of submerged objects. In 1850, Jean Leon Foucault conclusively demonstrated that the speed of light changes as it enters a medium having a different density from the medium in which it arrived. The speed of light decreases as it enters a higher density medium such as water, and will actually change direction as it slows down. This bending of light rays, called *refraction*, makes objects seem closer (and thus bigger) underwater. Refraction also accounts for our bad aim at a shell or fish when we poke a stick into the water surface while standing in shallow water. Not only does the untrained spear fisherman miss his target, but the spear appears to suddenly bend the moment it enters the water.

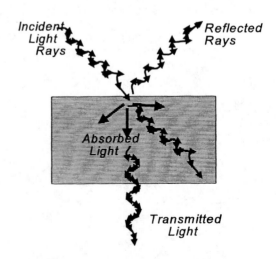

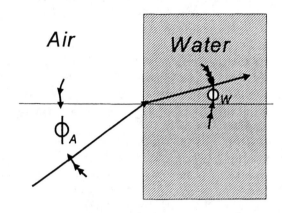

The refraction of light as it passes from one medium to another can be predicted by *Snell's Law*

$$\frac{\sin \phi_A}{\sin \phi_W} = \frac{N_W}{N_A} \qquad (2\text{-}47)$$

where ϕ_A is the angle at which the light strikes the water surface, i.e., the *angle of incidence*; ϕ_W is the angle at which the light is refracted into the water, i.e., the *angle of refraction*; N_A is the *index of refraction* of the medium through which the light arrives (air in this case); and N_W is the index of refraction of the refracting medium (water in this case), see Table 2-5.

Table 2-5: Optical Properties of Typical Substances

Medium	Index of Refraction, N_i
Glass (SiO_2)	1.544
Water @ 20° C	1.333
Air	1.000

We can use Snell's Law to predict how light is altered as it passes from air to water as follows:

$$\frac{\sin \phi_A}{\sin \phi_W} = \frac{1.333}{1.000} = \frac{4}{3}$$

This has the effect of making underwater objects appear to be larger, and closer, on a ratio of 4 (apparent size) to 3 (actual size). This effect is most pronounced when a diver is wearing a face mask of a helmet with a glass face-plate. The light rays reflected from an object first passes through the water, then through the glass, and finally travels through the air inside the mask or helmet before reaching the diver's eye. At each interface, the light ray is refracted as it enters a medium having a different density.

2.13 Sound Transmission in Water

Good communications between divers and surface tenders greatly improves safety and efficiency of underwater operations. Predictably, however, numerous obstacles are encountered when attempting to establish reliable voice communications underwater. In order that we may comprehend the factors which tend to disrupt and alter sound transmission underwater, a few basic principles of sound and speech behavior must be understood. Underwater acoustics is a much studied phenomenon with interest to all disciplines of undersea work and research. We will limit, however, our discussion to the concern of sound transmission for the working diver.

Sound behavior is similar to light behavior, in that sound and light are both wave phenomena. Sound waves, however, are waves of pressure rather than radiation. Vibrating objects produce sound which propagates in a wave pattern of moving molecules through the transmitting medium (air, seawater, etc). Since sound pressure is transmitted by molecules, the more closely packed, that is to say, the more dense the medium, the more efficiently the sound waves will be transmitted.

Water is an excellent conductor of sound because the molecular structure of water is more dense relative to that of air. The speed of sound underwater is about 5000 feet per second, compared to approximately 1,100 feet per second in air. Sound in water therefore travels more efficiently than in air-- sound emitted from a distance underwater will arrive at a diver over 4 times faster than sound emitted from the same distance on land. While this allows a diver to pick up sounds more easily underwater, it does present the diver with some difficulties.

Directional discrimination by the human ear is dependent upon the ability to detect the difference in time of arrival of sound in each ear. Sound is received, or detected, by vibration response to the sound that reaches the eardrum or microphone diaphragm (this is called sympathetic vibration). In air, we are able to discern the different times that sounds reach our two ears, allowing us to readily detect the direction from which the sound is originating. Since sound travels at a much higher speed underwater, however, the time interval between arrival at each ear is usually indiscernible by the diver. It is therefore difficult to determine the direction of any sound source underwater.

Another negative characteristic of sound travel underwater to the diver is the low attenuation of sound intensity over large distances. Low attenuation of sound underwater makes it difficult for divers to determine if the noise emitted from a power boat is coming directly overhead, or from several hundred feet away. The un-aided diver will be unable to tell what direction the power boat is traveling, or whether it is approaching or moving away.

Voice communications underwater are adversely affected for many reasons. First, sound originating in air will be highly attenuated as it enters water; likewise, sound originating in water will be highly attenuated as it enters air. Due to the large difference in densities of these two mediums, a sound wave will be mostly reflected at the air-water interface. Second, voice transmissions through water are inhibited since vocal chords and eardrums are adapted to transmit and receive vibrations in air. Talking underwater, therefore, is virtually impossible from diver to diver unless aided with electronic communications, or by eliminating the water interface between the divers (helmet to helmet contact has been used by divers to remove the water interface).

Other communications problems are encountered as a result of the life support equipment used by divers. Equipment worn by the diver for breathing purposes creates noise during operation. This equipment can also restrict the diver's vocal mechanisms, and alter the quality of the diver's voice sound by reverberation within the mask or helmet. Air intake jets in a diver's mast or helmet create noise as pressurized breathing gas expands and rushes into the mask or helmet. These inlet and exhaust valves can sometimes chatter as a result of vibrations induced by this gas flow.

Additionally, exhaust bubbles escaping into the water create noise. The effect of this noise is two-fold; first, it introduces a level of background noise which interferes with the diver's voice transmissions and sound receptions. Second, it interferes with the diver's ability to hear himself speak. Restricting the diver's ability to hear his own speech, tends to inhibit the diver's automatic self-regulating voice control mechanisms, causing him to shout or distort his speech.

Mouthpieces, face masks, and helmets will also tend to restrict the free movement of our vocal mechanisms. A mouthpiece inhibits the motion of our tongue and lips for articulating speech. A full face mask often presses the chin into the throat, making it difficult to move the jaw properly and placing pressure on the vocal chords. Some helmets use a neck ring assembly, or neckdam, which puts pressure on the throat area and affects the vocal chords. Demand air valves, incorporated in many mask and helmet designs, are designed to maintain a pressure inside the mask or helmet that is slightly higher than the surrounding seawater pressure. While this ensures that water does not enter the mask or helmet, it requires the diver to speak against a slightly elevated back pressure, causing some speech distortion.

The airspace within masks and helmets also act as an acoustic chamber where sound from the diver's voice will reverberate. A helmet usually offers greater air space and produces better sound quality than masks. In addition, helmets allow the diver's ears to remain dry, exposing the ears to sound from the diver's voice directly. This dry enclosure allows better auditory feedback, which contributes to an improved self-regulating speech. On the other hand, masks usually provide less air space for sounds to reverberate, resulting in greater distortion. Also, masks which do not enclose the ears do not allow the diver to directly hear the sound from his own speech; this sometimes causes the diver to shout, or elevate the volume of his speech.

Elevated pressures associated with deep diving operations also directly effect the quality of the diver's speech in two ways. First, high pressures have been shown to produce a steady decline in speech intelligibility. Voice levels tend to rise, with speech tones taking on a nasal quality. This may be partially due to the elevated back pressures present in breathing apparatuses which alter the vocal chords' response frequency. Second, as exposures increase in depth various gas mixtures are employed to satisfy the diver's physiological needs. These different respiratory gases tend to change the vocal sounds that a diver will make due to their increased densities, resulting in higher speeds of sound propagation. At depths beyond 190 FSW, mixtures of helium and oxygen are primarily used as the breathing medium, with higher percentages of helium used as depth increases. A 90% helium content in the breathing medium generally renders a diver's speech almost completely unintelligible.

Finally, another concern to the diver which results from the reduction in sound attenuation underwater is the increased risk of hearing loss. Physical pain and ear damage can occur from underwater operations producing dangerous noise levels, operations which would ordinarily be safe if conducted in air at the surface. The sound levels of some high-powered pneumatic tools approach pain threshold underwater. Most damaging to the ears are the shock effects caused by the pressure waves produced through underwater explosions.

2.14 Closure

The physical phenomena discussed in this chapter have critical influences on the way that the human body reacts to the high pressure environments that exist beneath the water's surface. The types and quantities of gases at elevated pressures must all be taken into consideration when designing life support equipment for diving and hyperbaric systems. The next two chapters will discuss many of the physiological concerns that we must face when breathing gases at high pressures.

3

Diving Physiology

Objectives

The objectives of this chapter are to
- gain a basic understanding of the circulatory and respiratory systems in the human body
- understand metabolic requirements as they relate to various activities
- understand the physiological concerns related to breathing gases at elevated pressures
- understand some of the mechanical effects of breathing gases at elevated pressures
- give an overview of the thermal concerns related to exposures to extreme environments

3.1   Introduction

The operators of manned submersibles, atmospheric diving systems, and deep-sea divers all require adequate support systems to maintain life in the hostile undersea environment. While the crew for submersibles and atmospheric diving systems are normally exposed to environments similar to that experienced on the surface, they must still have their atmospheres carefully maintained, with regards to gas composition and temperature, to prevent adverse physiological effects or excessive thermal losses.

The deep-sea diver's work capacity, on the other hand, is severely limited by the physiological effects of the high surrounding pressures and the bone-chilling seawater temperatures. Increased gas density has been shown to restrict the diver's ability to do useful work by limiting the maximum voluntarily ventilation (MVV) in his lungs by up to 50% when in dry chamber environments at 1000 feet of seawater (FSW) (U.S. Navy Diving Manual, 1991). The ability to breathe is further reduced when utilizing an underwater breathing apparatus (UBA) at elevated pressures due to the inherent resistance of the UBA to the dense gas medium. Water temperatures as low as -2°C, coupled with the thermal properties of the surrounding medium, necessitates reliable means to protect divers from excessive heat losses through their clothing and during respiration.

An equally important concern to divers is the increasingly tight control that must be maintained on the quality and composition of their breathing gas as depth increases. The very gas that we depend on to sustain life on the surface becomes toxic to the deep-sea diver (NOAA Diving Manual, 1991). Nitrogen in air becomes increasingly narcotic as depth increases, causing a rapid drop in performance and judgment. Air is generally replaced with a less narcotic helium-oxygen (heliox), or hydrogen-oxygen (hydrox), mixture when the partial pressure of nitrogen (P_{N2}) exceeds 81.5 psi (5.55 atmospheres), equivalent to a P_{N2} when breathing air at depths beyond 190 FSW (~58 meters).

Further refinements in the diver's breathing gas must be made to avoid the toxic behavior of oxygen when present at elevated atmospheric pressures. Acute exposures to oxygen partial pressures (P_{O2}) above approximately 23.5 psi (1.6 atm) cause a distinct possibility for divers to experience toxic reactions, ultimately leading to convulsions similar to those seen in epileptic seizures. This apparent poisoning of the central nervous system (see *CNS oxygen toxicity*) could occur when breathing pure oxygen at depths beyond 20 feet of seawater (6 meters), or when breathing air at depths beyond 213 FSW (65 meters). Even at a P_{O2} as low 7.4 psi (0.5 atm), severe irritation and damage can occur in the lungs during prolonged exposures (see *pulmonary oxygen poisoning*). Such a hazard is not likely to become a factor except during *saturation diving* (i.e., long duration exposures where decompression is no longer dependent on mission length).

And yet, sufficient oxygen must be present in the inspired gas mix to support life. Generally, a minimum oxygen partial pressure of 0.16 to 0.2 Ata is required to maintain normal oxygen levels in the blood. Due to the above considerations, and the fact that gas partial pressures increase directly with increases in the environmental pressure, divers are required to use multiple gas mixtures as they travel to variable depths. It is not uncommon for divers at depths of 1000 feet of seawater, or more, to breathe a gas mixture containing less than 1% oxygen by volume with the remaining 99+% being helium, or even a blend of helium and nitrogen. Even more critical is the minimal margin of error that can be tolerated with these gas mixes in deep dives; oxygen percentages above 1.6% could mean pulmonary oxygen poisoning during long missions at 1000 FSW, while the first signs of hypoxia would occur with oxygen percentages below 0.5%. This need for ever-increasing accuracy in the gas mix will continue as depths increase.

The above considerations must be well understood by the designer of life support equipment for use in hyperbaric environments. This chapter will discuss many of these critical concerns and give an overview of how these concerns are amplified in a subsea environment. We will first look at the basic physiological processes that are necessary to maintain human life, and then review some of the ways in which exposures to elevated pressures can adversely affect these physiological processes.

3.2   The Circulatory and Respiratory Systems

In engineering terminology, the human body can be thought of as an assemblage of well tuned systems and subsystems, all vitally interdependent. The 2 major systems of particular importance to the life support engineer are the *circulatory system* and the *respiratory system.*

3.2.1 Circulatory System

The circulatory system, shown schematically in Figure 3-1 actually consists of two separate circuits, connected to one another by the heart. The *systemic circuit* supplies oxygen enriched blood to the cells throughout the body's skeletal, muscular, and nervous systems, and removes the metabolically produced carbon dioxide from these cells for expulsion in the lungs. The *pulmonary circuit* supplies blood enriched with carbon dioxide to the lungs and returns oxygen enriched blood to the heart for a repeat circulation. Since the human body has no mechanism for storing oxygen, this circulation process must continue uninterrupted or cell damage will occur within minutes.

Each circuit consists of a vast network of *capillaries* where blood-gas exchanges take place within the lungs and the systemic systems. Blood is supplied from the heart to these capillaries in both circuits through *arteries* and returned to the heart through *veins*. The heart contains two upper chambers (*atriums*) which receive the returned blood from the veins, and two muscular lower chambers (*ventricles*) which pump the blood out through the arteries. The right side of the heart receives blood from the systemic circuit through the *vena cava* and pumps it to the pulmonary capillary bed to expel carbon dioxide and uptake oxygen. The left side of the heart receives oxygenated blood back from the pulmonary circuit and pumps it via the large elastic *aorta* to the systemic circuit.

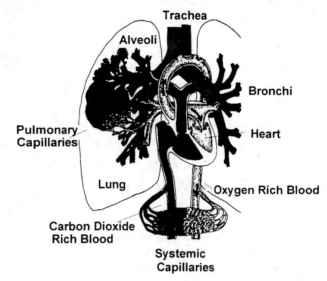

Figure 3-1: Cardio-pulmonary system.

At rest, a healthy human heart will pump approximately 5 liters of blood per minute. This *cardiac output* can increase to 35 liter/min for an individual at hard work. Considering that a blood volume of approximately 6 liters is typical (approximately 40 cc per pound of lean body weight), it is somewhat amazing that the entire volume of blood makes a complete circulation in slightly over a minute when at rest; this reduces to 8 seconds when at hard work! This circulating blood consists of approximately 50% plasma, 45% red cells containing the iron-rich hemoglobin, and approximately 5% white cells and platelets. The red cells have a high affinity for oxygen, and provide the major avenue for oxygen delivery to the cells. The white cells attack and consume bacteria in the body, and provide our major source of defense against disease. Platelets are involved in the important blood clotting process.

3.2.2 Respiratory System

The human respiratory system consists of the lungs, air passages, rib cage, and diaphragm. The lungs are made up of two elastic organs containing approximately 300 million tiny air sacs, called *alveoli* located at the ends of the air passages. The alveoli (each with an average diameter of 0.25 mm) present a large (estimated to be up to 750 square feet), moist surface area to facilitate the gas-exchange processes between medium and the pulmonary blood flow. The alveoli walls, although infiltrated with an almost solid network of interconnecting pulmonary capillaries, are extremely thin (averaging approximately 0.5 microns). Obviously, these gas-exchange membranes are extremely fragile and can tolerate only small pressure differentials across them without suffering damage. Breathing gases reach the alveoli by traveling through the nose or mouth into the trachea (the main wind pipe), into successively smaller branches including the *bronchi* and *bronchioles*.

The process of respiration can be divided into two distinct but interrelated categories:

1) pulmonary ventilation, or the inflow and outflow of breathing gases between the atmosphere and the alveoli,

and

2) the exchange of oxygen, carbon dioxide, and other inert gases which take place throughout the body as part of the metabolic process.

For clarification, the first category will be referred to as "*external respiration*" while the second category will be referred to as *internal respiration.*

3.2.2.1   *External Respiration*

The movement of gases in and out of the lungs results from the cyclic expansion and contraction of the lung volume. The lung volume expands as the diaphragm contracts and moves downward to lengthen the chest cavity, while the rib cage is elevated to increase the diameter of the chest cavity. We saw from Boyle's Law (see Diving Physics) that as a volume expands the pressure within that

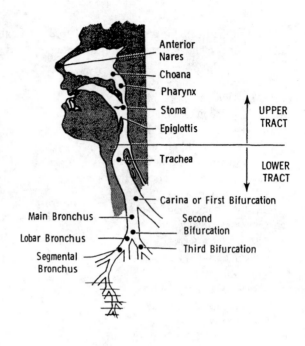

Figure 3-2: Human airways.

volume must fall. This reduction in pressure relative to atmospheric pressure causes additional gases to be drawn into the lungs (inspiration). During expiration, the diaphragm is relaxed, allowing it to move upward while the rib cage diameter decreases. The effect is to reduce the lung volume while increasing the intra-alveoli pressure above the atmospheric pressure, resulting in respiratory gases being forced out. During normal respiration, the rise and fall of alveoli pressure relative to the surrounding atmosphere is less than 1 mm Hg. During maximum expiratory efforts, however, the alveoli pressure can be increased to over 100 mmHg (slightly less than 2 psi) in a healthy male, and during maximum inspiratory effort it can be reduced to as low as -80 mmHg (approximately -1.5 psi) without damaging the delicate gas-exchange membranes. Following an expiration, the lungs will still maintain approximately 1.0 - 1.5 liters of gas no matter how hard we try to force all gases out. This volume, referred to as the *residual volume* provides gas in the alveoli to aerate the blood between breaths. Were it not for this residual volume the alveoli would collapse between expiration and inspiration and cause the concentrations of oxygen and carbon dioxide in the blood to rise and fall markedly with each breathing cycle.

The level of expansion and contraction of the lungs will vary to accommodate a wide range of activity levels. Figure 3-3 depicts how the volumes of our lungs change to deliver sufficient oxygen and remove the necessary carbon dioxide over this range of activity levels. Descriptions of these lung characteristics follow.

Tidal Volume

The amount of gas inspired and expired with each normal breath is referred to as the *tidal volume (TV).* This volume is directly related to the diver's activity level, varying from as low as 0.5 liters when at rest to as high as 3 liters for short durations of extremely hard work (Guyton, 1976).

Inspiratory Reserve Volume

The extra gas volume that can be inspired over and above a normal tidal volume is called the *inspiratory reserve volume (IRV)*. As shown in Figure 3-3, the healthy adult male can accommodate up to approximately 3 liters additional gas volume over resting during high activity or during a forced inhalation.

Expiratory Reserve Volume

The amount of gas that can still be forcefully exhaled at the completion of a normal expiration is called the *expiratory reserve volume (ERV)*. This normally amounts to about 1.1 liters in a healthy adult male.

Residual Volume

As discussed previously, following maximum expiration to the limits of the ERV, the lungs will still maintain approximately 1.0-1.5 liters of gas. This volume, called the *residual volume*, consists of the volume of gas in the bronchi, bronchioles, and the gas in the alveoli. Were it not for this residual volume the alveoli would collapse between expiration and inspiration, and be unable to aerate the blood between breaths. This would cause the concentrations of oxygen and carbon dioxide in the blood to rise and fall markedly with each breathing cycle.

Vital Capacity

Vital capacity (VC) is the maximum volume of gas that a person can forcefully expel from his lungs after first inflating the lungs to the maximum extent. Note that the vital capacity equals the sum of the resting tidal volume, the

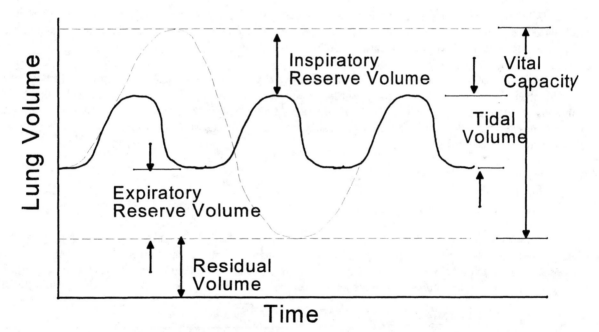

"Typical" Lung Volumes (Healthy Male Adult)

Residual Volume: 1.0 - 1.5 Liters
Tidal Volume: 0.5 L (Resting) - 3 L (Hard Work)
Inspiratory Reserve: 3.0 Liters
Expiratory Reserve: 1.1 Liters
Vital Capacity: 4.6 Liters

Figure 3-3: Volumes of the human lung during respiration.

inspiratory reserve volume, and the expiratory reserve volume, or

$$VC, \; liters \; = \; TV \; + \; IRV \; + \; ERV$$

In a healthy adult male, the vital capacity will nominally be about 4.6 liters (Guyton,1976); approximately 20-25% less in women. We will see later that in the design of a closed or semi-closed circuit breathing apparatus, the counter-lung must have a volume at least as big as the vital capacity to provide sufficient reserve volume in the circuit to satisfy all activity levels.

Dead Space

The volume of gas which enters the lungs at end of an inspiration never reaches the gas exchange membranes in the alveoli and thus does not directly participate in the blood oxygenation or carbon dioxide removal processes. At the end of an expiration, the CO_2- enriched gas occupying the air passages will remain to be mixed with fresh gas during the next inspiration. This volume of gas, occupying the upper airways, is called the *anatomical dead space* and consists of approximately 150 ml in a healthy male adult (about 1/3 of a resting tidal volume).

Since the volume of gas that actually reaches the alveoli with each breath equals the tidal volume minus the dead space, the larger the dead space, the more difficult it will be to eliminate CO_2. Although anatomical dead space is fixed, certain parts of a breathing apparatus, including the mouthpiece, oral-nasal mask, or full-face mask, will add an additional *engineering dead space* to the total lung/apparatus system. The wearer of these apparatus must compensate for this additional dead space by bringing in more gas with each breath; ie, he must increase his tidal volume by an amount equal to the added engineering dead space to provide the same level of ventilation to the alveoli. A failure to increase tidal volume will result in a build up of carbon dioxide within the lungs. This increase in tidal volume increases the energy that the user must expend to breathe, making it mandatory that the designer of breathing apparatus minimize this external dead space.

Respiratory Minute Volume

To satisfy the our body's requirements, oxygen is extracted from the respiratory gases as these gases travel through the lungs. The amount of gas that is processed through the lungs each minute to accomplish this oxygen delivery is referred to as the *respiratory minute volume (RMV)*[1], equal to the volume of gas moving in and out of the lungs per breath (lung *tidal volume (TV)*) times the *respiratory rate (f)*, the number of breaths taken per minute. That is

$$RMV \; (liters/min) \; = \; TV \; (liters/breath) \; x \; f \; (breaths/min) \qquad \textbf{(3-1)}$$

The normal respiratory rate for an adult is approximately 12 breaths per minute, but can go as high as 30 breaths per minute during heavy exercise. Therefore, RMV's ranging from a low of 6 liters per minute can be handled by the healthy adult when at rest, to a maximum of about 90 liters per minute during heavy work.

---

[1]RMV is generally expressed in units of liters per minute at conditions of *BTPS*, implying body temperature (98.6°F), ambient pressure, and saturated with water vapor.

3.2.2.2   *Internal Respiration*

Internal respiration for a person breathing air at 1 ATA is shown in the simplified diagram below. Dry air at 1 ATA (760 mm Hg) contains approximately 21% oxygen and 79% nitrogen with a trace (0.035%) of carbon dioxide. This gas mixture gives partial pressures for the inspired air of P_{O2} = 159 mmHg, P_{N2} = 600 mmHg, and P_{CO2} = 0.3 mmHg. Within the air passages the inspired gas mixes with residual gases in the lung and becomes fully humidified at body temperature (P_{H2O} = 47 mm Hg). Upon entering the alveoli the gas will have a P_{O2} = 100 mmHg, P_{CO2} = 40 mmHg, P_{H2O} = 47 mmHg, and P_{N2} = 573 mmHg. Rapid diffusion of oxygen occurs through the alveolus membrane into the pulmonary blood, raising the blood oxygen partial pressure from about 40 mmHg to 100 mmHg. Likewise, carbon dioxide diffuses almost instantaneously out across the alveolus membrane, reducing the blood P_{CO2} from 46 mmHg to about 40 mmHg. As a result of this mixing and exchange process within the lungs, the expired gas will show a P_{O2} of about 104 mmHg and P_{CO2} of 40 mmHg. Note that if the ambient pressure is higher or

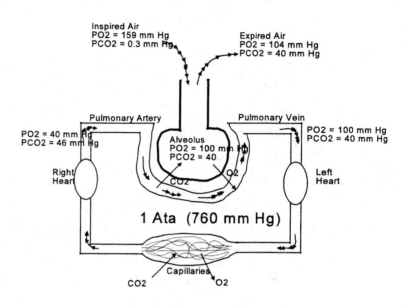

Figure 3-4: Gas exchange mechanisms in the cardiovascular/respiratory system at 1 Ata with air.

lower than 1 ATA, the partial pressures of each gas constituent will increase or decrease accordingly. Also, observe that since nitrogen does not participate in the cellular metabolic processes, no net exchange of nitrogen will occur across the alveoli membrane following equilibration with the bodies tissues.

3.3   Metabolic Needs

3.3.1 Oxygen Requirements

The entire gas exchange process at the alveolus - pulmonary blood flow interface occurs in our lungs such that oxygenated blood can be furnished to the systemic cells and metabolically-produced carbon dioxide can be removed. The amount of oxygen metabolized at the cells during the combustion of proteins, fats, and carbohydrates will vary with activity level; ranging from a low of 0.25 standard liters per minute (SLPM)[2] for a person while resting, to an excess of 3 SLPM for a short duration, hard activity. These rates of oxygen usage by the cells, referred to as the *oxygen consumption rate*, $\dot{V}_{O_2}$, are not effected by ambient pressure. That is, a diver working at 1000 FSW will consume the same amount of oxygen as a diver at the surface who is doing the same activity.

---

[2]A standard liter (SL) is specified at a temperature of 32°F (0°C) and a pressure of 1.0 atmosphere.

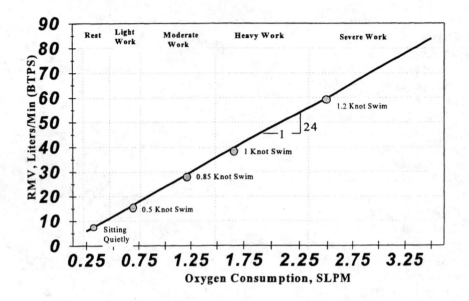

Figure 3-5: Oxygen Consumption and Respiratory Minute Volume At Varying Work Rates

Note that although the gas density passing through the diver's lungs will be affected by the ambient pressure in which the gas is being breathed, RMV will not be affected. Thus, we would expect that similar activities at varying depths will give similar values of RMV when recorded in units of BTPS. Figure 3-5 shows the relationships of oxygen consumption rate and respiratory minute volume to various underwater activities. This figure shows a nearly linear relationship between these two variables, observed experimentally as the following

$$\frac{RMV, \ LPM \ (BTPS)}{\dot{V}_{O_2}, \ SLPM} = 24 \qquad\qquad (3\text{-}2)$$

3.3.2 Carbon Dioxide Generation

Closely related to the oxygen consumption rate is the rate of carbon dioxide generation, $\dot{V}_{CO_2}$. As the cells burn oxygen and nutrients, carbon dioxide is generated as a by-product. The rate of carbon dioxide generation to oxygen uptake is called the *respiratory quotient (RQ)*. That is

$$RQ = \frac{\dot{V}_{CO_2}}{\dot{V}_{O_2}} \qquad\qquad (3\text{-}3)$$

Values for *RQ* change under different metabolic conditions. When a person is consuming carbohydrates entirely for body metabolism, *RQ* approaches 1.0. However, when a person utilizes fats almost entirely for metabolism, his *RQ* falls to approximately 0.7. On a normal diet of carbohydrates, fats and proteins a person will have an *RQ* of approximately 0.82. With this approximation we can calculate the rate at which carbon dioxide must be removed from a closed system, through ventilation or absorption, to prevent toxic levels of carbon dioxide to build up.

3.3.3 Control of Breathing

Respiratory centers in the brain and peripheral chemoreceptors on the aorta and carotid arteries, sensitive to the level of carbon dioxide in the blood, control the rate and volume of breathing. When the partial pressure of CO_2 becomes too high in the blood (a condition called *hypercapnia*) and the blood pH decreases, the centers trigger an increase in RMV until the carbon dioxide and acid levels are returned to normal.

The level of oxygen is also monitored by these peripheral receptors. A fall in oxygen partial pressure in the blood (a condition called *hypoxia*) will also cause signals to be sent to the respiratory centers in the brain. However, a low oxygen level, by itself, may not increase the breathing rate until a dangerously low P_{O2} occurs. Under these conditions, we may not be aware of impending danger.

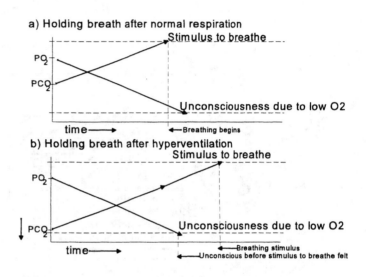

Figure 3-6: The dangers of hyperventilating prior to making a breath hold dive underwater.

Such are the dangers of *hyperventilation* in underwater environments as demonstrated graphically in Figure 3-6. Hyperventilation is a proven technique for prolonging a person's breathholding capability. By over-ventilating the lungs the partial pressure of carbon dioxide in the blood can be reduced below normal levels. This reduction in P_{CO2} removes the primary stimulus for breathing, allowing the diver to hold his breath longer until the carbon dioxide level builds. Meanwhile the P_{O2} in the blood may drop to dangerously low levels, causing unconsciousness, before the diver begins feeling air hunger or regains the stimulus to breathe.

3.4 Diving Maladies

Now that we are aware of the mechanisms in which our bodies carry on normal ventilation and circulatory functions, let us look at ways in which these mechanisms might break down when a person is subjected to different pressures and gas mixtures.

3.4.1 Hypoxia

As previously stated, hypoxia is a condition in which the cells fail to receive or utilize enough oxygen to support the metabolic process. Hypoxia can result from a number of reasons including:

- blockage or restriction of the airways
- diseased lungs which inhibit the diffusion processes which take place across the alveolar membranes
- circulatory restrictions such as those which occur in decompression sickness
- conditions in the blood which interfere with oxygen transport in the blood, and
- inadequate oxygen in the breathing mixture

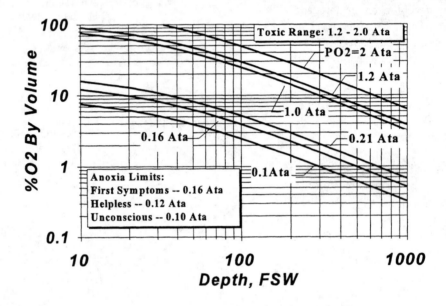

Figure 3-7: Oxygen requirements to avoid hypoxia and oxygen toxicity as depth varies.

As shown previously, the partial pressure of oxygen in dry inspired air at 1 Ata is approximately 0.21 Ata (159 mmHg). Under these conditions rapid diffusion of oxygen occurs at the alveolar membrane to raise the partial pressure of oxygen in the blood stream from about 40 mmHg to 100 mmHg. Sufficient oxygen can then be transported to the cells to support metabolic demands. However, if the P_{O2} being supplied to the lungs decreases, due to a reduction in oxygen concentration in the breathing mix or a decrease in environmental pressure (as in the case of mountain climbers or in other high altitude exposures) the diffusion of oxygen into the blood stream decreases.

Figure 3-7 shows the relationship between environmental pressure and minimum oxygen concentrations required to insure sufficient oxygen partial pressures to support life. Acceptable concentrations of oxygen can readily be found for any depth by using the expression

$$\%O_2 = \frac{P_{O_2}, Ata}{P_{Depth}, Ata} \times 100\%$$

Figure 3-7 shows that as the P_{O_2} drops from a normal level of 0.21 Ata to 0.16 Ata, the first symptoms of hypoxia appear. As this drop in atmospheric oxygen progresses, the subject becomes drowsy and unable to think clearly; similar to the effect of intoxication. As the level drops to 0.12 Ata the subject will begin rapid breathing and become quite helpless. Unconsciousness follows at 0.10 Ata, and death will quickly follow at 0.06 Ata unless higher P_{O_2} levels can be restored.

Effects of Various O$_2$ Partial Pressures on Humans
(Taken from U.S. Navy Diving and Manned Hyperbaric Systems
Safety Certification Manual, Oct 87)

Oxygen Partial Pressure, Ata	EFFECTS
0.18 - 0.21	No noticeable effect.
0.16 - 0.12	Increased breathing rate; lack of coordination.
0.14 - 0.10	Easily tired; easily upset emotionally; loss of sensitivity to pain or injury; abnormal fatigue from exertion.
0.10 - 0.06	Lethargic; apathetic; confused thinking; physical collapse; possible unconsciousness; nausea and vomiting.
0.06 or less	Convulsive movements; gasping; cessation of breathing

3.4.2 Oxygen Toxicity Concerns

As depth increases, the oxygen levels in a diver's breathing gas mixture must necessarily decrease to maintain the same oxygen partial pressure that we have acclimated to at the surface. P_{O_2} levels above approximately 1.6 atm have been shown to cause an acute toxic reaction to the diver. This level of oxygen partial pressure can be seen to occur at 1000 FSW with a gas mixture containing only 5% oxygen. Note in Figure 3-7 that the satisfactory oxygen concentrations in the breathing mix will vary with depth. That is, a mixture containing 5% oxygen may cause a toxic reaction when breathed at 1000 FSW but cause symptoms of hypoxia at depths less than 70 FSW.

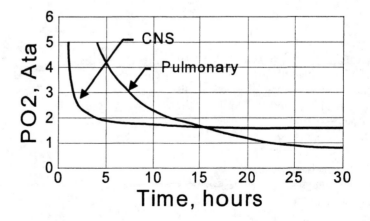

Figure 3-8: Time relationships for oxygen toxicity.

Acute oxygen toxicity appears to attack the central nervous system (CNS), thus frequently referred to as *CNS oxygen toxicity*. Muscle twitching, nausea, and even convulsions can occur with continued exposure to high levels of oxygen partial pressure. The acronym **VENTID** is often used to assist in remembering some of the symptoms common with CNS oxygen toxicity. This acronym stands for the following:

V	vision is impaired; tunnel vision
E	hearing is impaired; ringing in the ears
N	nausea
T	twitching
I	irritability
D	dizziness

Not to be confused with acute oxygen toxicity is *pulmonary oxygen toxicity*, a malady associated with prolonged exposures to elevated oxygen partial pressures in which cellular damage can occur in the airways. Figure 3-8 shows that both of these maladies are time related, in that divers can generally tolerate oxygen levels above 2.0 atm for short durations (less than 30 minutes) without experiencing CNS symptoms. On the other hand, oxygen exposures of less than 1.0 atm can cause tissue damage in the lungs after approximately 20 hours (U.S. Navy Dive Manual, 1977).

3.4.3 Hypercapnia

Defined as an excess of carbon dioxide in the blood, this condition can result from

a) an excessive level of carbon dioxide in the breathing gas
b) inadequate pulmonary ventilation, or
c) a failure of the carbon dioxide removal equipment used in either a closed or semi-closed breathing apparatus

As with oxygen toxicity, hypercapnia is time related as shown in Figure 3-9. For relatively short durations (up to 80 minutes), carbon dioxide partial pressures up to 0.015 atm can be tolerated without any perceptible physiological effects (U.S. Navy Diving-Gas Manual, 1971).

As carbon dioxide levels increase, or as the exposure durations increase, minor perceptive changes, including increased tidal volumes and small threshold hearing losses, can result (Zone II in Figure 3-9). In Zone III, headaches, tipsiness, nausea, "air hunger", tunnel vision, and mental depression might result. At carbon dioxide levels above 0.08-0.10 atm, a person could become helpless in less than 10 minutes (Zone IV), followed by unconsciousness unless the carbon dioxide level is reduced.

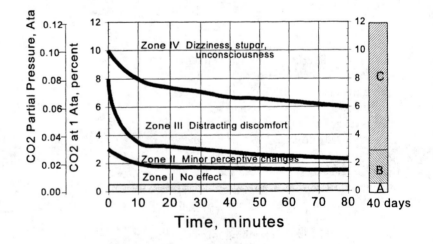

Figure 3-9: Relation Of Physiological Effects To Carbon Dioxide Concentration And Exposure Period (Taken from U.S. Navy Diving-Gas Manual, 1971).

During long duration exposures, carbon dioxide levels below 0.005 atm are required to cause no perceptible effects on a diver (Zone A). Note that this partial pressure of carbon dioxide represents a volume percentage of less than 0.016% when the diver is at a depth of 1000 FSW.

3.4.4 Asphyxia

Asphyxia is a term which describes the presence of both hypoxia and hypercapnia.

3.4.5 Carbon Monoxide Poisoning

The carbon monoxide molecule has an affinity for hemoglobin in the blood about 200 times stronger than does oxygen. Consequently, CO concentrations as low as 0.002 Ata (2000 parts per million) can be fatal as the primary transport mechanism for carrying oxygen in the blood will be critically inhibited (CO will be carried preferentially by the hemoglobin instead of O_2). Headache, nausea, vomiting, unnatural redness of the lips and fingernails are typical symptoms.

3.4.6 Nitrogen Narcosis

More romantically referred to as "rapture of the deep", nitrogen narcosis results due to the narcotic property of nitrogen when breathed at elevated partial pressures. While tolerances to nitrogen vary considerably, generally this narcotic behavior is first observed at about 100 FSW, although the diver is likely to be more relaxed at shallower depths. Narcosis can be extremely hazardous to the diver as depth increases; as the narcotic effect is magnified. Partial pressures of nitrogen greater than about 5.5 Ata (equivalent to breathing air at approximately 200 FSW) are not recommended. For deep dives beyond 200 FSW, nitrogen is generally replaced with a less narcotic inert gas such as helium or hydrogen.

3.4.7 High Pressure Nervous Syndrome (HPNS)

HPNS is a neurological and physiological dysfunction generally associated with hyperbaric exposures. Since symptoms of HPNS have normally been observed during high pressure exposures in heliox atmospheres (helium and oxygen mixtures), this malady has often been referred to as "helium tremors". Tremors, nausea, dizziness, and even convulsions may result from this poorly understood malady; however, these effects are generally attributed to the high pressure exposures rather than any physiological effect resulting from breathing helium. The addition of small levels of nitrogen (trimix) to the helium/oxygen mixture have been reported to lessen the severity of HPNS. Also, by slowing the rate of compression to reach a desired dive depth, the onset of HPNS has been shown to be minimized.

3.5 Injuries Due to the Mechanical Effects of Pressure (Barotrauma)

3.5.1 During Descent

3.5.1.1 Body Squeeze

When wearing dry suits in conjunction with a rigid helmet, excessive external pressure can build up on the diver if the pressure inside the helmet and suit are not equally increased as the diver descends. In the most severe accidents, such as when a diver falls from his diving platform or when the diver's gas umbilical from the surface was cut (prior to the introduction of non-return valves in helmets), a diver's body can be forced into his helmet.

3.5.1.2   Dry Suit Squeeze

Similarly, if the pressure inside a dry suit is not equilibrated with the surrounding water pressure, the suit material folds can pinch the diver's skin causing severe discomfort.

3.5.1.3   External   Ear   Squeeze

A tight fitting hood or ear plug will prevent the pressure on the outside of the ear drum to increase with increasing water pressure during a descent. Elevated pressures in the middle ear during the descent will cause the ear drum to be pressed outward causing pain, swelling, and possible rupture outward of the tympanic membrane.

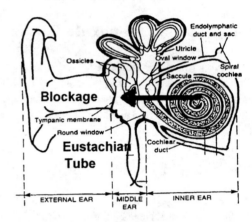

Figure 3-10: External Ear Squeeze.

3.5.1.4   Internal Ear Squeeze

A blocked eustachian tube connecting the middle ear with the diver's air passageway can become blocked due to swelling of the lining on this tube, or due to a buildup of mucous. Such blockage prevents the middle ear pressure from equilibrating with the surrounding water pressure. This can result in the ear drum being pressed inward causing pain, swelling, and possible rupture inward of the tympanic membrane.

3.5.1.5   Thoracic Squeeze

The increasing pressure during a descent while holding one's breath can cause the lung to be compressed to a volume less than the lung residual volume. Compression beyond the residual volume can cause body fluids (plasma, etc) to be forced into the airways. Thoracic squeeze is the primary limitation to the depth capability of breath hold diving (free diving).

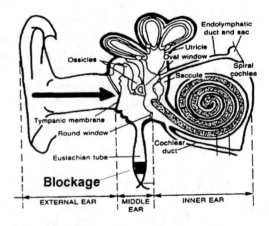

Figure 3-11: Internal Ear Squeeze

3.5.1.6   *Other Pressure Injuries During Descent*

Injuries which might result due to the failure to equalize pressures in the body's natural air spaces are

Eye Squeeze

Eye squeeze is common when using goggles or not equalizing mask during a descent.

Face Squeeze

Failure to equalize mask pressure may result in face Squeeze.

Tooth Squeeze

Tooth squeeze due to the presence of an internal void resulting from an improper tooth filling.

Sinus Squeeze

Sinus squeeze is commonly due to blockage from sinus congestion

3.5.2 Injuries During Ascent

Similarly, there are several injuries which might result as a direct consequence of the mechanical effects of pressure while making an ascent (decreasing pressure). These include

3.5.2.1 *Gas Embolism*

Gas embolism is caused by the blockage of blood flow in the arteries of the heart or brain due to gas bubbles. These bubbles generally result from an over-inflation injury to the alveolar membrane in the lungs while breath holding during ascent. Paralysis, unconsciousness, and death can result.

3.5.2.2 *Emphysema*

Emphysema is the abnormal swelling of body tissues by the accumulation of gases. Common forms of emphysema include

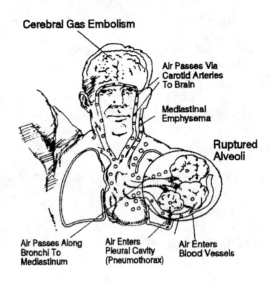

Figure 3-12: Over-inflation injuries occurring during ascent. (From NOAA Dive Manual, 1991)

<u>Interstitial Emphysema</u> Gas trapped in the lung tissues due to a tear in the gas exchange membranes.

<u>Subcutaneous Emphysema</u> Gas trapped beneath the skin generally in the region of the neck or shoulders. Gas released from a tear in the lungs will migrate upward into this region. This injury is generally associated with a change in the pitch of the diver's voice as the swelling applies pressure to the larynx.

<u>Mediastinal Emphysema</u> Gas trapped in the middle of the chest cavity, surrounding the heart, trachea, esophagus, and major blood vessels. This injury is associated with a tightness in the chest and difficulty in breathing.

3.5.2.3 *Pneumothorax*

Pneumothorax results from gas trapped between the lungs and the lining of the chest cavity. This injury results from gas leaking through torn lung tissue due to over-expansion of the lungs. Further ascent can cause the damaged lung to collapse.

3.6 Physiological Responses to Hot and Cold

3.6.1 Metabolic Heat Production

Our bodies produce heat as a by-product of our metabolic processes, including muscular efforts and the normal life sustaining processes such as digestion, respiration, blood circulation and purification processes in the kidneys and liver. The rate of heat production will vary with the level of muscular activity from a *basal metabolism* rate of approximately 82 watts (280 Btu/hr),

Table 3-1: Metabolic Heat Production Rates for Various Surface and Underwater Activities
(Taken from Penzias and Goodman, 1973)

Activity	Btu/hr	Watts
Surface		
Sleeping	280	82.0
Lying, relaxed	290	85.0
Seated, relaxed	400	117.2
Standing, relaxed	440	128.9
Writing, seated	430	126.0
Slow movement about room	600	175.8
Slow walking	900	263.7
Swimming crawl 1 mph	1670	489.3
Swimming backstroke 1 mph	1980	580.1
Cycling 13.2 mph	2380	697.3
Underwater		
Slow walking on hard bottom	693	203.0
Swimming 0.5 knot	924	270.7
Slow walking on mud bottom	1270	372.1
Swimming 0.85 knot	1618	474.1
Maximum walking speed hard bottom	1732	507.5
Swimming 1.0 knot	2080	609.4
Maximum walking speed mud bottom	2080	609.4
Swimming 1.2 knot	2890	846.8

which includes the heat produced by a resting individual to maintain normal body functions, to as high as 10 times that quantity when the individual is exerting high muscular efforts. Table 3.1 tabulates the approximate metabolic heat production rates for various activities.

These metabolic rates, $\dot{M}$, can be approximated from the oxygen consumption rate, $\dot{V}_{O_2}$ (see section 3.3.1), or the respiratory minute volume, RMV, using the following relationships:

$$\dot{M}, \frac{Btu}{hr} = 1143 \; \dot{V}_{O_2} = 47.6 \; RMV$$

$$\dot{M}, watts = 334.9 \; \dot{V}_{O_2} = 14.0 \; RMV$$

(3-4)

where $\dot{V}_{O_2}$ is given in standard liters per minute (SLPM), and *RMV* is given in liters per minute (BTPS).

3.6.2 Thermal Balance

Under normal circumstances this produced metabolic heat will be lost to the environment through several transfer modes, including conduction, convection and radiation from the body surface, and evaporation of moisture from perspiration and respiration. Or, expressed as a delicate energy balance

Energy Produced as Heat - Heat Lost = Stored Heat

$$\dot{M} - \dot{W} - (\dot{q}_C + \dot{q}_R + \dot{q}_K + \dot{q}_{Evap}) = \dot{S}$$

(3-5)

where the terms within the parentheses refer to the amount of heat loss, or gain, from convection, radiation, conduction and evaporation, respectively; $\dot{W}$ is the rate at which work is being done; and $\dot{S}$ is the rate at which heat is being stored, or depleted, from the body. A detailed discussion of each of these heat transfer mechanisms will follow later.

In keeping this energy balance in check, the body is maintained in a thermally stable condition, a condition referred to as *homeostasis*, with a *core temperature* (i.e., the temperature of such vital organs as the brain, heart, lungs, liver and upper digestive tract) of approximately 37°C (98.6° F), and an average skin temperature of approximately 33°C (91.3° F). A complex thermoregulatory system, controlled by the *hypothalamus* within the brain, attempts to maintain the body core at this constant temperature to maximize the efficiency of these complex biochemical systems. The remaining parts of the body, including the muscles, skeletal system, fat reserves and skin, do not depend on stable or uniform temperatures for optimal physiological performance. These body parts are treated as a defensive "shell" surrounding the vulnerable "core", which the thermoregulatory system manipulates to buffer and protect the core from thermally stressful environments.

This protection is accomplished in several different ways. First, the flow of warm blood into the shell is controlled to either increase or decrease convective heat losses between the environment and the skin surface. During cold exposures, blood flow is greatly reduced to the tissues that are adjacent to the body's surface, a regulatory action referred to as *vaso-constriction*. As a consequence, an effective increase in thermal insulation is achieved from this exterior shell, resulting in a net reduction of convective heat transfer between the skin and the cold environment. This regulatory mechanism is so powerful that, in very cold environments, the periphery of the shell, such as the hands and the feet, will be thermally sacrificed, causing severe cold injury such as frostbite. If the thermal response from vaso-constriction is insufficient to maintain a constant core temperature, the thermoregulatory system will further act by increasing muscular activity in the form of shivering. This increased activity elevates the metabolic heat production, as well as oxygen consumption, in an attempt to further offset the net heat loss from the core. Under normal conditions, the above defense mechanisms are sufficient to keep the core at a near constant temperature.

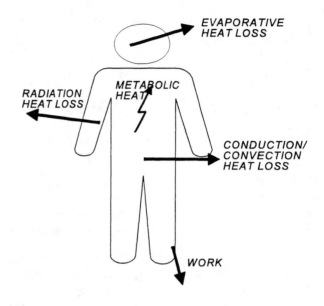

Figure 3-13: Thermal balance in the human body.

Under more severe cold stresses, however, the body's metabolic heat production is not able to keep up with the losses to the environment. As the core temperature drops below 35°C, a condition defined clinically as *hypothermia* results. A reduction in body heat content below this level is usually accompanied by mental confusion, an impairment of rational thought, and an inability to defend oneself from further danger. Table 3.2 indicates the resulting conditions of the body if a net loss in body temperature continues during prolonged, severe thermal stresses to the body.

Conversely, in severely warm environments *hyperthermia*, or an excessive increase in core temperature can result. Although not normally associated with underwater environments, this condition can be even more life threatening than is hypothermia. The thermoregulatory system's defense against hyperthermia starts as an increased blood flow from the core to the shell by complete opening of the surface blood vessels, referred to as *vasodilation*. This control mechanism maximizes the convective heat transfer between the skin and the environment by placing the warm blood in close proximity to the skin's surface, thereby reducing the insulation effect of the shell. Such a condition can usually be perceived as a "flushed" or reddened appearance of the skin.

A further defense against excessive heat buildup in the core is the introduction of perspiration from the sweat glands onto the surface of the skin. Evaporative cooling of this perspiration, in conjunction with vasodilation, is generally sufficient to maintain body core temperatures within a narrow fixed temperature range. Note, however, that evaporative cooling is most effective in relatively dry environments, and will be totally ineffective in environments that are already saturated with water vapor.

Table 3-2: Signs And Symptoms Of Dropping Core Temperature
(Taken from U.S. Navy Diving Manual, 1991)

Core Temperature		Symptoms
°C	°F	
37	98.6	●Cold sensations ●Skin vaso-constriction ●Increased muscle tension ●Increased oxygen consumption
36	97	●Sporadic shivering suppressed by voluntary movements ●Gross shivering ●Further increases in oxygen consumption ●Uncontrollable shivering
35	95	●Clinical hypothermia ●Voluntary tolerance limit in laboratory experiments ●Mental confusion ●Impairment of rational thought ●Decreased will to struggle
34	93	●Loss of memory ●Speech impaired ●Sensory function impaired ●Motor performance impaired
33	91	●Hallucination, delusions, clouding of consciousness ●Shivering impaired
32	90	●Heart rhythm irregularities ●Motor performance grossly impaired
31	88	●Shivering stopped
30	86	●Loss of consciousness ●No response to pain
27	80	●Death

3.6.3 Thermal Exposure Limits

Producing a state of complete thermal comfort in all diving modes is an extremely difficult, if not impossible, task. Researchers have proposed thermal limits to protect divers against the dangers implicit in hypothermia and hyperthermia (Webb *et al*, 1976), (Kuehn and Ackles, 1978). These limits were established to give design guidelines for the development of thermal protective systems, and give estimates of safe exposure limits for divers in severely harsh environments. Note that these limits were designed to insure that mental, motor and sensory functions will be minimally impaired so as not to jeopardize the performance and safety of the diver. These limits will not ensure that the diver will always be comfortable.

a) The diver net body heat loss should not exceed 200 kcal. (This has also been given as 3 kcal per kg of body mass to account for the range of diver body sizes.)

b) The diver body core temperature should not drop by more than 1°C.

c) Mean skin temperature should not go below 25°C, and individual skin temperatures should not go below 20°C, except that of the hands, which should not go below 15°C.

d) The diver's metabolic response from shivering should not exceed an incremental increase in oxygen consumption rate of 0.5 liters/minute above the metabolic cost of the diver's activity.

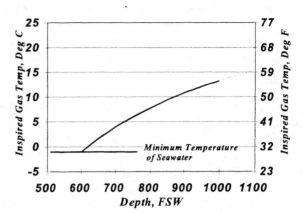

Figure 3-14: Minimum Inspired Gas Temperatures (Taken from Braithwaite, 1972).

e) The minimum inspired gas temperature should not fall below that specified by Figure 3-14.

To maintain safe exposures in hot water temperatures, the following limits have been recommended (Webb *et al*, 1976):

a) Core temperatures should not exceed 38.5°C.

b) Mean and individual skin temperatures should not exceed 42°C.

c) The maximum inspired gas temperature should be less than 45°C for a one-hour exposure and 40°C for indefinitely long exposures.

3.6.4 Thermal Endurance Limits

Based on the guidelines given above for cold exposures, acceptable cold exposure durations have been estimated (Nuckols *et al*, 1994) using the expression

$$t, hrs = \frac{-837}{(\dot{M} - \dot{q}_{RESP}) - \dfrac{22.04\ (77 - T_{AMB})}{CLO_{SUIT}}} \qquad (3\text{-}6)$$

where $\dot{M}$ is the metabolic heat production of the diver, given in Btu/hr; $\dot{q}_{RESP}$ is the respiratory heat loss from the diver, BTU/hr (a discussion of respiratory heat loss will follow later); T_{AMB} is the surrounding water temperature, °F; and CLO_{SUIT} is the insulation value of the diver's suit (suit insulation values will be discussed in detail in Chapter 7).

Example: A diver is dressed in a variable volume dry suit having an insulation value of 1.2 CLO. While being exposed to cold water temperatures of 34°F, the diver's oxygen consumption level was 0.5 SLPM and the heat loss from respiration was estimated as 150 Btu/hr. What is the estimated endurance limit for this diver, based on the safe exposure guidelines given above?

Solution: The diver's metabolic heat production can be estimated using Equation (3-4) to be

$$\dot{M} = 1143 \cdot \dot{V}_{O_2} = 1143 \,(0.5) = 571.5 \,\frac{Btu}{hr}$$

Substituting this into Equation (3-6) gives

$$t, \, hrs = \cfrac{-837}{(571.5 - 150) - \cfrac{22.04 \,(77 - 34)}{1.2}} = 2.27 \, hrs$$

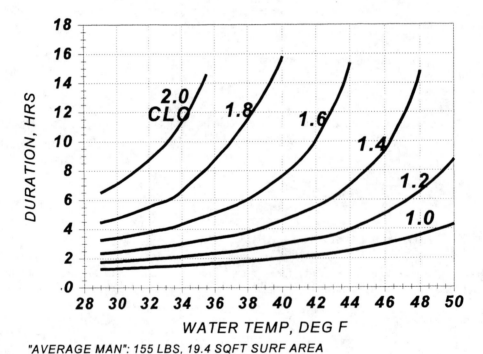

"*AVERAGE MAN*": 155 LBS, 19.4 SQFT SURF AREA

Figure 3-15: Estimated mission durations for a resting diver in cold water. Mission durations are based on the time to loose 5.4 BTU per pound of body mass.

    Figures 3-15 and 3-16 show estimated mission durations for a resting and lightly working diver, respectively, who are wearing garments with passive insulation levels varying between 1.0 and 2.0 CLO[3]. These estimates indicate that, theoretically, a resting diver (defined in this analysis as metabolic heat generation minus respiratory heat loss equal to 400 BTU/hr) in 34°F water could be expected to function properly for greater than 6 hours with a garment having an insulation level between 1.7 to 1.8 CLO. The diver who increases his activity only slightly, as shown in Figure 3-16, with metabolic minus respiratory heat rates equal to 600 BTU/hr, could function adequately with a suit insulation reduced to approximately 1.3 CLO in the same water temperature.

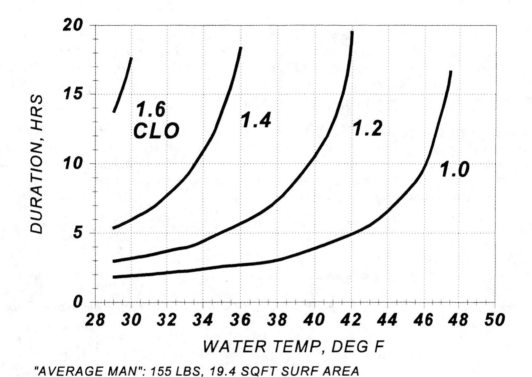

"AVERAGE MAN": 155 LBS, 19.4 SQFT SURF AREA

Figure 3-16: Estimated mission durations for a lightly working diver in cold water. Mission durations are based on the time to loose 5.4 BTU per pound of body mass.

---

[3] CLO as a unit of thermal protection can be characterized as the insulation inherent in a business suit when worn in air. It can be quantified as 1.136 divided by the suit conductance, where suit conductance is measured in BTU/ft²-hr-°F; ie

$$CLO = \frac{1.136}{\left(Suit\ Conductance,\ \dfrac{BTU}{ft^2-hr-{}^{\circ}F} \right)}$$ (3-7)

See Chapter 7 for a detailed discussion of suit insulation values and thermal protection suit designs.

3.6.5 Respiratory Heat Loss

3.6.5.1   Normal Respiration

The human respiratory system contains an elegant set of defense mechanisms to protect its internal environment. The human respiratory tract, with its intricate mucosal membrane, filters foreign matter and bacteria from inspired gases on their journey to the lungs. Additionally, the upper respiratory tract regulates the temperature and moisture content of the respired gases. In this way the delicate, gas exchange membranes in the lungs are protected from thermal injury and drying.

During inspiration, heat and moisture are added to the respiratory gases as they make their way from the nasal passages to the alveoli. This heat is taken from a moving mucus blanket covering the upper respiratory tract (nose to the trachea). Researchers have found that the relative humidity of inspired air reaches 80%, and the temperature 34°C, before the air reaches the pharynx under normal atmospheric conditions. By the time the air passes the trachea, the air generally reaches full body temperature and 100% relative humidity.

During expiration, the carbon dioxide enriched gas returning from the lungs again passes over the mucosal membrane, cooled during inspiration, and returns some of its heat and water vapor content. This causes a fall in the expiratory gas temperature, resulting in substantial (30-40%) recovery of body heat and water vapor. Hoke et al (1971) found that the expired gas temperatures can be predicted under most environmental conditions as a function to the inspired gas temperature according the following relationship:

$$T_E = 29.3 + 0.09 \ T_I + 0.004 \ T_I^2 \qquad\qquad \textbf{(3-8)}$$

where T_E and T_I are expiration and inspiration temperatures (°C), respectively.

The net heat lost from the lungs and respiratory tract due to heating and humidification of the breathing gas can then be found as

$$\dot{q}_{Resp} = \dot{m}_{gas} \cdot c_{P_{gas}} \cdot \left(T_E - T_I \right) + \dot{m}_{gas} \cdot h_{fg} \cdot \left(w_E - w_I \right) \qquad\qquad \textbf{(3-9)}$$

where $\dot{m}_{gas}$ is the mass rate of gas flow through the lungs, c_{pgas} is the specific heat of the breathing gas, h_{fg} is the latent heat of vaporization that goes into humidifying the breathing gas, and w_E and w_I are the humidity ratios (mass of water per mass of dry gas) of the expired and inspired gases, respectively (See Chapter 8).

During normal breathing of room air at 25°C and 50% relative humidity, man looses approximately 250 ml of water and 350 kcal of heat daily through respiration. This accounts for approximately 10-20% of the total body losses under resting conditions.

3.6.5.2   Conditioning of Inspired Gases At Hyperbaric Conditions

The costs in heat and water vapor when conditioning the inspired gases in divers airways increase substantially due to the effects of breathing dry, cold, dense gases at increased respiratory rates. Additionally, mandatory mouth breathing is somewhat of a disadvantage that the scuba diver must tolerate due to the relative inefficient conditioning capability of the oral cavity as compared to the nasal passageway. This deficiency is partially overcome by greater heat and moisture transfer taking place in the lower respiratory tract. Unfortunately, this decreased conditioning capability during mouth breathing reduces the heat and water recovery process during expiration.

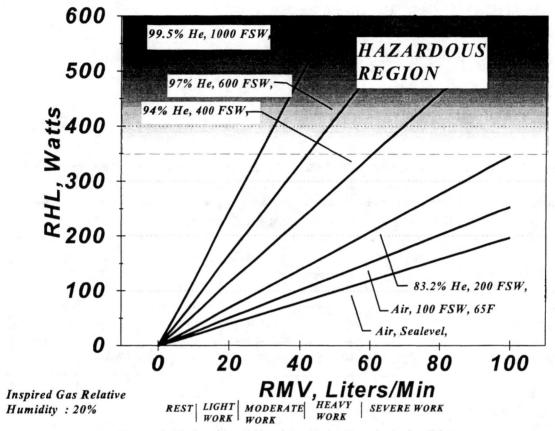

Figure 3-17: Respiratory Heat Loss Under Hyperbaric Conditions.

At depths greater than approximately 190 feet, helium makes up a large percentage of the respired gas. Helium, having a specific heat approximately five times that of air, requires a larger addition of heat to bring the inspired gas up to body temperature. The combination of this high heat capacity and increased gas densities as the diver goes deeper causes respiratory heat losses for divers to be an appreciable part of the total body heat loss. Fortunately, respiratory heat loss is proportional to metabolic heat production at the depths of current operational diving (Braithwaite, 1972), and thus the heat balance in the diver's body can normally be maintained. However, since the metabolic heat production is independent of ambient pressure while respiratory heat loss increases proportional to depth, eventually the heat balance will break down as the diver goes to further depths. Hoke et al (1971) concluded that conditions in which the respiratory heat loss of a diver surpassed 350 watts were hazardous and should be avoided. Figure 3-17, derived from the information tabulated in Table 3-3, shows when these hazardous conditions can be expected.

**TABLE 3-3: MOISTURE AND HEAT LOSSES
UNDER VARIOUS RESPIRATORY CONDITIONS**
(RMV given in liters/min, BTPS)

Heat Loss: $\quad \dot{q}_{RESP}, \dfrac{BTU}{min} = A * RMV \qquad\qquad \dot{q}_{RESP}, watts = B * RMV$

Moisture Loss: $\quad \dot{w}, \dfrac{lb\ H_2O}{min} = C * RMV$

GAS	DEPTH, FSW	CONDITIONS	A	B	C
Air	Sealevel	70°F, 50% RH	66.2	1163.4	0.050
Air	Sealevel	30°F, 20% RH	90.0	1581.1	0.055
Air	100	65°F, 20% RH	115.5	2028.8	0.058
83.2% He/16.8% O$_2$	100	65°F, 20% RH	101.3	1780.1	0.057
83.2% He/16.8% O$_2$	200	50°F, 20% RH	157.6	2769.4	0.053
94.0% He/6.0% O$_2$	400	45°F, 20% RH	262.1	4604.4	0.056
97.0% He/3.0% O$_2$	600	40°F, 20% RH	377.5	6633.0	0.054
99.5% He/0.5% O$_2$	1000	40°F, 20% RH	558.9	9820.1	0.049

3.7   Closure

The physiological concerns discussed in this chapter are critically important to the life support designer. A failure to design systems which will keep divers and hyperbaric workers within acceptable physiological limits will have catastrophic consequences. Human life is at stake!

The next chapter will deal with an equally important physiological concern--the absorption of excess inert gases into our bodies during hyperbaric exposures. Similar to the life threatening consequences that will result from inadequate thermal protection or the use of inappropriate breathing gas mixtures, properly dealing with these excess dissolved gases is essential to the safety of humans following exposures to high pressure atmospheres.

4

Decompression Theory and Practice

Objectives

The objectives of this chapter are to
- review some of the physical and physiological causes of decompression sickness
- understand the concept of gas diffusion and off-gassing from living tissues
- introduce the concept of tissue half-life and tissue saturation
- review the derivation of existing decompression tables for diving with either nitrogen or helium as the inert gas
- investigate how residual gases in tissues are treated during repetitive dives.

4.1   Introduction

We saw previously that the amount of gas that will be absorbed in our blood and other body tissues is directly proportional to the partial pressure of that gas that is in contact with our bodies (see Henry's Law in Chapter 2). If the excess gas, resulting from a high pressure exposure during a dive is not slowly brought out of solution during ascent, the excess dissolved gas can lead to the formation of bubbles in the blood stream and other body tissues. Symptoms from these bubbles can range from pain in the joints, resulting from pressure on nerve endings (*Type I, or Pain Only Decompression Sickness*), to paralysis or death, resulting from pressure on the central nervous system (*Type II, or CNS Decompression Sickness*) or a blockage of blood flow to the brain (*Gas Embolism*). While these physical phenomenon, and the consequences of inadequate decompression, are readily known today by even the most amateur of divers, this dangerous condition was basically unknown by divers until early this century.

In 1880, Paul Bert, a French physiologist, was the first person to propose that the cause of numerous illnesses experienced by caisson workers was excess dissolved gases in these workers bodies resulting from prolonged, high-pressure exposures during the construction of tunnels and bridge foundations. Bert observed that severe cases of "caisson disease", including paralysis and death, often occurred when these workers immediately returned to the surface following a lengthy period inside the caisson. He also recognized that "caisson disease" was identical to the problems experienced by deep sea divers, and suggested that it was caused by the release of dissolved nitrogen from the bloodstream. He suggested that caisson workers and deep sea divers be returned to the surface following their day's work by gradually reducing the surrounding pressure, i.e., *decompress* gradually following hyperbaric exposures.

The first systematic study of decompression requirements following exposures to elevated pressures was reported by Boycott, Damant and Haldane (1908). Following extensive exposures of small animals to high air pressures, these researchers developed a rational basis for the calculation of staged decompression schedules. The basic tenets of their procedure, which became popularly known as the "Haldane Method", relate to

a) the estimation of the percent of complete saturation or desaturation of the body tissues with inert gas during any pressure exposure time-course, and

b) the determination of the amount of excess gas pressure in the tissues related to the seawater pressure which can be tolerated without the symptoms of decompression sickness resulting during, or following, the reduction of pressure to 1 Ata.

4.2   Haldanian Theory of Decompression

Haldane attempted to quantify the amount of inert gas that is dissolved in our bodies during exposures to high-pressure environments, and particularly the rates at which these gases are absorbed and desorbed as these environmental pressures changed. He started by simplifying the gas uptake process at the interface between our blood and other body tissues, i.e., within the capillaries.

We saw earlier in Chapter 3 that the gases absorbed in our blood are rapidly brought into equilibrium with the gases which pass through our lungs (i.e., the partial pressures of the inert gases in the lungs will equilibrate rapidly with the inert gas pressures in the blood). This is due to the large, and efficient gas exchange mechanism that exists within the alveoli. These inert gases are transported to the capillaries by the blood flow, where they can be absorbed into the body tissues. Under normal conditions, equal partial pressures of this inert gas will exist in the blood and the other body tissues. The result--no net inert gas exchange within the capillaries will occur; the same quantity of inert gas that enters these tissues will also leave, resulting in zero net gain.

However, if the partial pressure of the inert gas in our breathing mixture is increased, either by increasing the atmospheric pressure or by increasing the percentage of the inert gas in this breathing mixture, an elevated partial pressure will be transported to the capillaries. The differential pressure that now exists at the blood-tissue interface within the capillaries will now result in a net increase in inert gas transfer into the tissues. This gas transfer, as illustrated in Figure 4-1, can be described by

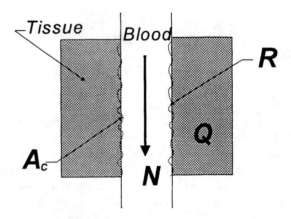

Figure 4-1: The Exchange of Inert Gases at the Blood/Tissue Interface.

Fick's Law, given as this simplified differential equation:

$$\frac{dQ}{dt} = \frac{A_c}{R} \cdot (N - Q)$$

(4-1)

where Q is defined as the partial pressure of the inert gas in the body tissue, N is defined as the partial pressure of the inert gas in the blood (assumed to be equal to the partial pressure of the inert gas in the breathing mixture), A_c is defined as the interface area that exists between the blood and the tissues, R is defined as the resistance to gas transfer at this blood-tissue interface, and t is time.

We can set an initial condition for this equation by noting that the initial inert gas pressure in the tissue will be equal to the initial gas pressure in the atmosphere that existed just prior to the elevated exposure (this assumes that the tissue has been previously exposed to the initial atmosphere for a time sufficient to reach a state of equilibrium).

That is,

$$Q = P \qquad @ \; t = 0 \qquad [\; Initial \; Condition \;]$$

where P is defined as the initial gas pressure in the tissue before the hyperbaric exposure.

This first-order, linear differential equation can be solved to give the following

$$Q = N - (N - P) \cdot e^{-\left(\frac{A_c}{R}\right)t}$$

(4-2)

a graphical solution of which is shown in Figure 4-2. As we would expect, this solution shows that the inert gas pressure in the body tissue will increase in an exponential manner, and reach a new equilibrium level with the elevated gas pressure that exists in the blood after some time period. After this new equilibrium has been reached, we say that the tissue has reached *saturation* with the elevated pressure exposure. Conceptually, this description of saturation is what happens to divers who remain under high pressures for extended periods--a special method of diving, referred to as *saturation diving* first implemented in the early 1960's.

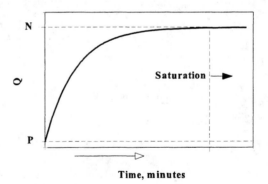

Figure 4-2: The exponential uptake of inert gas into a tissue. Gas uptake continues until the tissue reaches a new equilibrium with the inert gas pressure in the hyperbaric atmosphere, at which time the tissue is said to be saturated.

Unfortunately, Haldane found that this equation was limited in its ability to accurately predict quantitatively the uptake of inert gases into the diver's body. Although conceptually useful, unless he could quantify the area of the blood-tissue interface area, A_c, and the transfer resistance at this interface, R, he would be unable to predict the amount of gas dissolved in the body. To tackle this obstacle, Haldane simplified these unknown quantities by defining the tissue characteristics A_c/R in terms of the time that it would take the inert gas pressure in the tissue to go half way between the initial pressure and the new inert pressure in the blood--essentially a *tissue half-life*, analogous to the half-life characteristics of various radioactive elements.

As shown in Figure 4-3, Haldane defined this tissue half-life, H, such that

$$Q = \frac{N + P}{2} \qquad @ \quad t = H \qquad \textbf{(4-3)}$$

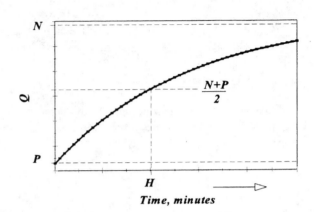

It is left to the reader to confirm that by substituting this definition of the tissue half-life in Equation 4-3 into Equation 4-2 we are able to quantify the unknown tissue characteristics, A_c/R, in terms of this tissue half-life, H; i.e.,

$$\frac{A_c}{R} = \frac{0.693}{H} \qquad \textbf{(4-4)}$$

Figure 4-3: Tissue half-life, defined as the time for a tissue to go half way toward saturating with a new inert gas pressure.

Combining Equations 4-2 and 4-4 now gives

$$Q = N - (N - P) \cdot e^{-0.693\left(\frac{t}{H}\right)} \qquad \textbf{(4-5)}$$

For simplifying computations, the above equation can be written as

$$Q - P = (N - P) \cdot \left[1 - e^{-0.693\left(\frac{t}{H}\right)} \right] \qquad \textbf{(4-6)}$$

We will find it advantageous to define the following shorthand form of Equation 4-6 to calculate tissue pressures that result during high pressure exposures:

$$S = F \cdot E \qquad \textbf{(4-6a)}$$

where we can see from Figure 4-3 that

$S = Q - P$ S is seen to be the change in tissue pressure that results from the exposure.

$E = N - P$ E is seen to be the initial driving force that causes gas uptake, or off gassing. (Note: If this driving force is positive, the tissues will absorb gas. If this driving force is negative, the tissues will off gas back to the blood.)

$$F = 1 - e^{-0.693\left(\frac{t}{H}\right)}$$

F is a time function which is only dependent on the tissue half-life.

Haldane recognized that our bodies are not homogeneous; that is, they can not be assumed to be characterized by a single tissue half-life. Rather, he proposed that the variable time-course of inert gas uptake for various parts of the body be simulated by use of a family of discrete hypothetical half-time tissues. He recognized that some tissues such as bone and cartilage will absorb and off gas inert gases more slowly than other, more blood perfused tissues. These "slow" tissues will have to be characterized necessarily with tissue half-lives that are much longer than those for blood or muscle, for instance. Rather than a single exponential curve as shown in Figure 4-3, the uptake of inert gases in our bodies can be more accurately represented by a family curves, each reaching saturation at different times as shown in Figure 4-4.

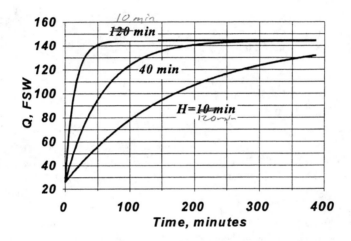

Figure 4-4: Exponential uptake of inert gas in various body tissues represented by different tissue half-lives based on a dive to 150 FSW on air.

Initially, Haldane chose hypothetical half-lives of 5, 10, 20, 40 and 75 minutes to represent the physiological processes of gas exchange in the whole body. Subsequent use of the Haldanian method to calculate decompression schedules for deep dives by the U.S. Navy revealed that these half-lives were inadequate for determining schedules for long, deep dives. Half-lives of 120 and 240 minutes were added to the initial family of tissues in the 1950's (Workman, 1965).

Today, the basic "Haldanian" algorithm is still being used by several navies to calculate decompression schedules, and dive equipment manufacturers to fabricate diver-carried decompression computers. The primary differences in all of their algorithms are the number of tissues being modeled and the range of tissue times being used. Half-lives of 480, and even 960, minutes are not uncommon.

Perhaps more important than the estimation of the uptake of inert gases in a diver's tissues is the concept of gas elimination through *stage decompression* during ascent that Haldane and his colleagues developed from their studies. This concept makes the fullest use of the permissible difference in gas pressure between that of the tissue and the blood to hasten the elimination of the inert gas from these tissues as the diver heads toward the surface. They initially applied a safe limit to the reduction allowable in surrounding seawater pressure to never allow the computed tissue inert pressure to be more than twice the ambient water pressure. This allowed the determination of the first decompression stop by simply halving the absolute pressure of the maximum diver depth (where the absolute pressure was expressed in equivalent feet of seawater).

Unfortunately, decompression schedules for divers based on this simple 2 to 1 ratio concept did not prove to be safe for long, deep exposures. Haldane himself recognized that some reduction in this pressure ratio would be required for air dives exceeding 6 Ata. Other studies also demonstrated that

a) tissues with faster half-lives sometimes control deep decompression stops even with high tissue pressure ratios.

b) pressure ratios can exceed the 2 to 1 estimate for the faster half-life tissues without jeopardizing the safety of the diver.

c) helium, having a low solubility in fat compared to nitrogen, may yield a shorter half-time than nitrogen in a tissue rich in fat; however,

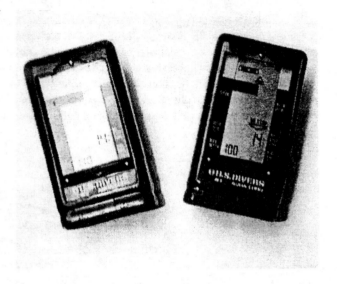

Figure 4-5: Diver-carried decompression computer which uses the concept of tissue half-lives for computing acceptable dive exposures. (Courtesy of U.S. Divers')

d) for helium diving, somewhat deeper decompression stops are required due to a more rapid rate of helium diffusion into the blood stream during ascent, which could cause bubble formation to be more likely if the early stages of decompression are too rapid.

Based on these studies, values for maximum tissue pressures, *M*, versus depth at 10-foot intervals were derived for a wide range of tissue half-lives with nitrogen or helium as the inert gas in the breathing mixture. The maximum tissue pressure, *M*, is defined as the greatest partial pressure of inert gas in a specific tissue which will not permit bubbles to form in the tissue at a given absolute pressure. Values of *M* for decompression stops up to 100 FSW are tabulated in Tables 4-1 and 4-2. Values of *M* for deeper stops can be easily calculated by adding the value ΔM for each added stop. For example *M* at 110 FSW for a 5 minute half-life tissue exposed to nitrogen is 266 + 18; or 284 FSW. Or in general, *M* values can be found as a function of stop depth as

$$M_D = M_{10} + \frac{D - 10}{10} \cdot \Delta M \qquad (4\text{-}7)$$

where M_D is the maximum tissue pressure for the decompression stop at depth *D*, FSW; M_{10} is the maximum tissue pressure for the 10-foot decompression stop; ΔM is the change in the maximum tissue pressure at each 10-foot interval; and *D* is the depth of the stop, FSW.

These maximum tissue pressures have been used with only slight modifications to develop the present Standard Air Decompression Tables used by the U.S. Navy (See Appendix C).

Table 4-1: Maximum Allowable Tissue Pressures (Equivalent FSW) For Nitrogen

H min	Depth of Decompression Stop, FSW										ΔM
	10 A=43	20 A=53	30 A=63	40 A=73	50 A=83	60 A=93	70 A=103	80 A=113	90 A=123	100 A=133	
5	104	122	140	158	176	194	212	230	248	266	18
10	88	104	120	136	152	168	184	200	216	232	16
20	72	87	102	117	132	147	162	177	192	207	15
40	56	70	84	98	112	126	140	154	168	182	14
80	54	67	80	93	106	119	132	145	158	171	13
120	52	64	76	88	100	112	124	136	148	160	12
160	51	63	74	86	97	109	120	132	143	155	11.5
200	51	62	73	84	95	106	117	128	139	150	11
240	50	61	72	83	94	105	116	127	138	149	11

Table 4-2: Maximum Allowable Tissue Pressures (Equivalent FSW) For Helium

H min	Depth of Decompression Stop, FSW										ΔM
	10 A=43	20 A=53	30 A=63	40 A=73	50 A=83	60 A=93	70 A=103	80 A=113	90 A=123	100 A=133	
5	86	101	116	131	146	161	176	191	206	221	15
10	74	88	102	116	130	144	158	172	186	200	14
20	66	79	92	105	118	131	144	157	170	183	13
40	60	72	84	96	108	120	132	144	156	168	12
80	56	68	80	92	104	116	128	140	152	164	12
120	54	66	78	90	102	114	126	138	150	162	12
160	54	65	76	87	98	109	120	131	142	153	11
200	53	63	73	83	93	103	113	123	133	143	10
240	53	63	73	83	93	103	113	123	133	143	10

4.3   Sample Decompression Calculations

A better understanding of how the Haldanian Method can be used to derive a decompression schedule is best obtained through a sample calculation. The following symbols will be used throughout this example:

D is the vertical distance below the surface at any phase of the dive, FSW.

A is defined as the absolute pressure at any depth expressed in equivalent feet of seawater, $(A = D + 33)$.

X is the oxygen volume fraction in the breathing mixture during each phase of the dive.

G is the volume fraction of the inert gas in the breathing mixture $(G = 1.0 - X)$.

N is the partial pressure of the inert gases in the breathing medium, FSW. It can be found as an expression of Dalton's Law

$$N = G \cdot A$$

P is the partial pressure of the inert gases in the tissue at the start of any particular time interval, given in FSW. When there has been no dive within 12 hours prior to the current dive, the initial tissue pressure at the surface at the start of the dive ($A = 33$ FSW) can be taken as that in air ($G = 0.79$). I.e., initially

$$P = 0.79 \cdot 33 = 26.1 \; FSW$$

Q is the final tissue pressure at the end of each step in the decompression calculation, FSW. Note that Q for one step becomes the initial tissue pressure P of the next step.

E was defined previously as the difference between the inert gas partial pressure of the breathing medium, N, and the initial tissue pressure, P. E represents the driving force for inert gas exchange between the blood and the tissue; if E is positive, the tissue absorbs inert gas; if E is negative, the tissue will off gas.

S was previously defined as the increase, or decrease, of tissue pressure during a time interval where the tissue is exposed to a differential pressure E. We derived an expression for calculating this change in Equation 4-6a.

t is the time interval for any phase of the dive. When calculating decompression schedules, we will divide the dive into multiple phases, including
   a) the initial exposure at depth; this will include both time of descent and time at depth
   b) the initial ascent from the bottom depth to the first decompression stop; in standard diving practice, the duration of this exposure is determined based on an ascent rate of 60 feet per minute or less
   c) the time of the first decompression stop, and
   d) the time of each subsequent decompression stop.

The time interval at each decompression stop depends on the length of time required to desaturate all the tissues to a final partial pressure, Q, that will be equal to, or less than, the maximum tissue pressure M for that depth. I.e., the time interval must be sufficient for the required change in tissue pressure S_{REQ} to equal the following:

$$S_{REQ} = M_D - Q \qquad \text{(4-8)}$$

where M_D is the maximum tissue pressure for that tissue at the present decompression stop.

F is a time function, dependent only on the time interval t and the tissue half-life H, and defined as

$$F = 1 - e^{-0.693\left(\frac{t}{H}\right)} \qquad \text{(4-9)}$$

Example: Using the Haldanian method, calculate the decompression schedule for a dive to a depth of 100 FSW for 80 minutes if the breathing gas consists of 60% nitrogen and 40% oxygen. Assume that the diver's body can be sufficiently represented by tissue half-lives of 5, 10, 20, 40, 80 and 120 minutes.

Solution: The dive is broken into several time intervals as discussed above.

4.3.1 Phase 1: Initial Exposure at Depth

We first calculate the final inert gas pressures Q in each of the six tissues at the completion of the 80 minute exposure at 100 FSW. These calculations are best made in tabular form as shown in Table 4-3:

D = 100 FSW $\qquad\qquad t$ = 80 minutes
A = 133 FSW
$N = G \cdot A = 0.6 \cdot 133 = 79.8$ FSW
$P = 0.79 \cdot 33 = 26.1$ FSW (Assuming that the diver was breathing air at the surface prior to the dive.)

Table 4-3: Tissue Pressures At The End Of The Bottom Exposure

H, minutes	$E = N - P$	F (Eq 4-9)	$S = F \cdot E$	$Q = S + P$	Comments
5	53.7	1.000	53.7	79.8	⟵ Saturated
10	53.7	0.996	53.5	79.6	
20	53.7	0.937	50.3	76.4	
40	53.7	0.750	40.3	66.4	
80	53.7	0.500	26.9	53.0	
120	53.7	0.370	19.9	46.0	

Observe that the final nitrogen pressure in the 5 minute tissue (Q = 79.8 FSW) has equilibrated with the level of nitrogen in the breathing gas (N = 79.8 FSW) after the initial 80 minute exposure at depth. The slower tissues have all absorbed some nitrogen from the breathing medium, but have not reached equilibrium by the time that the diver is prepared to begin surfacing.

At what depth, if any, does the diver need to make the first decompression stop? Note that the diver cannot ascend to a depth such that his final tissue pressures exceed the maximum pressures for nitrogen shown in Table 4-1.

We can see by inspection in this table that the final tissue pressure will exceed the maximum pressure for the 20 and 40 minute tissues at the 10 foot stop; i.e., $Q > M_{10}$ for the 20 and 40 minute tissues. Although the final pressures in the other tissues are all below their M_{10} values (indicating that it is safe to ascend to the surface), the diver would be required to stop at the 10 foot stop to satisfy the decompression requirements for the 20 and 40 minute tissues.

Another, more systematic, approach to arrive at the same decompression requirements is to calculate what will be defined as the *Trial First Stop (TFS)* for each tissue as follows:

$$TFS = \left(\frac{Q - M_{10}}{\Delta M} \right) \cdot 10 \qquad \textbf{(4-10)}$$

where Q is the final tissue pressure when the diver begins ascending to the surface, M_{10} is the maximum inert pressure at the 10 foot decompression stop (i.e., the maximum inert pressure allowable before the diver can safely ascend to the surface), and ΔM is the change in maximum pressures for each 10 foot stop interval, see Table 4-1. The quantity $Q - M_{10}$ can be interpreted as the total amount of inert gas that must be removed from the tissue between the time that the diver leaves the bottom until he reaches the surface. Dividing this amount of total inert gas removal by ΔM, the amount of gas removal per 10-foot stop, gives the required number of decompression stops for that tissue. Since each stop adds 10 feet to the diver depth, the depth of the 1st stop is found by multiplying the required number of stops by 10. We can calculate the Trial First Stop for each tissue in the table below:

Table 4-4: Determining The Depth Of The First Decompression Stop

H, minutes	Q	M_{10}	ΔM	TFS	Comments
5	79.8	108	18	-13.4	
10	79.6	88	16	-5.2	
20	76.4	72	15	2.9	← 10 FSW Stop
40	66.4	56	14	7.4	← 10 FSW Stop
80	53.0	54	13	-0.7	
120	46.0	52	12	-5.0	

Observe from the above table that the 20 and 40 minute tissues must stop prior to reaching the surface. Although stops shallower than 10 FSW are indicated for both tissues (2.9 FSW for the 20 minute tissue and 7.4 FSW for the 40 minute tissue), in practice we conduct decompression stops in 10-foot intervals; thus these tissues would be required to stop at the next deepest stop (10 FSW) to satisfy safe ascent practices. The negative TFS values shown for the other tissues indicate that these tissues could continue to ascend above sea level if desired with no harmful effects--a fact that is only important in allowing us to ignore these tissues during the ascent to the first stop. **Note: since the 40 minute tissue calls for the deepest decompression stop, all faster tissues (H = 5, 10, and 20 minutes) can be excluded from further decompression calculations. This will always be true--an observation that can reduce significantly other tedious calculations.**

4.3.2 Phase 2: Ascent to First Stop

Now that we are aware of the required depth of the 1st decompression stop we will look at the next phase of the dive exposure--the initial ascent from the bottom at 100 FSW to the first stop at 10 FSW. This exposure is treated in a similar manner as we used in the initial exposure at depth, except that

a) since depth is variable in this phase, the depth is assumed to be the average of the depths at the bottom and the 1st stop, and

b) the time interval of this exposure is calculated based on the time required to reach the first stop when traveling at a uniform ascent rate (in practice, an ascent rate of 60 feet per minute or less is assumed).

Thus

$$D_{AVG} = \frac{100 + 10}{2} = 55 \ FSW \qquad\qquad t = \frac{D - 10 \ FSW}{60 \ \dfrac{FSW}{min}} = 1.5 \ minutes$$

$$A_{AVG} = D_{AVG} + 33 = 88 \ \text{FSW} \qquad\qquad N_{AVG} = 0.6 \cdot 88 = 52.8 \ \text{FSW}$$

Below, we will calculate the tissue pressures upon arriving at the 10-foot decompression stop for only those tissues having half-lives greater, or equal, to the "controlling" (implying the most decompression requirement) tissue. **Note that the initial pressures used for this phase of the dive are the previous values of Q (final pressures in the previous phase of the dive) which were calculated above.**

Table 4-5: Change in Tissue Pressures During The Initial Ascent To First Stop

H Minutes	P (Previous Q)	N (Average)	$E=N-P$	F (for $t = 1.5$)	S	New Q
40	66.4	52.8	-13.6	0.0256	-0.35	66.1
80	53.0	52.8	-0.2	0.0129	-0.00	53.0
120	46.0	52.8	6.8	0.0086	0.06	46.1

Observe that the driving force E is negative for the 40 and 80 minute tissues, implying that these tissues are off gassing as the diver ascends to the 1st decompression stop. If enough inert gas comes out of the tissues as the diver ascends, such that the tissue pressure drops below the maximum tissue pressure for that stop (for all the tissues), the stop can be ignored. When this occurs for deep stops we must re-calculate this second phase of the dive using the next shallower decompression stop for the initial ascent calculations.

Observe also in Table 4-5 above that the slowest tissue continues to absorb inert gas even during the initial ascent. Continued gas uptake for these slower tissues often make them the "controlling" tissue during shallower decompression stops for deeper, longer dives.

4.3.3 Phase 3: Initial Decompression Stop

How long, if at all, would the diver be required to remain at the 10-foot stop in this example? Note that all tissue pressures, Q, after reaching the stop must be less than, or equal to, the M_{10} values before the diver can move on. A quick comparison of these new tissue pressures that exist upon arrival at the 10-foot stop with the maximum allowable pressures shown in Table 4-1 (M_{10}) reveals that the 40 minute tissue must remain at the 10-foot stop until the inert gas pressure in this tissue drops from the 66.1 FSW to the required maximum of 56 FSW (M_{10}). That is, the 40 minute tissue must remain at the 10-foot stop until a tissue pressure change, S_{REQ}, given by Equation 4-8 occurs:

$$S_{REQ} = M_{10} - Q = 56 - 66.1 = -10.1 \; FSW$$

Even though the gas pressures in the 80 and 120 minute tissues (as well as the tissues faster than 40 minutes) would allow them to immediately ascend to the next stop (i.e., the surface), the diver would be required to remain at the 10-foot decompression stop until the 40 minute tissue lost enough gas to equal the required M_{10} level. The time that would be required for this change to occur can be calculated from the time function, F, where F is derived after rearranging Equation 4-6a

$$F = \frac{S_{REQ}}{E} \tag{4-11}$$

Treating this stop as another exposure at a constant depth of 10 FSW for an unknown duration, we now have

$D = 10$ FSW $\qquad\qquad\qquad\qquad t = ?$
$A = 43$ FSW
$N = 0.6 \cdot 43 = 25.8$ FSW

Table 4-6: Determination Of The Required Time At Decompression Stop

H Minutes	P (Previous Q)	N	$E = N - P$	M_{10}	$S_{REQ} = M_{10} - Q$	$F = S_{REQ}/E$
40	66.1	25.8	-40.3	56	-10.1	0.2506
80	53.0	25.8	-27.2	54	(+1.0)	------
120	46.1	25.8	-20.3	52	(+5.9)	------

The negative values shown for E above indicate that all three tissues are off gassing during the decompression stop. The positive values shown for S_{REQ} for the 80 and 120 minute tissues indicate that these tissues do not require any off gassing prior to ascending to the next stop (in fact, these tissues could tolerate additional gas uptake). Thus, when calculating time functions for the two slower tissues, a negative value for F results-- meaningless values that should be ignored.

The required decompression time at the 10-foot stop is now found based on the definition of F

$$F = \frac{S_{REQ}}{E} = 1 - e^{-0.693\left(\frac{t}{H}\right)}$$

or for the 40 minute tissue

$$0.2505 = 1 - e^{-0.693\left(\frac{t}{40}\right)}$$

rearranging

$$e^{-0.693\left(\frac{t}{40}\right)} = 0.7494 \qquad implies \qquad -0.693\left(\frac{t}{40}\right) = \ln(0.7494) = -0.2885$$

We can now calculate the required stop time t as

$$t = \frac{-0.2885 \cdot 40}{-0.693} = 16.6 \ minutes$$

In practice, decompression stop times are rounded up to the next highest whole minute. Thus, the Haldanian method would propose a 17 minute stop at 10 feet after the initial 80 minute exposure to a depth of 100 feet when using a gas mixture of 60% nitrogen and 40% oxygen.

As a check, we can confirm that the "controlling" 40 minute tissue, and the other slower tissues, have off-gassed sufficiently at the end of the 17 minute stop so that all the final tissue pressures have dropped to levels equal to, or below, the M_{10} levels as shown below.

$$D = 10 \ FSW \qquad\qquad t = 17 \ minutes$$
$$A = 43 \ FSW$$
$$N = 0.6 \cdot 43 = 25.8 \ FSW$$

Table 4-7: Tissue Pressures At The Completion Of Decompression Stop

H Minutes	P (Previous Q)	N	E = N - P	F (for t = 17)	S = F · E	Q (New)
40	66.1	25.8	**-40.3**	0.2551	-10.3	55.8
80	53.0	25.8	**-27.2**	0.1369	-3.7	49.3
120	46.1	25.8	**-20.3**	0.0935	-1.9	44.2

4.3.4 Phase 4: Subsequent Decompression Stops

For longer, and deeper dives where the first stop may be deeper than 10 feet, the same procedure shown above in Tables 4-6 and 4-7 can be used to calculate successively shallower stops. The final gas pressures calculated for each stop, Q *(New)* above in Table 4-7, will be carried to the next stop to become the initial gas pressures (P) for this next shallower stop. **Note that the short ascent times between stops are generally ignored for these subsequent stop calculations.** This procedure can be repeated until the stop times for all decompression stops are found. At the completion of the final stop, all tissue pressures should be less than, or equal to, their respective M_{10} values, indicating that a safe ascent to the surface would be permitted.

The approach shown above is essentially the same approach that was used by the U.S. Navy to develop the

initial decompression tables for diving with air, except that the volume fraction for nitrogen in air was used instead of 60% as shown in the above example. It should be noted however, that the Standard Air Decompression Tables given in Appendix C, resulted from refinements of the Haldanian schedules after numerous verification dives by the U.S. Navy Experimental Diving Unit. Similar decompression schedules for heliox mixtures and nitrox mixtures have been developed and tested extensively for use in operational diving. **The generation of operational decompression tables for other gas mixtures using the Haldanian method should never be attempted without extensive verification trials in controlled testing.**

4.4 Repetitive Dives

Even though in the above example it is now safe to surface, notice that the tissues have not yet returned to the initial inert pressures that they contained prior to the dive. These tissue pressures, called *residual pressures*, will continue to decrease while the diver remains on the surface breathing air, eventually reaching equilibrium again with the nitrogen in this surface atmosphere (in practice, we assume that this equilibrium is completed within a 12 hour interval after surfacing). If the diver does not intend to make another dive prior to re-establishing this equilibrium, we need not concern ourselves with these *residual pressures*.

However, in the event that the diver will make a second dive prior to this new equilibrium, it will be necessary to determine the initial tissue pressures, *P*, at the start of the succeeding dive (note that we can not assume that these initial pressures are equal to 26.1 FSW, as we did in the first dive). These initial pressures could be computed in an identical manner as that described above, assuming another dive phase at surface conditions (i.e., breathing air at the surface) for a duration equal to the *surface interval*, i.e., the time between the diver surfacing from the first dive until the beginning of the second dive. The initial tissue pressures for this surface exposure would be the final tissue pressures upon surfacing from the preceding dive found above.

For repetitive dives using air, special dive tables shown in Tables 4-8 and 4-9 have been developed by the U.S. Navy which take into account these residual pressures for planning subsequent dives. When using these special tables, divers are cautioned to always enter the tables at the next deeper and next longer schedule if the dive is not listed separately.

4.4.1 No-Decompression Limits and Repetitive Group Designation Tables for Air

The No-Decompression Limits shown in Table 4-8 summarizes all depth and bottom time combinations for which no decompression is necessary when using air as the breathing gas. For instance, a diver at 60 FSW can have a bottom time of up to 60 minutes and return to the surface without decompressing; similarly, a diver at 100 FSW could remain for 25 minutes on the bottom without decompressing. Although decompression is not required if we stay within these limits, the residual nitrogen remaining in the diver's tissues after each dive must still be taken into consideration if a repetitive dive is going to be made within a 12-hour period.

Depth (FSW)	No-decom limits (min)	A	B	C	D	E	F	G	H	I	J	K	L	M	N	O
10		60	120	210	300											
15		35	70	110	160	225	350									
20		25	50	75	100	135	180	240	325							
25		20	35	55	75	100	125	160	195	245	315					
30		15	30	45	60	75	95	120	145	170	205	250	310			
35	310	5	15	25	40	50	60	80	100	120	140	160	190	220	270	310
40	200	5	15	25	30	40	50	70	80	100	110	130	150	170	200	
50	100		10	15	25	30	40	50	60	70	80	90	100			
60	60		10	15	20	25	30	40	50	55	60					
70	50		5	10	15	20	30	35	40	45	50					
80	40		5	10	15	20	25	30	35	40						
90	30		5	10	12	15	20	25	30							
100	25		5	7	10	15	20	22	25							
110	20			5	10	13	15	20								
120	15			5	10	12	15									
130	10			5	8	10										
140	10			5	7	10										
150	5			5												
160	5				5											
170	5				5											
180	5				5											
190	5				5											

Table 4-8: No-Decompression Limits and Repetitive Group Designation Table for No-Decompression Air Dives

Table 4-9: Residual Nitrogen Timetable for Repetitive Air Dives
(Source: U. S. Navy Diving Manual, 1985)

RESIDUAL NITROGEN TIMETABLE FOR REPETITIVE AIR DIVES

*Dives following surface intervals of more than 12 hours are not repetitive dives. Use actual bottom times in the Standard Air Decompression Tables to compute decompression for such dives.

Repetitive group at the beginning of the surface interval

Group	Surface interval ranges (hr:min) — top row start times / bottom row end times
A	0:10 / 12:00*
B	0:10 2:11 / 2:10 12:00*
C	0:10 1:40 2:50 / 1:39 2:49 12:00*
D	0:10 1:10 2:39 5:49 / 1:09 2:38 5:48 12:00*
E	0:10 0:55 1:58 3:23 6:33 / 0:54 1:57 3:22 6:32 12:00*
F	0:10 0:46 1:30 2:29 3:58 7:06 / 0:45 1:29 2:28 3:57 7:05 12:00*
G	0:10 0:41 1:16 2:00 2:59 4:26 7:36 / 0:40 1:15 1:59 2:58 4:25 7:35 12:00*
H	0:10 0:37 1:07 1:42 2:24 3:21 4:50 8:00 / 0:36 1:06 1:41 2:23 3:20 4:49 7:59 12:00*
I	0:10 0:34 1:00 1:30 2:03 2:45 3:44 5:13 8:22 / 0:33 0:59 1:29 2:02 2:44 3:43 5:12 8:21 12:00*
J	0:10 0:32 0:55 1:20 1:48 2:21 3:05 4:03 5:41 8:41 / 0:31 0:54 1:19 1:47 2:20 3:04 4:02 5:40 8:40 12:00*
K	0:10 0:29 0:50 1:12 1:36 2:04 2:39 3:22 4:20 5:49 8:59 / 0:28 0:49 1:11 1:35 2:03 2:38 3:21 4:19 5:48 8:58 12:00*
L	0:10 0:27 0:46 1:05 1:26 1:50 2:20 2:54 3:37 4:36 6:03 9:13 / 0:26 0:45 1:04 1:25 1:49 2:19 2:53 3:36 4:35 6:02 9:12 12:00*
M	0:10 0:26 0:43 1:00 1:19 1:40 2:06 2:35 3:09 3:53 4:50 6:19 9:29 / 0:25 0:42 0:59 1:18 1:39 2:05 2:34 3:08 3:52 4:49 6:18 9:28 12:00*
N	0:10 0:25 0:40 0:55 1:12 1:31 1:54 2:19 2:48 3:23 4:05 5:04 6:33 9:44 / 0:24 0:39 0:54 1:11 1:30 1:53 2:18 2:47 3:22 4:04 5:03 6:32 9:43 12:00*
O	0:10 0:24 0:37 0:52 1:08 1:25 1:44 2:05 2:30 3:00 3:34 4:18 5:17 6:45 9:55 / 0:23 0:36 0:51 1:07 1:24 1:43 2:04 2:29 2:59 3:33 4:17 5:16 6:44 9:54 12:00*
(Z row)	0:10 0:23 0:35 0:49 1:03 1:19 1:37 1:56 2:18 2:43 3:11 3:46 4:30 5:28 6:57 10:06 / 0:22 0:34 0:48 1:02 1:18 1:36 1:55 2:17 2:42 3:10 3:45 4:29 5:27 6:56 10:05 12:00*

NEW → GROUP DESIGNATION

Z	O	N	M	L	K	J	I	H	G	F	E	D	C	B	A

REPETITIVE DIVE DEPTH	Z	O	N	M	L	K	J	I	H	G	F	E	D	C	B	A
40	257	241	213	187	161	138	116	101	87	73	61	49	37	25	17	7
50	169	160	142	124	111	99	87	76	66	56	47	38	29	21	13	6
60	122	117	107	97	88	79	70	61	52	44	36	30	24	17	11	5
70	100	96	87	80	72	64	57	50	43	37	31	26	20	15	9	4
80	84	80	73	68	61	54	48	43	38	32	28	23	18	13	8	4
90	73	70	64	58	53	47	43	38	33	29	24	20	16	11	7	3
100	64	62	57	52	48	43	38	34	30	26	22	18	14	10	7	3
110	57	55	51	47	42	38	34	31	27	24	20	16	13	10	6	3
120	52	50	46	43	39	35	32	28	25	21	18	15	12	9	6	3
130	46	44	40	38	35	31	28	25	22	19	16	13	11	8	6	3
140	42	40	38	35	32	29	26	23	20	18	15	12	10	7	5	2
150	40	38	35	32	30	27	24	22	19	17	14	12	9	7	5	2
160	37	36	33	31	28	26	23	20	18	16	13	11	9	6	4	2
170	35	34	31	29	26	24	22	19	17	15	13	10	8	6	4	2
180	32	31	29	27	25	22	20	18	16	14	12	10	8	6	4	2
190	31	30	28	26	24	21	19	17	15	13	11	10	8	6	4	2

RESIDUAL NITROGEN TIMES (MINUTES)

The method used to keep account of the residual nitrogen levels qualitatively is through the use of *Repetitive Group Designations*, as shown in Table 4-8. These group designations, indicated as letters of the alphabet, are assigned to a diver after every dive to represent the quantity of residual inert gas remaining in the diver's body upon surfacing. For instance, after surfacing from a dive to 48 FSW with a bottom time of 33 minutes a diver will be assigned a Repetitive Group Designation of "F" (it is necessary to enter Table 4-8 using 40 minutes at 50 FSW to arrive at this appropriate designation). Note that longer bottom times at this depth, or the same bottom time at deeper depths, will result in a group designation further down the alphabet, indicating more residual nitrogen is present.

4.4.2 Residual Nitrogen Timetable for Repetitive Air Dives

After a diver surfaces from a dive, the residual nitrogen in the diver's tissues will continue to be off-gassed until these tissues return to equilibrium with surface air. As dissolved nitrogen passes out of the tissues and blood while on the surface, the repetitive group designation will change. This gradual return to normal levels will generally be completed within a 12-hour period after surfacing. If additional dives will be conducted within this 12-hour period, it will be necessary to keep track of the residual nitrogen in the diver's body at the time that the repetitive dive begins. The *Residual Nitrogen Timetable* given in Table 4-9 permits the new designation to be determined at any *surface interval* between two consecutive dives. It should be understood that the development of this table was obtained through a continued application of the exponential off-gassing model discussed above.

The upper portion of Table 4-9 is composed of various time intervals between 10 minutes (expressed as 0:10) and 12 hours (expressed as 12:00). Each interval has two limits, a minimum time (top limit)·and a maximum limit (bottom limit). Note that surface intervals for less than 10 minutes after surfacing are disregarded, and the dives before and after this short surfacing interval will be treated as a single dive. Likewise, dives after surface intervals of more than 12 hours are not considered repetitive dives. Just before a repetitive dive is initiated, the new repetitive group designation can be determined from Table 4-9 by entering the schedule on the diagonal slope using the group designation that was found after surfacing from the previous dive. We then read horizontally until the actual surface interval is found to be equal to, or between, the two limits in the schedule. The new repetitive group designation at the end of this surface interval can then be found by reading directly downward to the bottom of that column.

Example: If the "F" diver from above remained on the surface for 3 hours before making a second dive, what repetitive group designation would this diver have at the beginning of the second dive?

Solution: Enter the diagonal slope in the upper portion of Table 4-9 at group designation "F" and move horizontally to the column which covers surface intervals between 2 hours 29 minutes and 3 hours 57 minutes. Move vertically downward to find that this diver would have off-gassed enough nitrogen during this surface interval to have a new group designation of "C" before starting the second dive.

The new repetitive group designation indicates the level of nitrogen that the diver will begin the next dive, an excess which results as a residual from the previous dive. In effect, this residual nitrogen will reduce the diver's allowable exposure time during the second dive if the diver wishes to make a no-decompression dive. This penalty in allowable exposure time can be found in the bottom portion of Table 4-9 in the form of a *residual nitrogen time or RNT*. The RNT can be thought of as the time that a diver must consider that he or she has already spent on the bottom when the repetitive dive to a specific depth is started. If a diver is making a decompression dive, the RNT will be added to the actual bottom time to compute the exposure time that must be used to compute the decompression schedule.

Example: At the end of the 3 hour surface interval, the "C" diver above wants to make a second no-decompression dive to 48 FSW. What is the maximum bottom time for this repetitive dive?

Solution: The residual nitrogen time (i.e., bottom time penalty) can be found in the bottom portion of Table 4-9 by continuing down the column for a "C" group designation to the row corresponding to the depth of the second dive (note that the depth is rounded up to 50 feet). Where the "C" column and the 50 feet depth intersect we find an RNT of 21 minutes. Since the no-decompression limit for 50 FSW is 100 minutes (see Table 4-8), this diver can have a maximum bottom time for the repetitive dive of

$$Maximum\ Bottom\ Time\ (MBT) = No-Decompression\ Limit\ -\ RNT$$

$$MBT = 100\ minutes\ -\ 21\ minutes\ =\ 79\ minutes$$

Example: A diver wishes to make a 35-minute repetitive dive to 60 FSW after completing a 12-minute dive to 92 FSW. How long must the diver remain on the surface between dives to make the repetitive dive without the need to decompress?

Solution: After completing the dive to 92 FSW for 12 minutes, the diver will have a repetitive group designation of "E" (we must enter Table 4-8 at 100 FSW for 15 minutes). Since the no-decompression limit for the repetitive dive to 60 FSW is 60 minutes, the maximum allowable RNT can not exceed 25 minutes to allow a 35-minute bottom time for the second dive. Entering the bottom part of Table 4-9 at a repetitive dive depth of 60 FSW, and moving horizontally across until we find an RNT that is less than or equal to 25 minutes, we see that this diver must have a group designation "D" before the start of the repetitive dive (an RNT of 24 minutes is seen for a "D" diver at 60 FSW). In order for the diver to drop from an initial group designation of "E" (at the end of the first dive) to a group designation of "D" will require a minimum surface interval of 55 minutes as shown in the top portion of Table 4-9.

4.5 Decompression After Saturation Diving

In the example above in Section 4-3, only the fastest tissue was seen to reach equilibrium with the inert gas in the breathing mixture before the diver began his initial ascent. For longer exposures, even the slowest tissues would reach equilibrium, at which point this dive exposure would be called a *saturation dive*. Once saturation is reached, the diver can remain at depth without experiencing any additional decompression obligation.

Calculations of decompression schedules following a *saturation dive* are simplified considerably due to the fact that the "controlling" tissue during decompression from saturation will always be the slowest tissue. Thus, all faster tissues can be ignored during these calculations and only the single, slowest tissue need be considered when satisfying maximum tissue pressures.

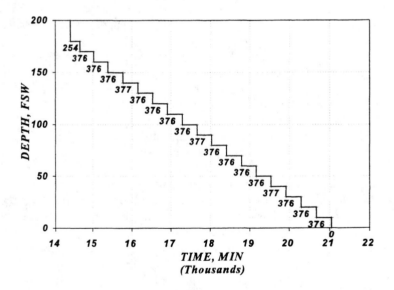

Figure 4-6: Conceptual decompression schedule following a saturation dive to 200 FSW for 10 days when a heliox mixture is used with 84% He/16% oxygen (based on H = 480 minutes). Stop dives are shown beneath each stop.

When using the Haldanian model to calculate saturation decompression schedules, it is only imperative that a tissue half-life be assumed that will cover the slowest, least blood-perfused tissues in the diver's body. Figure 4-6 shows the decompression schedule predicted for a diver saturated at 200 FSW when using a heliox breathing mixture consisting of 84% helium and 16% oxygen. This schedule is based on a single tissue half-life, H, of 480 minutes. Based on this exposure, nearly 6600 minutes (110 hours) is estimated as the required time to reach the surface. This decompression schedule can be accelerated considerably by increasing the oxygen partial pressure as the diver approaches the surface.

In practice, the U.S. Navy uses a more simplified approach to decompressing divers following saturation exposures. Rather than decompressing the divers in 10-foot intervals as indicated above, the pressures in decompression chambers are continuously reduced according the following *standard saturation decompression schedule*:

Table 4-10: U.S. Navy Standard Helium-Oxygen Saturation Decompression Rates
(taken from U.S. Navy Diving Manual, Vol 2, 1991)

From Depths of	To Depths of	Use Decompression Rate
1000 FSW	200 FSW	4 FSW per hour
200 FSW	50 FSW	2.5 FSW per hour
50 FSW	Surface	2 FSW per hour

4.6   Closure

Eliminating inert gases from body tissues when going from a high pressure environment at depth to reduced pressures at the surface is essential to the safety of a diver. Similarly, an astronaut, protected by his space suit with an internal pressure of approximately 4 psia, would suffer the same consequences as the diver unless the inert gases in his body have been safely reduced prior to exposures to the near vacuum of space. This is accomplished in space applications by breathing oxygen prior to the space walk to flush out nitrogen from the astronaut's tissues. In both applications, the same principles apply. The solubilities of inert gases in our body tissues depend on the environmental pressure acting on our bodies. A sudden reduction in this pressure, whether locking out of a space capsule or rapidly returning to the ocean's surface after a dive, will cause these gases to come out of solution at an rate that is excessive for our normal exchange mechanisms to handle. Proper development of decompression schedules to control this pressure reduction will allow these gases to be carried by the blood to the lungs for removal during normal respiration.

5

Carbon Dioxide Removal Methods

Objectives

The objectives of this chapter are to
- review alternative chemical and physical methods for removing carbon dioxide from respiratory gases, and to gain an appreciation for the applications of regenerative systems and expendable systems
- determine the theoretical capacities of various chemicals for removing carbon dioxide
- determine the oxygen production capacities of certain dual-purpose chemicals
- present a systematic approach for designing carbon dioxide scrubbers
- be able to calculate the flow resistances in chemical scrubbers and know their influences on human breathing characteristics.

5.1   Introduction

The removal of metabolically-produced carbon dioxide is an absolute necessity in any closed environment in which human, or any animal life is being supported. Left unchecked, the carbon dioxide content of our expired breath will contaminate our surrounding atmosphere, leading to the symptoms of carbon dioxide poisoning discussed previously in Chapter 3. Removal of expired carbon dioxide can be achieved by simply ventilating the closed environment with fresh gas---the proper ventilation rates will be discussed in Chapter 6---or removed with one of several different methods discussed below.

5.2   Carbon Dioxide Absorption Methods

The conventional methods used for removing carbon dioxide from diving gases deal with the chemical absorption of carbon dioxide with alkali metal hydroxides; ie, calcium hydroxide, sodium hydroxide, lithium hydroxide, and barium hydroxide. However, there are numerous other techniques which the designer of carbon dioxide scrubber systems should be aware. These techniques can be divided into two fundamental groups; chemical and physical removal methods as outlined in the Table 5-1.

TABLE 5-1: ALTERNATE CARBON DIOXIDE REMOVAL METHODS

CHEMICAL		PHYSICAL
HYDROXIDES		MOLECULAR SIEVES
PEROXIDES		CRYOGENIC
SUPEROXIDES	OXYGEN GENERATORS	
OZONIDES		MEMBRANE SEPARATION
AMINES	REGENERATIVE	ELECTRO-CHEMICAL
METAL OXIDES		
SABATIER		
BOSCH REACTOR		

5.2.1 Chemical Removal of Carbon Dioxide

The entire family of alkali and alkaline earth metal hydroxides, peroxides, superoxides, and ozonides react chemically with carbon dioxide and water to form carbonates, bicarbonates, or hydrates. These chemical processes are normally thought of as irreversible, the chemical absorbent being replenished with a fresh supply after a predetermined interval. On the other hand, various metal oxides and organic amines have been used as regenerative absorbent systems in atmospheres which remain sealed for prolonged durations; e.g., submarines, submersibles, and one-atmosphere diving systems. A brief description of these processes is given below.

5.2.1.1 *Hydroxides*

Because of the ease in handling and low cost, this group of absorbents is the most commonly used in diving systems. Their overall chemical reaction[4], as typified by the following equations is exothermic and requires that the carbon dioxide is initially dissolved in water to produce carbonic acid before absorption will occur.

---

[4] M in these reactions represents an alkali metal from Group IA or IIA of the Periodic Table of Elements; ie, IA includes lithium, sodium, potassium; IIA includes magnesium, calcium, or barium.

IA	IIA	IIIB	IVB	VB	VIB	VIIB	VIII			IB	IIB	IIIA	IVA	VA	VIA	VIIA	0
1 H 1.00797																1 H 1.0079	2 He 4.0026
3 Li 6.939	4 Be 9.012											5 B 10.811	6 C 12.011	7 N 14.007	8 O 15.9994	9 F 18.998	10 Ne 20.183
11 Na 22.990	12 Mg 24.312											13 Al 26.98	14 Si 28.086	15 P 30.97	16 S 32.064	17 Cl 35.453	18 Ar 39.95
19 K 39.102	20 Ca 40.08	21 Sc 44.96	22 Ti 47.90	23 V 50.94	24 Cr 52.00	25 Mn 54.94	26 Fe 55.85	27 Co 58.93	28 Ni 58.71	29 Cu 63.54	30 Zn 65.37	31 Ga 69.72	32 Ge 72.59	33 As 74.92	34 Se 78.96	35 Br 79.91	36 Kr 83.80
37 Rb 85.47	38 Sr 87.62	39 Y 88.91	40 Zr 91.22	41 Nb 92.91	42 Mo 95.94	43 Tc 99	44 Ru 101.07	45 Rh 102.91	46 Pd 106.4	47 Ag 107.87	48 Cd 112.40	49 In 114.82	50 Sn 118.69	51 Sb 121.75	52 Te 127.60	53 I 126.90	54 Xe 131.30
55 Cs 132.90	56 Ba 137.34	57-71 La series*	72 Hf 178.49	73 Ta 180.95	74 W 183.85	75 Re 186.2	76 Os 190.2	77 Ir 192.2	78 Pt 195.1	79 Au 196.97	80 Hg 200.59	81 Tl 204.37	82 Pb 207.19	83 Bi 208.98	84 Po 210	85 At 210	86 Rn 222
87 Fr 223	88 Ra 226	89- Ac series†															

58 Ce 140.12	59 Pr 140.91	60 Nd 144.24	61 Pm 147	62 Sm 150.35	63 Eu 151.96	64 Gd 157.25	65 Tb 158.92	66 Dy 162.50	67 Ho 164.93	68 Er 167.26	69 Tm 168.93	70 Yb 173.04	71 Lu 174.97
90 Th 232.04	91 Pa 231	92 U 238.03	93 Np 237	94 Pu 239	95 Am 241	96 Cm 242	97 Bk 249	98 Cf 252	99 Es 254	100 Fm 253	101 Md	102 No	103 Lw

Metals — Nonmetals

Periodic Table of Elements. The atomic number and the atomic weight (carbon = 12.000) are shown for each element.

$$2\,M\,OH + CO_2 \rightarrow M_2CO_3 + H_2O \qquad (Alkali\ Metals\ --\ I\ A)$$

$$M(OH)_2 + CO_2 \rightarrow MCO_3 + H_2O \qquad (Alkali\ Earth\ Metals\ --\ II\ A)$$

(5-1)

Table 5-2 lists the absorption capacities and relative causticities for common metal hydroxides. Note that in general, the alkali metal hydroxides, group IA on the Periodic Table of Elements, have higher absorption capacities than the alkali earth hydroxides, group IIA. However, as a rule, this advantage is offset somewhat by the relatively high causticity inherent with the alkali metals. Also, the apparent advantage of LiOH in absorption capacity over sodalime (primarily $Ca(OH)_2$) is lost when determined on a volumetric basis.

When low operating temperatures are a concern, as is usually the case in diving application, LiOH has a decided advantage over other common absorbents. At temperatures as low as 5° C, LiOH has been shown to undergo only small reductions in efficiency, while calcium hydroxide and other alkali earth hydroxides suffer major reductions.

TABLE 5-2: PROPERTIES OF METAL HYDROXIDES

Compound	Chemical Formula	Molecular Weight	Capacity gm CO_2/gm
ALKALI METAL HYDROXIDES			
Potassium Hydroxide	KOH	56.1	.392
Sodium Hydroxide	NaOH	40.0	.55
Lithium Hydroxide	LiOH	23.9	.919
ALKALI EARTH METAL HYDROXIDES			
Barium Hydroxide	Ba(OH)$_2$	171.4	.257
Calcium Hydroxide	Ca(OH)$_2$	74.1	.594
Magnesium Hydroxide	Mg(OH)$_2$	58.3	.755

5.2.1.2   Peroxides

Alkali metal peroxides have found use as carbon dioxide absorbents, but unlike the hydroxides, release oxygen concurrently according to the general reaction

$$M_2O_2 + CO_2 \Rightarrow M_2CO_3 + 0.5\ O_2 \qquad\qquad (5\text{-}2)$$

The most common compound in this category, lithium peroxide (Li_2O_2), can theoretically remove 0.96 kg of carbon dioxide with each kilogram of lithium peroxide while at the same time, release 0.35 kg of oxygen. Its *system respiratory quotient (SRQ)*, defined as the ratio of the volumes of carbon dioxide absorbed to oxygen produced, equals 2.0 as can be seen from the above reaction. This SRQ would require that an additional source of oxygen be used to meet the desired human respiratory quotient, RQ, of approximately 0.8 (see Chapter 3). However, the theoretical absorption capacity of lithium peroxide is approximately 4 percent greater than lithium hydroxide. On this basis lithium peroxide is an attractive chemical for consideration in a mixed, active chemical system where its high carbon dioxide absorption capacity could be used while supplemented with an auxiliary oxygen supply. Table 5-3 lists other metal peroxides and superoxides used in air revitalization systems.

TABLE 5-3: CAPACITIES OF PEROXIDE AND SUPEROXIDE COMPOUNDS

Compound	Chemical Formula	Molecular Weight	Capacity gm CO_2/gm	Available O_2 gm O_2/gm
Lithium Superoxide	LiO_2	38.9	.566	.617
Sodium Superoxide	NaO_2	55.0	.40	.436
Potassium Superoxide	KO_2	71.1	.309	.338
Lithium Peroxide	Li_2O_2	45.8	.96	.349
Sodium Peroxide	Na_2O_2	78.0	.564	.205

5.2.1.3   Superoxides

Like peroxides, superoxides release oxygen concurrently with the absorption of carbon dioxide. However, unlike the peroxides, the reactions with superoxides potentially can be controlled to match the human respiratory quotient of approximately 0.8. The generalized equation governing superoxide reactions with carbon dioxide

$$2\ MO_2 + CO_2 \Rightarrow M_2CO_3 + 1.5\ O_2 \qquad\qquad (5\text{-}3)$$

yields a respiratory quotient of 0.67. However, a competing reaction with carbon dioxide and water forms a bicarbonate as follows:

$$2 \ MO_2 \ + \ H_2O \ + \ 2 \ CO_2 \ \rightarrow \ 2 \ MHCO_3 \ + \ 1.5 \ O_2 \qquad\qquad \textbf{(5-4)}$$

Here the SRQ is 1.33. It can be seen that by properly controlling the proportion of carbonate and bicarbonate formation, the respiratory quotient can be make to approach that required for human metabolism. Studies have indicated that the superoxide reactions can be potentially controlled to produce SRQs equal to 0.8 by controlling the inlet carbon dioxide/water mole ratio at 2:1. Additional studies have shown that the desired formation of carbonates and bicarbonates can be controlled by accurately maintaining the proper bed temperature (bicarbonate formation is favored if bed temperature is kept low). In practice however, the accurate control of these reactions has been found to be extremely difficult. Systems in the past have opted for parallel canisters of potassium superoxide and lithium hydroxide to remove carbon dioxide to avoid over-, or under-producing oxygen. Table 5-3 lists the theoretical carbon dioxide absorption capacities and oxygen generation capacities for various superoxide compounds. Lithium superoxide has not been successfully manufactured and is probably unstable. The high temperature and pressure at which sodium superoxide must be produced makes its cost unattractive. The most commonly used compound, potassium superoxide, has found applications in USSR manned spacecraft, submersibles, and multi-person environmental control systems.

5.2.1.4   Ozonides

Ozonides, shown in Table 5-4, have the highest theoretical oxygen release capacities of all known carbon dioxide absorbents. Like the superoxides, competing reactions between carbonate formation

$$2 \ MO_3 \ + \ CO_2 \ \rightarrow \ M_2CO_3 \ + \ 2.5 \ O_2 \qquad\qquad \textbf{(5-5)}$$

and bicarbonate formation

$$2 \ MO_3 \ + \ H_2O \ + \ 2 \ CO_2 \ \rightarrow \ 2 \ MHCO_3 \ + \ 2.5 \ O_2 \qquad\qquad \textbf{(5-6)}$$

produce SRQs between 0.4 and 0.8. Notice that if bicarbonate formation could be forced continually when using this chemical, a SRQ compatible with the normal human metabolic needs could be met without the need for dual canister systems that are required in superoxide applications.

TABLE 5-4: CAPACITIES OF OZONIDE COMPOUNDS

Compound	Chemical Formula	Molecular Weight	Capacity gm CO_2/gm	Available O_2 gm O_2/gm
Lithium Ozonide	LiO_3	54.9	.401	.729
Sodium Ozonide	NaO_3	71.0	.31	.563
Potassium Ozonide	KO_3	87.1	.253	.459

Unfortunately, these materials are difficult to synthesize, making their costs excessive. Additionally, they are likely to ignite and even explode when put in contact with many materials. Exposure to an excessive supply of water will cause a violent reaction, with generation of a large quantity of oxygen and toxic byproducts.

5.2.1.5   *Oxides*

Metal oxides received some attention during the early 1970s as carbon dioxide absorbents with regenerative capability. Silver oxide, the most popular of these compounds, was first investigated by the US Navy in the 1940s as a reversible carbon dioxide absorbent. Absorption efficiencies of better than 60 percent were reported when silver oxide was present in a form that displayed a large surface area. In fact, it appears that the large surface area requirement is the primary obstacle to making this a practical alternative, due to the limited rate of diffusion of carbon dioxide gas through a silver carbonate surface layer. The metal oxide can easily be regenerated by heating the carbonate byproduct to 185° C or prolonged heating at 99° C with no caustic or toxic effects reported.

Table 5-5 lists various metal oxides and their respective absorption capacities. The metal oxide possessing the highest capacity for carbon dioxide, lithium oxide, is extremely unstable in the presence of water.

TABLE 5-5: ABSORPTION CAPACITIES OF METAL OXIDES

Compound	Chemical Formula	Molecular Weight	Capacity gm CO_2/gm
Lithium Oxide	Li_2O	29.8	1.477
Sodium Oxide	Na_2O	62.0	.71
Potassium Oxide	K_2O	94.2	.467
Silver Oxide	Ag_2O	231.8	.19
Magnesium Oxide	MgO	40.3	1.092
Calcium Oxide	CaO	56.1	.784
Strontium Oxide	SrO	103.6	.425
Barium Oxide	BaO	153.3	.287
Zinc Oxide	ZnO	81.4	.541

5.2.1.6 Amines

Another class of carbon dioxide absorbents with regenerative capability is represented by aqueous solutions of ethanolamines. The most common of these liquid amines, monoethanolamine (MEA), is used extensively in industrial applications and on submarines. These solutions readily absorb carbon dioxide when cooled and are easily reversed by boiling to give up carbon dioxide. Used in a system shown schematically in Figure 5-1, liquid amines have found widespread use in carbon dioxide removal systems onboard nuclear powered submarines. The major shortcoming of these systems deals with the tendency for the aqueous solutions to release toxic gases such as ammonia during operation. That, along with the requirement for a substantial power supply to repeatedly heat and cool the liquid, limits their applications to large, multi-person environmental control systems.

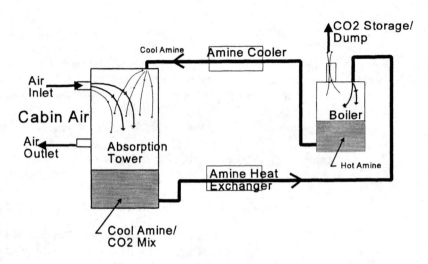

Figure 5-1: Schematic Representation Of A Liquid Amine Carbon Dioxide Absorption System.

5.2.1.7 Sabatier

An additional chemical process which can be used to revitalize atmospheric gases is referred to as the Sabatier process. Concentrated carbon dioxide is mixed with hydrogen at a molar ratio of approximately 4.35 parts hydrogen to 1 part carbon dioxide and passed over a ruthenium-on-alumina catalyst at 400 to 700° C. Methane, which can be used to produce energy, and water vapor, for replenishing water supplies, are the reactants; see Figure 5-2.

5.2.1.8 Bosch Reactor

Water at high pressure is used commercially in a Bosch reactor to absorb carbon dioxide. Unfortunately, the efficiency of this process is reduced considerably at low pressures and low carbon dioxide concentrations.

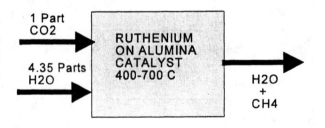

Figure 5-2: Sabatier Process For Converting Carbon Dioxide Into Useful Resources.

5.2.2 Physical Systems For The Removal Of Carbon Dioxide

5.2.2.1   *Molecular Sieves*

Molecular sieves, normally consisting of synthetic crystalline zeolites, are the most commonly used physical means for the removal of carbon dioxide from a life support system. The molecular sieve, in the form of pellets of beads, is formed by bonding the zeolite, in the form of a fine white powder, with 20 percent clay. The pore size of the molecular sieve is selected to adsorb carbon dioxide and toxic impurities from the breathing gas onto the large surface areas of the pellets or beads. The zeolites have a relatively high affinity for polarized molecules such as carbon dioxide, but unfortunately, a still higher affinity for the polarized water molecule. Thus, the air stream is commonly dried by passing it through silica gel prior to being introduced into the zeolite beds. When exhausted, the molecular sieve can be regenerated either by the application of a vacuum to the sieve bed or by increasing the bed temperature. In addition to the zeolites, silica gel, activated charcoal, and alumina can be used for adsorbing carbon dioxide from breathing gases. However, these materials are far less efficient than the zeolites.

5.2.2.2   *Membrane Separation*

The use of semi-permeable membranes has been proposed to enrich various components of breathing gas mixtures by allowing selective diffusion between the breathing gas and the surrounding seawater. By so doing, carbon dioxide can diffuse across the membrane to be expelled into seawater while oxygen is diffused into the breathing gas. Cascade systems have been proposed to complete this diffusion process in a multistage operation with each step further enriching or depleting the gas stream of the selected component. The major shortcomings of such systems pertain to the fragility of the thin membrane films and to the large surface areas required to meet the gas diffusion needs (as shown in Figure 5-3, approximately 35 square meters of dimethyl silicone membrane 0.025 mm thick would be required to supply 2.0 SLPM of oxygen to a diver and remove his exhaled carbon dioxide). However, the recent advances in thin membrane technology are moving this separation technique into the realm of being feasible.

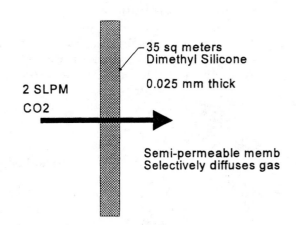

Figure 5.3: Membrane Separation Technique For Removing Carbon Dioxide From Respiratory Gases.

5.2.2.3   *Cryogenic Removal*

Carbon dioxide can be selectively removed from exhaled gases by lowering the gas stream below the freezing point of carbon dioxide (-78°C) while remaining above the freezing points of the other constituents (oxygen, nitrogen, and helium all freeze at temperatures below -180°C). The most attractive system freezes both carbon dioxide and water, which are then removed by sublimating the solids in a vacuum. Similar systems for the recovery of helium in saturation diving are presently operational. These systems require a substantial power supply to produce the cold temperatures and are thus limited in application.

5.2.2.4   *Electrochemical*

Various electrochemical systems have been proposed for the removal of carbon dioxide from respiratory gases. However, they also require large power sources, limiting their potential applications to situations where such energy sources are available.

5.3   Carbon Dioxide Scrubber Design

Acceptable levels of carbon dioxide can be maintained in an underwater breathing apparatus or an enclosed space through ventilation or by using one of the removal techniques discussed above. When designing a carbon dioxide scrubber for a closed or semi-closed circuit system the key issues that must be addressed by the designer are

a) What is the rate at which carbon dioxide is being produced metabolically?
b) What is the theoretical capacity of the chemical to remove carbon dioxide?
c) What is the theoretical life of an absorption canister?
d) What is the expected utilization of the chemical during a diving mission?
e) How long can we expect a scrubber design to operate effectively?

5.3.1 Metabolic Load

The answer to the first question is necessarily tied to the expected activity level of the diver during the underwater mission. We saw previously in Equation 3-3 that the rate at which carbon dioxide is being produced, $\dot{V}_{CO_2}$, is directly related to the *oxygen consumption rate*, $\dot{V}_{O_2}$, by the *respiratory quotient* (RQ) as

$$\dot{V}_{CO_2}, \; SLPM \; = \; \dot{V}_{O_2} \; * \; RQ \tag{5-7}$$

The *metabolic load*, $\dot{m}_{CO_2}$, for the scrubber will be defined as the mass generation rate of carbon dioxide during the

mission, given in pounds of carbon dioxide per hour. This metabolic load can be found by multiplying the carbon dioxide generation rate by the density of carbon dioxide at conditions of 32°F and 1.0 Ata, or

$$\dot{m}_{CO_2}, \; lb/hr \; = \; \frac{\dot{V}_{CO_2}, \; SLPM}{28.3 \; lit/ft^3} \; * \; \rho_{CO_2}, \; lb/ft^3 \; * \; 60 \; \frac{min}{hr} \tag{5-8}$$

Example: Calculate the metabolic load for a UBA scrubber which must support a diver at 200 FSW in 50°F water when the diver activity is characterized by an oxygen consumption rate of 1.25 SLPM. Assume that the diver has a respiratory quotient of 0.85.

Solution: When calculating the mass generation rate of carbon dioxide **it is critical that the same conditions be observed** when multiplying the carbon dioxide generation rate by the gas density. Since the carbon dioxide rate is specified in SLPM (ie, 32°F and 1 Ata) we should find the density of carbon dioxide at these same conditions using the expression

$$\rho_{CO_2} \; = \; 144 \; \frac{P}{R_{CO_2} \; T} \tag{5-9}$$

where ρ_{CO_2} is the density of carbon dioxide, given in lb/ft³; P is the gas pressure expressed in lb/in²; R_{CO_2} is the gas constant for carbon dioxide given as 35.1 ft-lbf/lb-°R, and T is absolute temperature, °R.

At the conditions specified, the density of carbon dioxide can be calculated as

$$\rho_{CO_2} @ \ 32°F, \ 1 \ ATA \ = \ 144 \ \frac{in^2}{ft^2} \ \frac{14.7 \ lbf/in^2}{35.1 \ \frac{ft-lbf}{lb-°R} \ 492°R} \ = \ 0.123 \ lb/ft^3$$

Using Equation (5-8), the metabolic load for this scrubber can be found as

$$\dot{m}_{CO_2}, \ lb/hr \ = \ \frac{\dot{V}_{O_2} \ * \ RQ}{28.3 \ liters/ft^3} \ * \ \rho_{CO_2} \ * \ 60 \ \frac{min}{hr}$$

$$\dot{m}_{CO_2}, \ lb/hr \ = \ \frac{1.25 \ * \ 0.85}{28.3} \ * \ 0.123 \ * \ 60 \ = \ 0.28 \ lb \ CO_2/hr$$

5.3.2 Theoretical Scrubber Capacity

The next step in sizing the scrubber design is to select the method in which carbon dioxide will be removed from the circuit. Generally, this step will involve the selection of a chemical absorber from one of the chemicals discussed previously. We can then either calculate the theoretical amount of chemical that will be required for a particular mission, or determine the theoretical duration of a scrubber with a known amount of absorbent.

Example: Calculate the *theoretical absorption capacity*, defined as the mass of carbon dioxide absorbed per mass of chemical absorbent, of a scrubber which contains 4 pounds of lithium hydroxide when it is being used to support the mission given above.

Solution: We saw previously that lithium hydroxide reacts with carbon dioxide to form lithium carbonate and water according to the chemical reaction

$$2 \ LiOH \ + \ CO_2 \ \Rightarrow \ Li_2CO_3 \ + \ H_2O$$

Notice that in this reaction, 2 moles of lithium hydroxide combines with one mole of carbon dioxide to produce one mole of lithium carbonate and one mole of water. We can use this chemical reaction to determine the *theoretical absorption capacity* of the absorbent by multiplying the ratio of moles of CO_2 to moles of LiOH by the ratios of their molecular weights; ie

$$Theoretical \ Absorption \ Capacity \ = \ \frac{Moles \ CO_2}{Moles \ Absorbent} \ * \ \frac{Mol \ Wt \ CO_2}{Mol \ Wt \ Absorbent} \qquad (5\text{-}10)$$

When using LiOH as the chemical absorbent, we can see that Equation 5-10 gives a theoretical capacity for LiOH of

$$Theoretical\ Capacity = \frac{1\ lb\text{-}mol\ CO_2}{2\ lb\text{-}mol\ LiOH} \times \frac{44\ \dfrac{lb\ CO_2}{lb\text{-}mol\ CO_2}}{23.94\ \dfrac{lb\ LiOH}{lb\text{-}mol\ LiOH}} = 0.92\ \frac{lb\ CO_2}{lb\ LiOH}$$

which confirms the capacity tabulated previously in Table 5-2. Note that lithium hydroxide can almost absorb its weight in carbon dioxide, making it one of the most efficient chemical absorbers on a per weight basis. The 4 pounds of LiOH in this scrubber could theoretically absorb 3.68 pounds of carbon dioxide provided that all of the chemical reacted completely to form lithium carbonate.

Also, note that moisture is produced as a product of this reaction, which can similarly be shown to be related to the absorption of carbon dioxide as

$$Water\ Production\ Rate = \frac{Moles\ H_2O}{Moles\ CO_2} * \frac{Mol\ Wt\ H_2O}{Mol\ Wt\ CO_2} \qquad \text{(5-11)}$$

Note that the water production rates for all alkali metal and alkali earth metal hydroxides will be the same since their reactions all produce one mole of water for every mole of carbon dioxide to give

$$Water\ Production\ Rate = \frac{1\ lb\text{-}mol\ H_2O}{1\ lb\text{-}mol\ CO_2} \times \frac{18.02\ \dfrac{lb\ H_2O}{lb\text{-}mol\ H_2O}}{44\ \dfrac{lb\ CO_2}{lb\text{-}mol\ CO_2}} = 0.41\ \frac{lb\ H_2O}{lb\ CO_2}$$

During a theoretical mission, water production from the chemical reaction would amount to

$$Water\ Production\ Rate = 0.28\ \frac{lb\ CO_2}{hr} \times 0.41\ \frac{lb\ H_2O}{lb\ CO_2} = 0.11\ \frac{lb\ H_2O}{hr}$$

This water production is coupled with moisture condensation which results when recirculated gases, saturated with water vapor in the diver's lungs, come in contact with the cold walls of the breathing circuit during a cold water dive. These two sources of moisture can become significant, particularly during cold water dives, and methods must be devised to contain or remove this moisture to prevent "caking" of the chemical absorbent, resulting in loss in its absorption capacity.

5.3.3 Theoretical Bedlife (TBL)

The theoretical useful life of a canister can be obtained by dividing its theoretical adsorption capacity found in 5.3.2 by the metabolic load derived in 5.3.1. This *theoretical bedlife*, *TBL*, can be used as an upper limit approximation for the mission duration that this canister could support under ideal conditions.

Example: What theoretical mission duration could the above canister support?

Solution: A canister containing 4 pounds of lithium hydroxide could theoretically remove 3.68 pounds of carbon dioxide (4 lb of LiOH x 0.92 lb CO_2/lb LiOH). Based on a metabolic load given above of 0.28 lb CO_2/hr, we can expect a theoretical bedlife for this scrubber as

$$TBL, \ hrs \ = \ \frac{Theoretical \ Absorption \ Capacity}{Metabolic \ Load} \qquad\qquad (5\text{-}12)$$

or for this example LiOH scrubber

$$TBL \ = \ \frac{3.68 \ lbCO_2}{0.28 \ \dfrac{lbCO_2}{hr}} \ = \ 13.1 \ hrs$$

5.3.4 Scrubber Efficiency (η)

Unfortunately, no chemical absorbent will react with carbon dioxide completely in an operational environment. Many factors, some of the more significant which are listed in Table 5-6, play a major part in determining whether gaseous carbon dioxide will react with the chemical scrubber as the respiratory gases travel through the canister.

Table 5-6: Factors Affecting CO_2 Absorption

a.	Gas flow velocity
b.	Canister geometry
c.	Gas residence time
d.	Gas diffusivity
e.	CO_2 concentration
f.	Absorbent particle size
g.	Absorbent porosity
h.	Moisture content
i.	Gas temperature

Factors such as the gas flow rate and canister geometry will impact the time in which the carbon dioxide is allowed to dwell within the canister (Nuckols,Purer,Deason, 1983). Given the right conditions and unlimited residence time, most or the chemical will react with carbon dioxide. However, the reaction products which result during the absorption of carbon dioxide, lithium carbonate in the above example, will form on the outside surfaces of the granular chemicals. Further reactions between the chemical and carbon dioxide must be preceded by the diffusion of carbon dioxide molecules through these reaction produces. At some point in the life of the scrubber these reaction products become too restrictive to the carbon dioxide diffusion, resulting in incomplete absorption as the gases pass through the canister. Generally, we define the termination of a canister's useful life, referred to as the canister *breakthrough time* *(t$_b$)*, when the canister effluent levels of carbon dioxide reach or exceed 0.5% by volume at 1.0 ATA (defined as 0.5% surface level equivalent, SEV), or P_{CO2} of 0.005 Ata. This useful canister life, or breakthrough time, is generally related to the theoretical bedlife TBL by defining a canister efficiency η such that

$$\eta = \frac{t_b}{TBL} \qquad (5\text{-}13)$$

Smaller absorbent particles and greater particle porosity will contribute to higher surface area for carbon dioxide diffusion to take place, resulting in higher absorption efficiencies. As seen above, excess moisture that becomes trapped in the canister could also impede the diffusion process as a result of chemical compaction, or "caking".

Temperature can also play a major role in determining the rate at which the chemical reaction occurs once the carbon dioxide comes in contact with the absorbent. Generally, the more reactive chemicals, characterized by the alkali metals (see section 5.2.1.1), are less impacted by temperature than the less caustic alkali earth metals. These alkali metals are generally characterized by higher absorption efficiencies at cold temperatures than the alkali earth metals. However, the advantages of these higher efficiencies at cold temperatures must be weighed against the increased risks to potential diver injury when using the more caustic chemicals.

A complete characterization of the efficiencies of carbon dioxide absorbents under all environmental conditions does not exist. It would literally be impossible to quantify the effects of the numerous factors listed above, as well as others, on absorption efficiency. Generally, the designer is forced to size a prototype canister based on theoretical performance and then perform extensive canister testing to confirm that the design has adequate absorption capability over the range of environmental conditions anticipated during his mission.

However, numerous studies have been conducted in recent years to only partially characterize chemical efficiencies for the most common absorbents under realistic operational conditions. One such study (Post, 1985) characterized the absorption efficiency of lithium hydroxide according to the relationship

$$\eta = 0.693 \ e^{-0.0128 \ Re_p} \qquad (5\text{-}14)$$

where Re_p is the particle Reynolds number defined as

$$Re_p = \frac{\rho \ \overline{V_s} \ e_p}{\mu} \qquad (5\text{-}15)$$

where ρ is the density of the gas mixture passing through the canister, lb/ft^3; μ is the viscosity of the gas mixture passing through the canister, lb/ft-sec; $\overline{V_s}$ is the superficial flow velocity (defined as the volumetric gas flow rate divided by the cross sectional area of the flow path), ft/sec; and e_p is the average absorbent particle diameter, ft, shown in Table 5-7.

Table 5-7: Typical Particle Mesh Sizes For Carbon Dioxide Chemicals

Tyler Mesh Range	Mesh Opening inches	Mean Particle Diameter, feet
4 - 8	0.187 - 0.093	1.167×10^{-2}
8 - 20	0.093 - 0.033	0.525×10^{-2}
10 - 20	0.067 - 0.033	0.417×10^{-2}
20 - 60	0.033 - 0.010	0.183×10^{-2}
32 - 60	0.020 - 0.010	0.125×10^{-2}

Example: What absorption efficiency can be predicted for a lithium hydroxide scrubber when supporting a dive mission to 200 FSW in 50°F water. Scrubber design parameters and gas properties for the respiratory mixture at bottom conditions are: gas density is 0.441 lb/ft³, gas viscosity is 1.17×10^5 lbm/ft-sec, average particle diameter (14 mesh) is 0.056 inches, volumetric flow rate is 30 liters/minute, canister cross-sectional area is 102 in².

Solution: The superficial gas velocity through the scrubber is found by dividing the volumetric flow rate by the canister cross-sectional area

$$\overline{V}_s = \frac{30 \ \frac{liters}{min} \ x \ \frac{ft^3}{28.3 \ liters} \ x \ \frac{min}{60 \ sec}}{102 \ in^2 \ x \ \frac{1 \ ft^2}{144 \ in^2}} = 0.025 \ \frac{ft}{sec}$$

resulting in a particle Reynolds number of

$$Re_p = \frac{0.441 \ \frac{lb}{ft^3} \left(0.025 \ \frac{ft}{sec} \right) \left(\frac{0.056 \ inch}{12 \ \frac{inch}{ft}} \right)}{1.17 \ x \ 10^{-5} \ \frac{lb}{ft-sec}} = 4.39$$

These conditions give an absorption efficiency as predicted by Equation (5-14) of

$$\eta = 0.693 \ \exp \ (-0.0128 \ x \ 4.39) = 0.655$$

Typical absorption efficiencies for lithium hydroxide are shown in Table 5-8 to range between 0.5 and 0.8. Efficiencies for calcium hydroxide, a less caustic alkali earth metal hydroxide, have been seen to range between 0.2 and 0.5, with the lower efficiencies generally occurring at cold temperatures.

TABLE 5-8: TYPICAL ABSORPTION EFFICIENCIES

Absorbent	Efficiency Range
Lithium hydroxide	0.5 - 0.8
Calcium hydroxide	0.2 - 0.5

5.3.5 Predicted Scrubber Duration (t_b)

The useful scrubber life is generally defined as the time that is required before the effluent carbon dioxide levels from the scrubber to reach 0.5% SEV (equivalent to a partial pressure of carbon dioxide of 0.005 ATA). Although, generally there exists a fair quantity of unreacted absorbent when this exhaust level of CO_2 occurs, the scrubber is no longer considered capable of providing a safe breathing mixture to the diver. The time to reach this "breakthrough" level of carbon dioxide is found either experimentally, using identical environmental conditions as the mission requirements, or estimated as the product of the canister efficiency found in 5.3.4 and the theoretical bedlife found in 5.3.3.

Example: What is the predicted scrubber duration for the canister defined above, containing 4 pounds of lithium hydroxide, when supporting a moderately hard working diver at 200 FSW in 50°F water?

Solution: With a theoretical bedlife TBL found previously as 13.1 hours and an expected absorption efficiency of 0.655, according to Equation 5-14, we would expect this sample lithium hydroxide scrubber to support the diver at 200 FSW for

$$t_b = \eta * TBL$$

$$t_b = 0.655 \ (\ 13.1 \ hours \ ) = 8.6 \ hours$$

5.4   Pressure Drop Through Chemical Scrubbers

When carbon dioxide canisters are used in a closed or semi-closed breathing circuit, it is necessary to minimize the added breathing resistance and added energy that the diver will need to expend in breathing. Flow resistances in canisters will become subjectively discomforting during inhalation at magnitudes exceeding 7-7.5 cm H_2O per liter per second (Silverman *et al*, 1951). Likewise, exhalation resistance should not exceed 2.9 cm H_2O per liter per second, and in no case should exhalation resistance exceed inhalation resistance.

The pressure drop through an absorbent bed will depend upon the rate of gas flow, bed length, absorbent particle size, and the physical properties of the gas stream. A satisfactory level of success has been obtained in predicting this pressure drop by treating the canister as being made up of uniform solid particles. In such a treatment, *modified friction factors, f_m* , have been derived from a correlation of available pressure drop data for flow through solid granular beds (Perry and Chilton, 1973). The correlation of available data on pressure drop through beds of solid particles can be presented in the form of this modified friction factor versus the *particle Reynolds number, Re_p* , given previously in Equation 5-15.

The modified friction factor can be calculated from one of two expressions covering laminar and turbulent flow, the transition of which has been experimentally determined to occur at a particle Reynolds number of approximately 40. For $Re_p < 40$ (laminar)

$$f_m \approx \frac{850}{Re_p} \qquad (5\text{-}16)$$

and for $Re_p > 40$ (turbulent)

$$f_m \approx \frac{38}{Re_p^{0.15}} \qquad (5\text{-}17)$$

After finding the appropriate friction factor, pressure drop across an absorbent canister can be predicted as

$$\Delta P = \frac{4 f_m L \rho \overline{V^2} A_f}{2 g_c e_p} \qquad (5\text{-}18)$$

where ΔP is the canister pressure drop, lbf/ft²; L is the canister bed length, ft; A_f is a dimensionless *wall effect factor* which depends on the ratio of the particle diameter to the canister diameter, see Figure 5-4; and g_c is the dimensional constant 32.174 lbm-ft/lbf-sec².

Equation 5-18 can be broken into laminar and turbulent regions by substituting Equations 5-16 and 5-17 for f_m, giving for $Re_p < 40$

$$\Delta P = \frac{53 \, \mu \, L \, \overline{V_s} \, A_f}{e_p^2} \qquad (5\text{-}19)$$

and for $Re_p > 40$

$$\Delta P = \frac{2.36 \, \mu^{0.15} \, L \, \rho^{0.85} \, \overline{V_s}^{1.85} \, A_f}{e_p^{1.15}} \qquad (5\text{-}20)$$

Equations 5-19 and 5-20 have been shown to give satisfactory agreement with experimental measurements for pressure drop across calcium hydroxide canisters (where e_p was approximately 0.01167 feet) in hyperbaric environments varying from 1 to 8 Ata with air (Riegel and Caudy, 1982). Figure 5-5 show the relationship of pressure drop to superficial velocity, pressure, and bed depth for air and helium

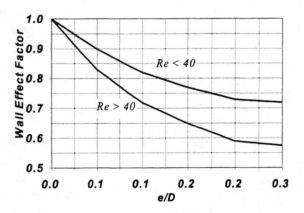

Figure 5-4: Wall Effect Factor (Note: For most canisters with internal diameters greater than 6 inches, A_f ranges from 0.9 to 1.0.)

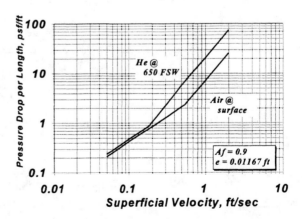

Figure 5-5: Pressure Drop Across Absorbent Canisters at Various Depths

passing through a bed of 4 to 8 mesh absorbent particles (e_p = 0.01167 feet) as predicted by Equations 5-19 and 5-20. These equations are also applicable for predicting pressure drops when using other gases at varying ambient conditions.

One other consideration that must be included when predicting canister flow resistance is how this resistance will vary as the absorbent bed is being depleted of active chemical. Absorption by-products, including carbonates and water, could tend to increase the flow resistances of the bed as the reactions progress. Purer *et al* (1982) observed less than 5 to 10 percent increase in bed resistance at canister breakthrough when water saturated, CO_2-laden gases were tested. During dry gas runs, pressure increases of less than 5 percent were observed. Riegel and Caudy (1982) likewise observed negligible changes in flow resistance during their experiments. Both investigations used particle mesh sizes of 4 to 8 mesh Tyler (see Table 5-7). For this size particle, the added resistance due to chemical by-products can generally be ignored. However, as absorbent particles become smaller, it is conceivable that this added flow resistance could become appreciable.

Example: An axial flow canister 10 inches in length, with a 6-inch diameter, is filled with 4 to 8 mesh calcium hydroxide. What will be the pressure drop across this canister when 6 ACFM of 97% helium/3% oxygen flow through this canister at an ambient pressure of 650 FSW?

Solution: At 650 FSW, we can find the properties of a 97% helium/3% oxygen mixture are (see Gas Properties, Chapter 2)

$$\rho = 0.256 \text{ lbm/ft}^3$$

$$\mu = 1.359 \times 10^{-5} \text{ lbm/ft-sec}$$

The superficial velocity of the gas flow (based on the cross-sectional area of the empty canister) can be calculated by dividing the volumetric flow rate by the cross-sectional area of the empty canister, giving

$$\overline{V}_s = \frac{6 \; \dfrac{ft^3}{min}}{\dfrac{\pi}{4}\left(\dfrac{6}{12}\right)^2 ft^2} = 30.6 \; \frac{ft}{min} = 0.51 \; \frac{ft}{sec}$$

Based on a mean particle diameter of 0.01167 feet for 4 to 8 mesh absorbent, the particle Reynolds number can be calculated as

$$Re_p = \frac{\rho \, \overline{V}_s \, e_p}{\mu} = \frac{\left(0.256 \; \dfrac{lbm}{ft^3}\right)\left(0.51 \; \dfrac{ft}{sec}\right)(0.01167 \; ft)}{1.359 \times 10^{-5} \; \dfrac{lbm}{ft\text{-}sec}} = 111.9$$

The modified friction factor can be found for this particle Reynolds number using Equation 5-17 (turbulent flow) as

$$f_m = \frac{38}{111.9^{0.15}} = 18.7$$

and the corresponding canister pressure drop is calculated using Equation 5-18, assuming a wall effect factor $A_f = 0.9$ (see Figure 5-4)

$$\Delta P = \frac{4 \ (18.7) \ \left(\frac{10}{12}ft\right) \ \left(0.256\frac{lbm}{ft^3}\right) \ \left(0.51\frac{ft}{sec}\right)^2 \ (0.9)}{2 \ \left(32.174\frac{lbm-ft}{lbf-sec^2}\right) \ (0.01167 \ ft)} = 4.98 \ \frac{lbf}{ft^2} = 0.035 \ \frac{lbf}{in^2}$$

An alternate solution to this problem would be directly obtained from Equation 5-20, giving

$$\Delta P = \frac{2.36 \ (1.359 \ x \ 10^{-5})^{0.15} \ \left(\frac{10}{12}\right) \ (0.256)^{0.85} \ (0.51)^{1.85} \ (0.9)}{(0.01167)^{1.15}} = 4.98 \ \frac{lbf}{ft^2} = 0.035 \ psi$$

5.5 Closure

Since World War I, when chemical absorbing agents were being investigated for gas masks, engineers have been asking how the absorption efficiencies of their carbon dioxide scrubbers can be optimized. What are the most favorable environmental conditions for efficient operation of the absorption canister? How does the geometry of the canister affect this efficiency? Can we predict the performance of the carbon dioxide scrubber under one flow condition based on our observations of its performance under different flow conditions.

The design of carbon dioxide absorption systems even today is an inexact process, based on initial design estimates, followed with extensive testing at the same environmental conditions that the systems will be used. This process is frequently iterative in nature, with much trial and error. However, by following the basic procedures described in this chapter, the designer of a carbon dioxide absorption system should find greater success in achieving his design goals.

Figure 5-6: Experimental carbon dioxide scrubber design (cylindrical canister shown on diver's back). (U.S. Navy photo.)

6

Gas Ventilation

Objectives

The objectives of this chapter are to
- derive methods to determine the ventilation requirements necessary to maintain safe exposures within a closed environment
- be able to estimate the time required to build up excessive carbon dioxide levels within a closed environment
- be able to estimate the time required to deplete oxygen levels within a closed environment to result in unsafe exposures

6.1   Introduction

Without proper ventilation, oxygen will be slowly depleted from an enclosed atmosphere while at the same time dangerously high levels of carbon dioxide will build up. How long does it take for the enclosed space to reach unsafe levels of these gases? Let's look at the enclosed atmosphere represented by a diver's helmet as an example. It should be noted however that the analysis given below is applicable to any enclosed space (ie, underwater habitat, submersible, hyperbaric chamber, etc).

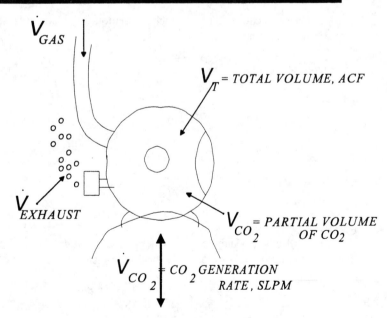

$\dot{V}_{GAS}$

V_T = TOTAL VOLUME, ACF

$\dot{V}_{EXHAUST}$

V_{CO_2} = PARTIAL VOLUME OF CO_2

$\dot{V}_{CO_2}$ = CO_2 GENERATION RATE, SLPM

Figure 6-1: Carbon dioxide removal concerns from a helmeted diver.

6.2   Carbon Dioxide Buildup

For a helmet, as shown in Figure 6-1, with a total system volume (excluding the diver head) of V_T, we can define the partial volume fraction of carbon dioxide in that helmet, V_{CO_2}, as

$$V_{CO_2} = X_{CO_2} * V_T \tag{6-1}$$

where X_{CO_2} is the volume fraction of carbon dioxide in the helmet.

If the carbon dioxide being generated by the diver is expired into the helmet and **mixed uniformly** with the gas inside the helmet, we can say that the time rate of change of the partial volume of carbon dioxide in the helmet can be equated to the diver's CO_2 generation rate as follows

$$\dot{V}_{CO_2} = \frac{dV_{CO_2}}{dt} \tag{6-2}$$

where

$\dot{V}_{CO_2}$ *is the carbon dioxide generation rate, slpm* $= \dot{V}_{O_2} * RQ$

$\dot{V}_{O_2}$ *is the oxygen consumption rate, slpm*

and RQ = Respiratory Quotient (see Chapter 3)

We can call the time at which ventilation to the helmet is stopped t_o, and integrate the above expression from time equal t_o to t, with V_{CO_2} equal to $V_{CO_{2i}}$ at $t_o = 0$, we have

$$\int_0^t \dot{V}_{CO_2} \, dt = \int_{V_{CO_{2i}}}^{V_{CO_2}} dV_{CO_2} \tag{6-3}$$

The change in partial volume of carbon dioxide in the helmet at any time t can be written

$$V_{CO_2} - V_{CO_{2i}} = \dot{V}_{CO_2} * t = \dot{V}_{O_2} * RQ * t \tag{6-4}$$

But we also know that the volume fraction of carbon dioxide in the helmet can be written as the ratio of the partial pressure of carbon dioxide to the total pressure, such that

$$X_{CO_2} = \frac{P_{CO_2}}{P_T} = \frac{V_{CO_2}}{V_T} \tag{6-5}$$

$$\text{where} \quad V_{CO_2} = \frac{P_{CO_2}}{P_T} * V_T \tag{6-6}$$

$$\text{and} \quad V_{CO_{2i}} = \frac{P_{CO_{2i}}}{P_T} * V_T \tag{6-7}$$

In the expressions above, P_{CO_2} is the partial pressure of carbon dioxide at any time t, Ata (defined as atmospheres, absolute); $P_{CO_{2i}}$ is the initial partial pressure of carbon dioxide; and P_T is the total system pressure, Ata. Therefore, we can write

$$(P_{CO_2} - P_{CO_{2i}}) * \frac{V_T}{P_T} = \dot{V}_{O_2} * RQ * t \tag{6-8}$$

If the helmet volume is given in actual cubic feet (ACF), we can convert all units to standard conditions[5] by multiplying V_T by the total pressure and making any temperature adjustment necessary; i.e.

$$V_T (SCF) = V_T (ACF) * P_T * \left(\frac{530}{T, °R}\right) \tag{6-9}$$

By also noting that standard liters per minute (SLPM) can be converted to standard cubic feet per minute (SCFM) by dividing oxygen consumption rate by 26.3 (this conversion includes the temperature difference between standard liters and standard cubic feet), we can then solve for the time it takes for carbon dioxide levels to reach any value of P_{CO_2} as

$$t, \min = \frac{26.3 * V_T * (P_{CO2_{Final}} - P_{CO2_{Initial}})}{\dot{V}_{O_2} * RQ} \left(\frac{530}{T, °R}\right) \tag{6-10}$$

where $P_{CO_{2Final}}$ is the partial pressure of carbon dioxide after some time t, Ata; $P_{CO_{2Initial}}$ is the initial level of carbon dioxide in the enclosed atmosphere, Ata; V_T is the enclosed volume, ACF; $\dot{V}_{O_2}$ is the oxygen consumption rate, SLPM; and T is the temperature of the enclosed space, °R.

Use of this derived expression for determining the time required to buildup an excessive level of carbon dioxide in any atmosphere can best be illustrated with the following example.

---

[5]A standard cubic foot (SCF) is defined at conditions of 70°F and 1.0 atmospheres. This contrasts with the definition used previously for a standard liter (SL) which had conditions of 32°F and 1.0 atmosphere.

Example: An underwater habitat is to contain 6 diver-scientists at a depth of 250 FSW. The total internal volume, which is pressurized to the ambient pressure at depth and is maintained at 75° F , is 750 ACF. The average oxygen consumption level of each man is 0.35 SLPM and their respiratory quotient is 0.85. If ventilation of this habitat is accidentally stopped, how long will it take before the divers get into trouble due to carbon dioxide buildup? The carbon dioxide level was being maintained at 0.5% SEV (0.005 ATA) prior to ventilation shutdown. Assume symptoms of carbon dioxide poisoning are first noticed at 2% SEV; unconsciousness will occur at 6% SEV.

Solution:

At 2% SEV: First symptoms

$$P_{CO_{2_{Final}}} = 0.02 \ ATA; \qquad\qquad P_{CO_{2_{Initial}}} = 0.5\% \ SEV = 0.005 \ ATA$$

$$t = \frac{26.3 \ \frac{SLPM}{SCFM} * 750 \ (ACF) * (0.02 - 0.005) \ ATA}{(6 * 0.35) \ SLPM * 0.85}\left(\frac{530}{535}\right)$$

$$t = 164.2 \ minutes \qquad (2.74 \ hours)$$

At 6% SEV: Unconsciousness

$$P_{CO_{2_{Final}}} = 0.06 \ ATA \qquad \Rightarrow \qquad t = 602 \ minutes \qquad (10 \ hours)$$

6.3   Oxygen Depletion

Similar to the previous analysis with carbon dioxide, we can solve for the time it takes for oxygen levels to reach any value of P_{O_2} as

$$t, \ min = \frac{26.3 * V_T * \left(P_{O_{2_{Initial}}} - P_{O_{2_{Final}}}\right)}{\dot{V}_{O_2}}\left(\frac{530}{T, \ °R}\right) \qquad (6\text{-}11)$$

where P_{O_2} is the partial pressure of O_2, Ata; V_T is the total system volume, ACF; $\dot{V}_{O_2}$ is the oxygen consumption rate, SLPM; T is the temperature of the enclosed volume, °R.

Again, an example will be used to illustrate the time required to deplete the oxygen in a closed atmosphere to a critical level.

Example: In the habitat of the previous example, how long does it take before the oxygen level is reduced where the first symptoms of hypoxia occur if no ventilation exists in the enclosed space? Assume the initial atmosphere contained a partial pressure of oxygen of 0.21 ATA before ventilation shutdown. How long before unconsciousness occurs?

Solution:

At P_{O_2} = 0.16 ATA: First symptoms

$$t = \frac{26.3 \; \dfrac{SLPM}{SCFM} \; * \; 750 \; (ACF) \; * \; (0.21 \; - \; 0.16) \; ATA}{(6 \; * \; 0.35) \; SLPM} \left(\frac{530}{535} \right)$$

$$t \; = \; 465 \; minutes \qquad (7.75 \; hours)$$

At P_{O_2} = 0.10 ATA: Unconsciousness

$$t = 1023 \; minutes \qquad (17.1 \; hours)$$

The subjects inside the chamber would have long since succumbed to carbon dioxide poisoning before hypoxia became a problem. Note that the time for carbon dioxide poisoning and oxygen depletion are both directly proportional to the system volume. In the case of a diver's helmet, we would expect these times to be significantly shortened. For instance, a person inside a helmet with a volume of 0.5 ACF, having the same initial atmosphere as in the above chamber, unconsciousness due to carbon dioxide poisoning would be predicted in a matter of 2-1/2 minutes; unconsciousness due to hypoxia, in 4 minutes!

6.4   Ventilation Requirements

As designers of life support equipment, we would generally not design an enclosure without providing an adequate means of ventilating the enclosed atmosphere. With the proper ventilation we would not have to concern ourselves with carbon dioxide buildup or oxygen depletion. Rather, we generally are interested in maintaining the input of sufficient fresh gas to provide a stable atmosphere which is always safe to breathe. What rates of gas flow are necessary to provide adequate ventilation?

Referring back to Figure 6-1 of the helmeted diver, we are now concerned with determining the flow rate of fresh gas into the enclosed space to maintain a prescribed and stable level of oxygen and carbon dioxide. If we **assume**

perfect mixing within the helmet, we can write a mass balance for carbon dioxide in the helmet as

$$CO_2 \ (in) + CO_2 \ (added \ lungs) - CO_2 \ (exhausted) = CO_2 \ accumulation \ rate \tag{6-12}$$

The carbon dioxide being added from the incoming gas is

$$CO_2 \ (in) = X_{CO_2} \ (input) * \dot{V}_{gas}$$

$$= \frac{P_{CO_2} \ (input)}{P_T} * \dot{V}_{gas} \tag{6-13}$$

Also, the carbon dioxide leaving the helmet in the exhaust gas can be written as

$$CO_2 \ (exhaust) = \frac{V_{CO_2}}{V_T} * \dot{V}_{exhaust} \tag{6-14}$$

In Chapter 3, we defined the rate at which carbon dioxide is being removed from the lungs as

$$CO_2 \ (added \ from \ lungs) = \dot{V}_{CO_2} = CO_2 \ generation \ rate \tag{6-15}$$

and the rate at which carbon dioxide builds up in the helmet can be written as

$$CO_2 \ accumulation \ rate = \frac{dV_{CO_2}}{dt} \tag{6-16}$$

Substituting Equations 6-13 through 6-16 into the carbon dioxide mass balance (Equation 6-12)gives

$$\frac{dV_{CO_2}}{dt} + \left[\frac{\dot{V}_{gas}}{V_T} \right] V_{CO_2} = \left[\dot{V}_{CO_2} + \frac{P_{CO_2} \ (input)}{P_T} \dot{V}_{gas} \right] \tag{6-17}$$

This is a first order, linear differential equation which can be solved, substituting the equality between partial volume and partial pressure shown before, to give the partial pressure of carbon dioxide at any time *t* as

$$P_{CO_2} = \left[\frac{\dot{V}_{CO_2} * P_T}{\dot{V}_{gas}} + P_{CO_2} \ (input) \right] \left[1 - \exp\left(\frac{-\dot{V}_{gas} * t}{V_T} \right) \right] \tag{6-18}$$

The above expression can be divided into two solutions; one describing the transient behavior when ventilation is first initiated, and the other describing the steady state value for the partial pressure of carbon dioxide after equilibrium has been reached. The transient solution is of interest if we want to know the response time that will be required for a ventilation system to reach a designated carbon dioxide level. We can think of the ratio $V_T / \dot{V}_{gas}$ as the characteristic time constant for the ventilation system. That is, as time t approaches the value of $V_T / \dot{V}_{gas}$ (taking care to use consistent units for these measurements), the system will have caused the atmosphere in the enclosed space to reach 63% of equilibrium; at time t equal to twice the value of $V_T / \dot{V}_{gas}$ (2 time constants), 87% of equilibrium is reached; 95% at 3 time constants; 98% at 4 time constants; and so forth. As t approaches ∞, the last term in Equation 6-18 goes to zero, and we are left with a steady value of P_{CO_2} given by

$$P_{CO_2} = \frac{\dot{V}_{CO_2} * P_T + P_{CO_2} \ (input) * \dot{V}_{gas}}{\dot{V}_{gas}} \qquad (6\text{-}19)$$

This equation can be rearranged to solve for the required ventilation rate $\dot{V}_{gas}$ to maintain a steady, prescribed partial pressure of carbon dioxide within a perfectly mixed enclosed space. (Note again the need to convert oxygen consumption rate to SCFM by dividing by 26.3).

$$\dot{V}_{gas} = \frac{P_T * \dot{V}_{O_2} * RQ}{26.3 \left[P_{CO_{2_{Design}}} - P_{CO_{2_{Input}}} \right]} \qquad (6\text{-}20)$$

where $P_{CO_{2_{Design}}}$ is the partial pressure of carbon dioxide that we desire to maintain in the enclosed atmosphere, ATA; $\dot{V}_{O_2}$ is the oxygen consumption level, SLPM; $\dot{V}_{gas}$ is the required ventilation rate, SCFM; P_T is the total pressure, ATA; and *RQ* is the respiratory quotient. Notice that the ventilation rate is not a function of the system volume.

6.4.1 Effects Of Incomplete Mixing

You may recall that Equation 6-20 was derived assuming complete mixing of carbon dioxide within the enclosed atmosphere. Depending on the flow paths of the incoming ventilation gases and the exhaust gases, complete mixing may not always exist. For example, a poorly designed helmet may have the diver's exhalation gases pass directly into the path of the incoming ventilation flow. This would result in unnecessarily high concentrations of CO_2 being inspired by the diver unless ventilation flow rates were increased to dilute the exhaled carbon dioxide. On the other hand, a well designed helmet might include ducting to direct the diver's exhalation gases toward the exhaust valve to minimize its mixing with the incoming ventilation. This could result in a reduction in ventilation flow to maintain the prescribed carbon dioxide level in the helmet.

It is customary to introduce a *mixing effectiveness factor, F,* to account for the variations of flow paths within different enclosures. This factor is usually of much greater concern when dealing with small enclosures, such as helmets, and their deviations from complete mixing must be characterized. By defining *F* as

$$F = Mixing\ Effectiveness\ Factor = \frac{\%CO_2\ in\ inspired\ gas}{\%CO_2\ in\ exhausted\ gas} \tag{6-21}$$

we can calculate the required ventilation rates for any enclosure as

$$\dot{V}_{gas}\ (SCFM) = \frac{P_T * \dot{V}_{O_2} * RQ * F}{26.3 \left[P_{CO_{2_{Design}}} - P_{CO_{2_{Input}}} \right]} \tag{6-22}$$

where

$F = 1$ Mixing is complete
$F < 1$ Mixing is intentionally incomplete; exhaled CO_2 is directed out the exhaust; minimizes ventilation requirement
$F > 1$ Mixing is incomplete (poor design); exhaled CO_2 is directed into the incoming vent

The following example illustrates the calculation of gas ventilation rates within a closed hyperbaric atmosphere. The same approach could be used to determine the ventilation rates within a manned submersible, an atmospheric dive system, or any other closed system.

Example: (a) For the underwater habitat described in the previous examples, what ventilation flow rate is required to maintain the partial pressure of carbon dioxide in the enclosure at 0.5% SEV (0.005 ATA) if the incoming flow has been fully "scrubbed" of carbon dioxide? Assume a mixing effectiveness factor of 1.0.

Solution:

At a depth of 250 FSW:

$$P_T = \frac{Depth,\ FSW\ +33}{33} = \frac{250\ = 33}{33} = 8.58\ ATA$$

$$and\quad \dot{V}_{gas} = \frac{8.58\ ATA\ (\ 6\ *\ 0.35\ SLPM\ )\ (\ 0.85\ )\ (\ 1.0\ )}{26.3\ \dfrac{SLPM}{SCFM}\ (0.005\ -\ 0\ )\ ATA}$$

$$\dot{V}_{gas} = 116.5\ SCFM \qquad (\ 13.7\ ACFM\ )$$

Example: How long would it take for steady state conditions to be reached in the habitat?

Solution: As seen previously, 95% of steady state conditions will be reached after 3 time constants, $V_T / \dot{V}_{gas}$. By converting the units of the total system volume to standard cubic feet, this variable will have consistent units with those for $\dot{V}_{gas}$, allowing us to solve for the time to reach steady state conditions. I.e.,

$$t = 3 \frac{V_T \cdot P_T}{\dot{V}_{gas}} \left[\frac{530}{T, \, °R} \right]$$

where the total pressure and temperature correction were included in the time constant to give consistent units for habitat volume, V_T (ACF), and the ventilation rate, $\dot{V}_{gas}$ (SCFM). Under these conditions, 95% of steady state will be reached at

$$t = 3 \frac{750 \; ACF}{116.5 \; SCFM} \cdot \left[8.58 \frac{530}{535} \right] \left(\frac{SCF}{ACF} \right)$$

$$t = 164.2 \; minutes \qquad (2.7 \; hrs)$$

6.5 Closure

The preceding analyses provided a method for us to determine the ventilation rates and reaction times necessary to maintain safe atmospheres within an enclosed living space. It is always prudent to minimize these ventilation flow rates as much as possible, consistent with the requirements for acceptable carbon dioxide and oxygen levels, due to the high noise levels usually associated with high gas flow rates. This is particularly true at elevated pressures and within metallic enclosures, typical of the surrounding materials associated with pressure vessels.

Reduced ventilation rates additionally minimize the pressure requirements and the associated compressor requirements to deliver these gases via piping systems and gas supply hoses. Detailed analyses of the pressure drops in these piping systems and compressor requirements to maintain these ventilation flow rates will be covered in Chapter 9.

7

Thermal Protection

OBJECTIVES

The objectives of this chapter are to
- present a basic overview of the heat transfer mechanisms that are applicable to diving and hyperbaric atmospheres
- discuss active and passive options for protecting a diver in extremely cold or hot environments
- investigate the feasibility of delivering warm liquids and gases to divers via umbilicals.
- investigate critical thermal considerations in the design of divers' garments

7.1 Introduction

Inadequate protection during cold water exposures severely limits a diver's ability to accomplish his mission. Providing this protection in an underwater setting is particularly difficult due to the thermal properties of the medium making up this underwater environment. Water has the ability to conduct heat away from the human body approximately 25 times faster than air. Additionally, water is capable of absorbing this lost body heat in quantities approximately 3500 times greater than air before a similar unit increase in temperature is recorded (the heat capacity of the medium can be determined as the product of its density and specific heat). As a result, unprotected divers can find a net heat drain from their bodies even in moderate (80°F or 26.7°C) water temperatures.

Advances in diving life support systems now permit divers to conduct long duration mission in moderate water temperatures. However, a diver's physical and mental performance can be impaired in cold water, resulting in significantly reduced safe dive durations (see Chapter 3). This can be a severe limitation for underwater activities which preclude surface support, due to remote locations or the clandestine nature of the operation. In the same token, severe heat stresses can similarly limit safe exposures, particularly when divers are undergoing decompression, or recompression, stages inside hyperbaric chambers having inadequate thermal control.

7.2   Active vs Passive Protection

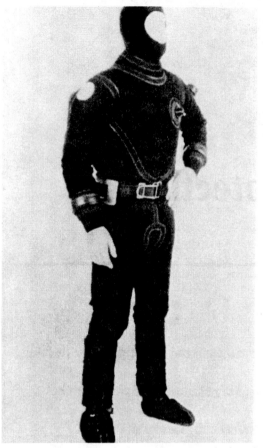

Figure 7-1: Dry suit thermal garment designed to prolong diver exposures in cold water with passive insulation.

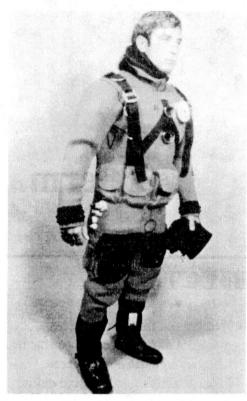

Figure 7-2: Hot water suit designed to prolong diver exposures in cold water with warm water supplied from the surface.

Active and passive methods of thermally protecting divers during long, cold water missions have been sought since man first began to work and explore in the seas[6]. With active protection, heat sources in the order of 0.5 kW have been shown to be adequate to extend the performances of free swimming divers' in shallow water missions at temperatures as low as 40°F (4.4°C); a submerged heat source with a capacity of 1 kW has been shown to accommodate deep dives where the limitation of a surface-supplied hot water source and a long hot water umbilical pose an unacceptable burden (Lippitt and Nuckols, 1983). Invariably, any active heating method used by divers will tend to handicap their performance by restricting mobility, and are generally not suited for remote missions where minimal surface support is available.

Passive methods of protecting divers, either using wet or drysuits, share one common advantage over their active heating counterparts; that is, no requirement for energy storage or energy distribution. This advantage tends to make passive protection less complex and usually less expensive. Unfortunately, in severe cold water, passive systems have customarily required that divers use thick, layered insulating garments, usually worn beneath waterproof dry suits

---

[6]Passive protection is defined here as any method which derives its effectiveness from the inherent insulation value of the materials used in the protection garment which tends to restrict the loss of body heat; in contrast, active protection derives its effectiveness from some external, heat source such as electric heating or a source of circulating warm water which creates a warm "micro-climate" adjacent to the diver's body.

to reduce the loss of excessive body heat to the surrounding water. These suits are typically bulky, excessively buoyant, and difficult to keep waterproof. Additionally, both wet and dry suits have been found to be only minimally effective in protecting the diver's feet and hands from the cold.

This chapter will discuss the three distinct modes for heat transmission: *radiation, conduction* and *convection.* Each of these modes of heat transfer will be described separately. However, it should be emphasized that, in most situations occurring in nature, heat is transmitted not by one, but by two or more of these mechanisms acting simultaneously. The application of these mechanisms for heat transfer from underwater and hyperbaric environments will be highlighted, with a focused discussion of the design of active and passive thermal protection systems.

7.3   Radiation Heat Transfer

Radiation heat transfer is a process by which heat flows via electromagnetic waves from a high temperature body to a low temperature body. Heat transmission between these two separated bodies can occur even when a vacuum exists between them. Heat transfer by radiation becomes increasingly important as the temperature difference between the two bodies increases. However, in most underwater environments where the surface temperature of a diver's suit approaches that of the surrounding water temperature, radiant heat loss from the suit will be minimal and can usually be neglected. Radiation heat transfer can also be minimized on the surface by removing a body from direct exposure to a high temperature sources; for example, an awning can be used to shade a recompression chamber onboard a ship from direct exposure to the sun.

In applications where the surface temperatures of these two bodies is not the same, as in the case of a diver surrounded by a gaseous environment inside a diving bell or a hyperbaric chamber, the net quantity of energy leaving the diver's body as radiant heat will depend upon the difference in the fourth power of the absolute temperatures of the body and the surrounding chamber wall, and nature of these surfaces (Kreith, 1960). When we assume that both surfaces act as perfect *radiators* or *black bodies* (defined as a body whose surface absorbs all the radiant energy incident upon it), the amount of radiant heat transmitted from the diver's *black body* surface to the chamber walls, whose surface is also assumed *black*, is given by the following:

$$\dot{q}_R = \sigma \, A_S \, (T_S^4 - T_W^4) \tag{7-1}$$

where $\dot{q}_R$ is the net rate of radiant heat transfer between the diver's surface and the chamber walls, Btu/hr; A_S is the surface area of the diver's suit, ft^2; T_S is the absolute temperature of the surface of the diver suit, °R; T_W is the absolute surface temperature of the chamber inside wall, °R; and σ is the *Stefan-Boltzmann constant*, with a value of 0.1714 x 10^{-8} Btu/hr-ft^2-°R^4.

In general, most real surfaces do not emit radiant energy as an ideal black body, but will transfer heat at some lower level than black bodies at an equal temperature. These bodies, which will transmit a constant fraction of black-body emission at some equal temperature, are called *gray bodies*, and the net rate of heat transfer from these gray surfaces at a temperature T_S to a black enclosure at T_W can be found as

$$\dot{q}_R = \sigma \, A_S \, \epsilon_S \, (T_S^4 - T_W^4) \tag{7-2}$$

where ϵ_S is the *emissivity* of the gray surface, defined as the fraction of the actual emission from the gray surface compared to that from a perfect black body. Note that most materials which are typically used for divers' suits, such as black rubber, will have surface emissivities in the 0.9-0.95 range (Gebhart, 1971), which makes errors when making assumptions of black body radiation relatively small.

Example: A diver is being transported to a deep dive site inside a personnel transfer capsule (PTC). The surrounding capsule wall temperatures are 40°F and the surface temperature of the diver's suit is 80°F. What is the net rate of radiant heat transfer from the diver to the PTC walls if the surface area of the diver's suit is 20 ft²? Assume that the capsule walls behave as a black body and the surface of the diver's suit has an emissivity of 0.9.

Solution: From Equation (7-2) above, we have

$$\dot{q}_R = 0.1714 \times 10^{-8} \, A_S \, \epsilon_S \, (T_S^4 - T_W^4)$$

and we are given $T_S = 80°F = 540°R$; $T_W = 40°F = 500°R$

$A_S = 20 \text{ ft}^2$; $\epsilon_S = 0.9$

Thus, we can solve for the net rate of radiant heat loss from the diver to the PTC walls as

$$\dot{q}_R = 0.1714 \times 10^{-8} \left(\frac{Btu}{hr\text{-}ft^2\text{-}°R^4} \right) 20 \, ft^2 \cdot 0.9 \cdot \left[540^4 - 500^4 \right] °R^4$$

or

$$\dot{q}_R = 0.1714 \cdot 20 \cdot 0.9 \cdot \left[\left(\frac{540}{100} \right)^4 - \left(\frac{500}{100} \right)^4 \right] = 695 \, \frac{Btu}{hr} \quad [\, 0.2 \, kW \,]$$

7.4   Conduction Heat Transfer

Heat transfer by conduction is a process whereby heat flows from a region of higher temperature to a region of lower temperature within a solid, liquid or gas, or between different mediums in direct contact with one another. The rate of heat conduction through a homogeneous section of material in a single direction is described by Fourier's Law as

$$\dot{q}_K = -K \, A \, \frac{dT}{dx} \qquad (7\text{-}3)$$

where K is the thermal conductivity of the material (see Appendix A for K values for typical materials used in divers' suit designs); A is the area of the section through which heat flows by conduction (this area is measured perpendicularly to the direction of heat flow); and

$\frac{dT}{dx}$ is the temperature gradient at the section in the

direction of the heat flow.

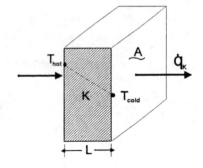

Figure 7-3: Conduction heat transfer through a single material layer.

At steady-state conditions, the rate of heat transfer by conduction per unit area through a section of material having one surface hotter than the other, can be written as

$$\dot{q}_K = A \, \frac{K}{L} \left(T_{hot} - T_{cold} \right) \tag{7-4}$$

where L is the thickness of the material, and T_{hot} and T_{cold} are the temperatures of the hot and cold surfaces, respectively. Equation (7-4) is analogous to the relation for the conduction of electricity, $I = \Delta V/R$ (Ohm's Law), where $\dot{q}_K$ is analogous to the flow of electrical current, the temperature difference is analogous to the voltage drop across a resistor, and $\dfrac{L}{A\,K}$ is analogous to electrical resistance. We can thus define an equivalent *thermal resistance* R_K for heat conduction through a section of material as

$$R_K = \frac{L}{A\,K} \tag{7-5}$$

and rewrite Fourier's Law as

$$\dot{q}_K = \frac{T_{hot} - T_{cold}}{R_K} \tag{7-6}$$

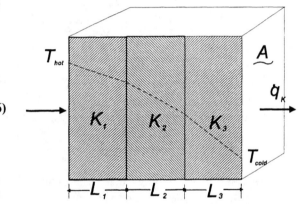

When heat is being conducted through multiple layers of materials in contact with one another, as shown for the composite, we can utilize the electrical analogy by recalling that the total resistance to current flow through resistors in series is equal to the sum of the all the individual resistors, i.e

$$R_{Total} = \Sigma \, R \tag{7-7}$$

Figure 7-4: Conduction heat transfer through a composite.

For the composite shown in Figure 7-4, the total thermal resistance can be written

$$R_{K_{Total}} = R_1 + R_2 + R_3$$

$$R_{K_{Total}} = \frac{L_1}{K_1\,A} + \frac{L_2}{K_2\,A} + \frac{L_3}{K_3\,A} \tag{7-8}$$

where the subscripts indicate the properties and dimensions for the corresponding composite layer, or in general

$$R_{K_{Total}} = \sum_{i=1}^{n} R_i \qquad (7\text{-}9)$$

where *n* is the number of layers in the composite. The heat transfer through this composite by conduction is written

$$\dot{q}_K = \frac{T_{hot} - T_{cold}}{\sum_{i=1}^{n} R_i} = \frac{T_{hot} - T_{cold}}{\dfrac{L_1}{K_1 A} + \dfrac{L_2}{K_2 A} + \dfrac{L_3}{K_3 A}} \qquad (7\text{-}10)$$

or, in general

$$\dot{q}_K = \frac{A (T_{hot} - T_{cold})}{\dfrac{L_1}{K_1} + \dfrac{L_2}{K_2} + \dfrac{L_3}{K_3} + \cdots + \dfrac{L_n}{K_n}} = \frac{A (T_{hot} - T_{cold})}{\sum_{i=1}^{n} \left(\dfrac{L}{K}\right)_i} \qquad (7\text{-}11)$$

Example: A diver is wearing a thin (1/16 inch thick), rubber-coated nylon drysuit over a set of 1/16-inch thick cotton underwear and a 0.3-inch thick Thinsulate thermal undergarment. If the average skin temperature of a diver having a surface of 19 ft^2 is 91°F, how much heat will be lost from the diver's drysuit if the surrounding water has chilled the outside surface of the drysuit to 40°F? The thermal properties of the suit materials can be found in Table 7-6 at the end of this chapter.

Solution: We will assume that the temperature on the inside of the suit is equal to the average skin temperature of the diver, and that the suit can be approximated as a flat plate for calculating suit heat loss. The drysuit can be modeled as a three layered composite having the following properties:

Layer	Thickness (ft)	Thermal Conductivity (Btu/ft-hr-°F)
Cotton underwear	0.0052	0.046
Thinsulate	0.025	0.019
Rubber, Nylon	0.0052	0.120

Using Equation (7-11) we get

$$\dot{q}_K = \frac{A (T_{hot} - T_{cold})}{\sum_{i=1}^{n} \left(\dfrac{L}{K}\right)_i} = \frac{19 \ ft^2 \ (91 - 40) \ °F}{\dfrac{5.2 \times 10^{-3} \ ft}{0.046 \ \dfrac{Btu}{ft-hr-°F}} + \dfrac{0.025 \ ft}{0.019 \ \dfrac{Btu}{ft-hr-°F}} + \dfrac{5.2 \times 10^{-3} \ ft}{0.120 \ \dfrac{Btu}{ft-hr-°F}}}$$

$$\dot{q}_K = 658.3 \ \frac{Btu}{hr} \qquad [\ 0.193 \ kW \ ]$$

7.5 Convection Heat Transfer

Convection heat transfer is the combined action of heat conduction, energy storage, and mixing as a fluid transfers energy with a solid at the interface of the solid and the fluid. For instance, if a solid has a surface temperature that is higher than an adjacent fluid, heat will first flow by conduction from the surface to particles of fluid within the *thermal boundary layer*[7] δ_T adjacent to the surface, see Figure 7-5. The transferred energy will then increase the temperature of these adjacent fluid particles, and as they are swept away by the motion of the fluid these particles will mix with, and transfer their increased energy content to other, lower temperature fluid particles.

The physical mechanism of convective heat transfer is thus actually one of heat conduction through the stationary fluid layer at the solid/fluid interface, which could be expressed by Fourier's Law as

$$\dot{q}_C = A \, \frac{K}{\delta_T} \, (\, T_W - T_\infty \,) \qquad (7\text{-}12)$$

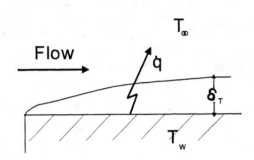

where $\dot{q}_C$ is the rate of heat transfer by convection, K is the thermal conductivity of the fluid, δ_T is the thermal boundary layer, T_W is the surface temperature and T_∞ is the fluid free stream temperature.

Unfortunately, the magnitude of the boundary layer thickness is difficult to predict since it is dependent on a number of variables, including

Figure 7-5: Convection heat transfer at solid/fluid interface.

        a) the fluid velocity,
        b) the geometry of the solid/fluid interface,
and
        c) the physical and thermal properties of the fluid.

Customarily, an empirically obtained *film heat transfer coefficient, h,* is defined instead such that

$$h = \frac{K}{\delta_T} \qquad (7\text{-}13)$$

and the heat transfer due to convection is expressed as *Newton's Law of Heating or Cooling*, given by

$$\dot{q}_C = h \, A \, (\, T_W - T_\infty \,) \qquad (7\text{-}14)$$

---

[7]The thermal boundary layer is defined as the relatively narrow layer of fluid thickness adjacent to the solid surface where 99% of the difference between the temperature of the fluid free stream and the surface temperature occurs.

Using a similar electrical analogy as above to define an equivalent thermal resistance for convection, we can write

$$\dot{q}_C = \frac{(T_W - T_\infty)}{R_C} \qquad where \qquad R_C = \frac{1}{h\,A} \tag{7-15}$$

It is beyond the scope of this text to describe methods to find values for the convective film coefficient h for all surface shapes and conditions. However, most applications of convection in life support design deal with only a few geometries which will be addressed below.

Similar to the practice of dimensional scaling used in fluid mechanics, convective film coefficients are commonly expressed in dimensionless groups to make experimentally derived convective heat transfer data applicable to a wide range of fluid flow conditions and fluid properties. This data is conventionally presented in general correlations in one of two forms, depending on whether the fluid is actively flowing past a surface (*forced convection*), or if the motion results from a change in buoyancy of the fluid adjacent to a surface as it changes in temperature due to the heat transfer at the fluid/surface interface (*natural or free convection*). These general correlations are presented in the following forms:

$$Forced\ Convection: \qquad \overline{Nu} = f\,(Re\,,\,Pr) \tag{7-16}$$

$$Natural\ or\ Free\ Convection: \qquad \overline{Nu} = f\,(Gr\,,\,Pr) \tag{7-17}$$

where the dimensionless groups commonly used in these correlations are the following:

Nusselt Number, $\overline{Nu}$, is the average dimensionless convective heat transfer coefficient, defined as

$$\overline{Nu_D} = \frac{h\,D}{K} \qquad or \qquad \overline{Nu_L} = \frac{h\,L}{K} \tag{7-18}$$

where D and L are characteristic dimensions; D is customarily given as a diameter used in the definition for Nusselt number when we are looking at flow around, or through, cylinders or spheres; L is customarily given as the surface length used in the definition for Nusselt number when we are looking at flow along flat surfaces. The subscript used with the Nusselt number definition will identify which of these two dimensions that the data is being based.

Reynolds Number, Re, is the dimensionless flow parameter which relates the inertia forces to viscous forces, defined as

$$Re_D = \frac{\rho\,V\,D}{\mu} \qquad or \qquad Re_L = \frac{\rho\,V\,L}{\mu} \tag{7-19}$$

where V is the free stream velocity, ρ is the fluid density, and μ is the fluid viscosity.

Prandtl Number, *Pr* , is a dimensionless flow parameter which relates the diffusion of momentum to the diffusion of heat, and defined as

$$Pr = \frac{\mu \; c_p}{K}$$
(7-20)

and

Grashof Number, *Gr* , is a dimensionless group used in the correlation of free convection data, which relates buoyancy forces to viscous forces. Grashof number can be calculated as

$$Gr = \frac{g \; \beta \; (T_W - T_\infty) \; L^3}{\nu^2}$$
(7-21)

where g is the acceleration of gravity, β is the *volume coefficient of expansion* where

$$\beta = \frac{1}{T_\infty} \quad \textit{for ideal gases}$$

ν is kinematic viscosity (μ divided by density), L is a characteristic length for the surface (this should be defined with the correlation equation), T_W is the surface temperature, and T_∞ is the fluid temperature. Free convection heat transfer coefficients are relatively low compared to forced convection applications. However, free convection is often the dominant heat flow mechanism for the stationary human body in a quiescent atmosphere. A simple way of determining the relative magnitudes of free or forced convection heating or cooling, and which convective mode will dominate in any application is to look at the ratio $\dfrac{Gr}{Re^2}$

$$\textit{if} \quad \frac{Gr}{Re^2} \ll 1 \quad \Rightarrow \quad \textit{Forced Convection Dominates (Ignore Free Convection)}$$

$$\textit{if} \quad \frac{Gr}{Re^2} \gg 1 \quad \Rightarrow \quad \textit{Free Convection Dominates (Ignore Forced Convection)}$$

Tables 7-1 and 7-3 give forced and free convection correlation equations for typical geometries that are of interest to designers of life support equipment.

Table 7-1: Correlation Equations for Forced Convection Heat Transfer

Geometry/Flow Conditions	Correlation	Restrictions
Gases Flowing Around a Single Cylinder 	$\overline{Nu}_D = C_1\ Re_D^{\ n}$ (See Table 7-2 for values for C_1 and n)	• Gas flow • Characteristic length is the cylinder diameter • Flow properties evaluated at film temperature $T_f = \dfrac{T_\infty + T_W}{2}$
Liquids Flowing Around a Single Cylinder	$\overline{Nu}_D = C_2\ Re_D^{\ n}\ Pr^{0.33}$ (See Table 7-2 for values for C_2 and n)	• Liquid flow • Applicable for $0.2 < Pr < 1000$ • Flow properties evaluated at film temperature $T_f = \dfrac{T_\infty + T_W}{2}$
Flow Around Spheres	$\overline{Nu}_D = 0.37\ Re_D^{0.6}$	• Applicable for $25 < Re_D < 100{,}000$ • Flow properties evaluated at film temperature $T_f = \dfrac{T_\infty + T_W}{2}$
Flow Inside Tubes	$\overline{Nu}_D = 0.023\ Re_D^{0.8}\ Pr^{\ n}$	**Heating Conditions:** $n = 0.4$ if $T_W > T_\infty$ **Cooling Conditions:** $n = 0.3$ if $T_W < T_\infty$

Table 7-2 : Constants and Exponents Used In Correlations for Forced Convection Heat Transfer

Re	C_1	C_2	n
1 - 4	0.891	0.989	0.33
4 - 40	0.821	0.911	0.385
40 - 4000	0.615	0.683	0.466
4000 - 40000	0.174	0.193	0.618
40000 - 250000	0.0239	0.0266	0.805

Table 7-3: Correlation Equations for Free Convection Heat Transfer

Geometry/Flow Conditions	Correlation	Restrictions
Horizontal and Vertical Planes, Pipes and Spheres (Laminar Flow)	$\overline{Nu} = 0.56 \, (Gr \cdot Pr)^{0.25}$	$10^4 < Gr \cdot Pr < 10^8$ **Characteristic Lengths:** L=Height for vertical planes and pipes L=Length for horizontal plates L= Diameter for horizontal pipes L=0.5 Diameter for spheres
Horizontal and Vertical Planes, Pipes and Spheres (Turbulent Flow) 	$\overline{Nu} = 0.13 \, (Gr \cdot Pr)^{0.33}$	$10^8 < Gr \cdot Pr < 10^{12}$ **Characteristic Lengths:** L = Height for vertical planes and pipes L = Length for horizontal plates L = Diameter for horizontal pipes L = 0.5 Diameter for spheres

Example: Estimate the convective heat transfer coefficient on the inside of a hose, having an inside diameter of 0.25 inches, when delivering warm water at 0.5 gallons per minute.

Solution: In this example, we will assume the following properties for warm water flowing inside the hose

$$\rho_w = 64 \text{ lb/ft}^3$$
$$c_w = 1 \text{ BTU/lb-}°\text{F}$$
$$\mu_w = 0.658 \times 10^{-3} \text{ lb/ft-sec}$$
$$K_w = 0.347 \text{ BTU/ft-hr-}°\text{F}$$

Table 7-1 gives the dimensionless heat transfer coefficient for flow inside a tube when the fluid temperature is greater than the inside wall temperature as

$$\overline{Nu_D} = 0.023 \ Re_D^{0.8} \ Pr^{0.3} \tag{7-22}$$

We can calculate the mean flow velocity inside the hose as

$$\overline{V} = \frac{\dot{V}}{A_{cs}} = \frac{0.5 \ \dfrac{Gal}{min}}{\dfrac{\pi}{4}\left(\dfrac{0.25}{12}ft\right)^2} \cdot \frac{1 \ ft^3}{7.48 \ gal} \cdot \frac{1 \ min}{60 \ sec} = 3.27 \ \frac{ft}{sec}$$

where $\dot{V}$ is the volumetric flow rate, and A_{CS} is the inside cross-sectional area of the hose.

This flow corresponds to a Reynolds number, based on the inside diameter of

$$Re_D = \frac{\left(64 \ \dfrac{lb}{ft^3}\right) \cdot \left(3.27 \ \dfrac{ft}{sec}\right) \cdot \left(\dfrac{0.25}{12}ft\right)}{0.658 \times 10^{-3} \ \dfrac{lb}{ft\text{-}sec}} = 6622$$

and the Prandtl number can be found using the thermal properties given in the problem statement as

$$Pr = \frac{\mu_w \ c_{p_w}}{K_w} = \frac{\left(0.658 \times 10^{-3} \ \dfrac{lbm}{ft\text{-}sec}\right)\left(1.0 \ \dfrac{Btu}{lbm-°F}\right)\left(3600 \ \dfrac{sec}{hr}\right)}{0.347 \ \dfrac{Btu}{ft\text{-}hr\text{-}°F}} = 6.82$$

Substituting into Equation (7-22) gives

$$\overline{Nu_D} = 0.023 \cdot 6622^{0.8} \cdot 6.82^{0.3} = 46.7 = \frac{h_i\,D_i}{K_w}$$

from which we can find the convective heat transfer coefficient on the inside of the hose as

$$h_i = \frac{\overline{Nu_D}\,k_w}{D_i} = \frac{46.7\left(0.347\ \dfrac{BTU}{ft\text{-}hr\text{-}^\circ F}\right)}{\dfrac{0.25}{12}ft} = 777\ \frac{BTU}{ft^2\text{-}hr\text{-}^\circ F}$$

Example: Estimate the convective heat transfer coefficient on the outside of the water supply hose when it is submerged in seawater. Assume that the hose has an outside diameter (OD) of 0.75 inches and it is wrapped in a neoprene insulation that is 0.1 inch thick.

Solution: For liquid flow around cylinders, we can use the dimensionless heat transfer correlation given in Table 7-1

$$\overline{Nu_D} = C\,Re_D^{\,n}\,Pr^{0.33} \qquad\qquad (7\text{-}23)$$

where C and n are constants which depend on Reynolds number, as shown in Table 7-2.

We will arbitrarily assume that the flow around the outside surface of the hose is generated by a water current equal to 0.5 knots (0.84 ft/sec). The tubing outside diameter is 0.75-inch plus a wrapping of foam neoprene 0.1-inch thick. Therefore, the outside diameter $D_o = 0.75 + 0.2 = 0.95$ inches.

The Reynolds number for flow around this cylinder can be calculated as follows:

$$Re_D = \frac{\rho_w\,\overline{V}\,D_o}{\mu_w} = \frac{\left(64\ \dfrac{lb}{ft^3}\right)\left(0.84\ \dfrac{ft}{sec}\right)\left(\dfrac{0.95}{12}ft\right)}{0.658\ x\ 10^{-3}\ \dfrac{lb}{ft\text{-}sec}} = 6468$$

From Table 7-2, for $4000 < Re_D < 40000$, a constant coefficient of $C = 0.193$ and $n = 0.618$ are found. Therefore, the dimensionless heat transfer coefficient for flow around this hose is

$$\overline{Nu_D} = 0.193 \cdot 6468^{0.618} \cdot 6.82^{0.33} = 82.9 = \frac{h_o\,D_o}{K_w}$$

from which we can find the convective heat transfer coefficient on the outside of the hose as

$$h_o = \frac{82.9 \left(0.347 \; \frac{BTU}{ft-hr-F}\right)}{\left(\frac{0.95}{12} ft\right)} = 363 \; \frac{BTU}{ft^2-hr-{}^\circ F}$$

7.6   Combined Conduction and Convection with Constant Temperature Differences

Most practical applications involve more than one mode of heat transfer. For instance, take the example of a flat layer of material which separates two different gaseous or liquid environments that are at different temperatures. This example might represent the wall of a diving bell which has a gaseous breathable atmosphere on the inside and seawater on the outside. Or, it might represent the thickness of a dry suit which has the inflation gas on the inside and water surrounding the outside. In either case, if a temperature differential exists between the inside and outside atmospheres heat will be transferred by convection on the inside surface to the wall. This heat will then be transferred by conduction to the outside of the wall where it will be lost to the colder outside environment via convection.

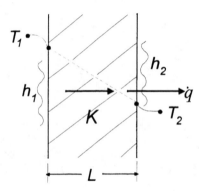

Using our previous electrical analogy, we can find the total resistance for heat transfer between these two environments as the sum of the two convective thermal resistances existing on each surface, Equation (7-15), and the thermal resistance due to conduction through this wall, Equation (7-5), giving

Figure 7-6: Combined conduction and convection through a single layer.

$$R_{Overall} = \frac{1}{h_1 \, A} + \frac{L}{K \, A} + \frac{1}{h_2 \, A} \qquad (7\text{-}24)$$

where h_1 and h_2 are the convective heat transfer coefficients on the inside and outside surfaces, respectively, L is the thickness of the wall, K is the thermal conductivity of the wall, and A is the area of the wall perpendicular to the direction of heat flow. Or in general, the overall thermal resistance of a composite wall having multiple layers of material would be

$$R_{Overall} = \frac{1}{h_1 \, A} + \sum_{i=1}^{n} \left(\frac{L_i}{K_i \, A}\right) + \frac{1}{h_2 \, A} \qquad (7\text{-}25)$$

where *n* is the number of layers making up this wall.

If the temperatures remain fixed, we can calculate the amount of heat that will be transferred between these two environments under steady state conditions, as

$$\dot{q} = \frac{T_{hot} - T_{cold}}{R_{Overall}} = \frac{T_{hot} - T_{cold}}{\dfrac{1}{h_1 A} + \sum\limits_{i=1}^{n}\left(\dfrac{L_i}{K_i A}\right) + \dfrac{1}{h_2 A}} \qquad (7\text{-}26)$$

It is convenient to pull the constant surface area out of the denominator and to define an *overall heat transfer coefficient, U,* such that

$$\dot{q} = U A \left(T_{hot} - T_{cold}\right) \qquad (7\text{-}27)$$

For flat walls, made up of multiple material layers, we can define this *overall heat transfer coefficient, U,* as

$$U = \frac{1}{\dfrac{1}{h_1} + \sum\limits_{i=1}^{n}\left(\dfrac{L_i}{K_i}\right) + \dfrac{1}{h_2}} \qquad [\text{ For Flat Plates }] \qquad (7\text{-}28)$$

For cases where the separating wall between these two environments is cylindrical, the total amount of heat that will be transferred between these constant temperature environments can similarly be calculated using a modified form of Equation (7-27). Since the surface area of the cylindrical wall varies from inside to outside, we must define whether the area *A* will be based on the inside surface of the cylinder or the outside surface. Based on the inside surface area, A_i, Equation (7-27) becomes

$$\dot{q} = U_i A_i \left(T_{hot} - T_{cold}\right) \qquad (7\text{-}29)$$

where the inside surface area for a cylinder with a length *L* can be written

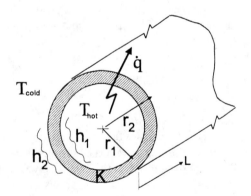

Figure 7-7: Combined conduction and convection heat transfer through a cylinder.

$$A_i = 2 \pi r_1 L \qquad (7\text{-}30)$$

The over heat transfer coefficient based on this inside area can be written in cylindrical coordinates as

$$U_i = \cfrac{1}{\cfrac{1}{h_i} + \cfrac{r_1}{K}\left(\ln\cfrac{r_2}{r_1}\right) + \cfrac{r_1}{r_2}\cfrac{1}{h_o}} \qquad [\textit{ For Cylinders Based Inside Area}]$$

(7-31)

When the overall heat transfer coefficient is based on the outside area, equation (7-27) becomes

$$\dot{q} = U_o \, A_o \left(T_{hot} - T_{cold}\right)$$

(7-32)

where the outside surface area for a cylinder with length L can be written

$$A_o = 2 \, \pi \, r_2 \, L$$

and

$$U_o = \cfrac{1}{\cfrac{r_2}{r_1}\cfrac{1}{h_i} + \cfrac{r_2}{K}\left(\ln\cfrac{r_2}{r_1}\right) + \cfrac{1}{h_o}} \qquad [\textit{ For Cylinders Based Outside Area}]$$

(7-33)

As in the case of composites for flat walls, the thermal resistances for additional layers in a cylindrical wall can be accounted for by adding terms in the denominators of Equations (7-31) and (7-33) for each conducting layer as follows

$$R_i = \frac{r_b}{K_i}\left(\ln\frac{r_{i+1}}{r_i}\right)$$

(7-34)

where R_i is the thermal resistance due to conduction through the ith layer of the composite, r_b is the radius for which the surface area is based (i.e., either the inside or outside surface radius), K_i is the thermal conductivity of the ith layer, r_{i+1} and r_i are the outside and inside radii of the ith layer, respectively. Table 7-4 summarizes the above relationships for combined conduction and convection heat transfer between two constant temperature environments.

Table 7-4: Summary of Combined Conduction and Convection Heat Transfer with Constant Environmental Temperatures

Configuration	Surface Area	Overall Heat Transfer Coefficient
Flat Walls $$\dot{q} = U\,A\left(T_{hot} - T_{cold}\right)$$	Width times height of wall section	$$U = \cfrac{1}{\cfrac{1}{h_1} + \sum_{i=1}^{n}\left(\cfrac{L_i}{K_i}\right) + \cfrac{1}{h_2}}$$
Cylinders: Based on Inside Surface Area $$\dot{q} = U_i\,A_i\left(T_{hot} - T_{cold}\right)$$	$$A_i = 2\,\pi\,r_1\,L$$	$$U_i = \cfrac{1}{\cfrac{1}{h_i} + \cfrac{r_1}{K}\left(ln\,\cfrac{r_2}{r_1}\right) + \cfrac{r_1}{r_2}\cfrac{1}{h_o}}$$
Cylinders: Based on Outside Surface Area $$\dot{q} = U_o\,A_o\left(T_{hot} - T_{cold}\right)$$	$$A_o = 2\,\pi\,r_2\,L$$	$$U_o = \cfrac{1}{\cfrac{r_2}{r_1}\cfrac{1}{h_i} + \cfrac{r_2}{K}\left(ln\,\cfrac{r_2}{r_1}\right) + \cfrac{1}{h_o}}$$

7.7   Combined Conduction and Convection with Varying Temperature Differences--Active Thermal Protection

It is frequently necessary to pump warm water to divers to be used as a heat source for protection from the extreme cold surrounding water temperatures. As this water is being pumped to the diver, heat losses will occur between the hose and the surrounding seawater. As a result, the temperature differences between the inside of the hose and the seawater surrounding the umbilical will vary over the entire length of the umbilical. These losses must be taken into account when deciding what water temperatures must be delivered at the surface in order that the diver does not receive excessively hot, or cold, supplies.

The following discussion is directed at a method of calculating these heat losses and estimating fluid delivery temperatures.   An example of warm water delivery will be used in this discussion which includes a hose supplying warm water from a surface heat source to a diver beneath the surface. The outside of the hose is surrounded by cold seawater which serves as an excellent heat sink. While this discussion involves only an application of water delivery, the same approach could be applied to the delivery of other fluids and gases as well.

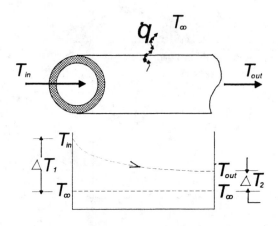

Figure 7-8: Heat transfer through a hot water hose having variable temperature difference along the length of the hose.

Example: We would like to deliver warm water at a rate of 0.5 gallons per minute to a diver at 60 FSW via the umbilical described in the previous two examples, such that the water arrives at the dive site at 100°F. Assume that the thermal conductivity of the hose wall, K_h, is 0.12 BTU/ft-hr-°F and the thermal conductivity of the neoprene insulation wrapping, K_n, is 0.03 BTU/ft-hr-°F. Eighty feet of this umbilical is used to supply the water at depth. Assume that the entire length of this umbilical is surrounded by seawater at 29°F. What temperature does the water need to enter the hose at the surface?   What total amount of heat is lost from the umbilical to the surrounding seawater?

Solution: Since we are no longer dealing with a constant temperature differential across the wall of the hose, the heat loss from the hose which will supply the water between the diver and a surface heat source must be written:

$$\dot{q}_{Hose} = U_o A_o \Theta_M = U_i A_i \Theta_M \qquad (7\text{-}35)$$

where $\dot{q}_{Hose}$ is the heat loss through the walls of the hose to the outside environment; U_o and U_i are the overall heat transfer coefficients for the hose based on the outside and inside surface area of the hose, given previously by Equations (7-33) and (7-31), respectively and, Θ_M is the log mean temperature of the water in the hose, defined as

$$\Theta_M = \frac{\Delta T_1 - \Delta T_2}{\ln\left(\dfrac{\Delta T_1}{\Delta T_2}\right)} \qquad (7\text{-}36)$$

where ΔT_1 and ΔT_2 are the temperature differentials across the wall of the hose at the inlet and exit of the hose. With T_∞ generally expressed as the surrounding seawater temperature

$$\Delta T_1 = T_{in} - T_\infty \qquad and \qquad \Delta T_2 = T_{out} - T_\infty \qquad (7\text{-}37)$$

The convective heat transfer coefficients on the inside and outside of the hose surface where found in two previous examples, such that

$$h_i = 777 \ \frac{Btu}{ft^2 - hr - °F} \qquad and \qquad h_o = 363 \ \frac{Btu}{ft^2 - hr - °F}$$

With the inside and outside convective heat transfer coefficients of the hose identified in this example, we can now find the overall heat transfer between the hose and the surrounding environment as

$$U_o = \frac{1}{\dfrac{r_3}{r_1 h_i} + \dfrac{r_3}{K_h} \ln\left(\dfrac{r_2}{r_1}\right) + \dfrac{r_3}{K_n} \ln\left(\dfrac{r_3}{r_2}\right) + \dfrac{1}{h_o}} \qquad (7\text{-}38)$$

where K_h and K_n are defined as the thermal conductivity of the hose wall and the neoprene insulation wrapping respectively. Note the added term in the denominator of the above equation, when compared to Equation (7-33), to account for the additional heat transfer resistance offered by the neoprene wrapping. Similarly, the effect on U_o due to other layers that might be added to this hose composite could be seen by adding additional resistance terms for each layer. An overall heat transfer coefficient for the present hose, based on the inside surface of the hose could likewise be determined as

$$U_i = \frac{1}{\dfrac{1}{h_i} + \dfrac{r_1}{K_h} \ln\left(\dfrac{r_2}{r_1}\right) + \dfrac{r_1}{K_n} \ln\left(\dfrac{r_3}{r_2}\right) + \dfrac{r_1}{r_3 h_o}} \qquad (7\text{-}39)$$

and noting the following identity must be observed, based on Equation (7-35)

$$U_o A_o = U_i A_i$$

A common dimensional error shows up in the calculation of overall heat transfer coefficients due to the presence of feet in thermal conductivity, and the hose radii expressed in inches. Additionally, take particular notice that hose radii are used in these calculations, rather than hose diameters. To avoid this common mistake, we will first convert all radii into units of feet. Based on the geometry of this supply hose described above, we have

$$r_1(in) = \frac{D_i \ (in)}{2} \qquad or \qquad r_1(ft) = \frac{D_i \ (in)}{24}$$

Therefore, we have for this example

$$r_1 = \frac{0.25}{24} ft, \qquad r_2 = \frac{0.75}{24} ft, \qquad r_3 = \frac{0.95}{24} ft$$

which will result in an overall heat transfer coefficient, based on the outside surface area of

$$U_o = \cfrac{1}{\cfrac{\frac{0.95}{24}}{\frac{0.25}{24}(777)} + \cfrac{\frac{0.95}{24}}{0.12} \ln\left(\cfrac{\frac{0.75}{24}}{\frac{0.25}{24}}\right) + \cfrac{\frac{0.95}{24}}{0.03} \ln\left(\cfrac{\frac{0.95}{24}}{\frac{0.75}{24}}\right) + \cfrac{1}{363}}$$

$$U_o = 1.47 \frac{BTU}{ft^2 - hr - {}^\circ F}$$

What temperature must the water, flowing at 0.5 gallons per minute, enter the 80-foot length of insulated hose described above to reach the diver at a desired temperature of 100°F? Assume that the hose is surrounded by seawater at 29°F.

Equation (7-35) gives us one expression which equates the amount of heat loss from the water supply hose to inlet temperature, T_{in}. The outside surface area of an 80-foot length of this hose with an outside diameter of 0.95 inches is

$$A_o = \pi D_o L = \pi \left(\frac{0.95}{12} ft\right)(80 \ ft) = 19.9 \ ft^2$$

The log mean temperature is calculated assuming the outside water temperature, T_∞, is 29°F and the supply temperature received by the diver, or exit temperature from the hose, T_{out} is 100°F. I.e.,

$$\Theta_M = \frac{\left(T_{in} - T_\infty\right) - \left(T_{out} - T_\infty\right)}{\ln\left[\dfrac{T_{in} - T_\infty}{T_{out} - T_\infty}\right]} = \frac{T_{in} - 100}{\ln\left[\dfrac{T_{in} - 29}{71}\right]}$$

Substituting the above into Equation (7-35), we have

$$\dot{q}_{Hose} = 1.47 \ \frac{BTU}{ft^2-hr-°F} \ (19.9 \ ft^2) \left[\frac{T_{in} - 100}{\ln\left(\frac{T_{in}-29}{71}\right)} \right] °F$$

$$\dot{q}_{Hose} = 29.2 \left[\frac{T_{in} - 100}{\ln\left(\frac{T_{in}-29}{71}\right)} \right] \frac{BTU}{hr} \qquad (7\text{-}40)$$

This gives us one expression with two unknowns since we don't know the amount of heat loss through the hose, and we are looking for T_{in}. However, the heat loss from the supply hose can also be shown to equal the total energy lost from the warm water as it flows through the supply hose, such that

$$\dot{q}_{Hose} = \dot{q}_{Water} \qquad (7\text{-}41)$$

where

$$\dot{q}_{Water} = \rho_w \ \dot{V}_w \ c_w \left(T_{in} - T_{out}\right) \qquad (7\text{-}42)$$

with $\dot{V}_w$ defined as the volumetric flow rate of the water, ρ_w is the density of the water, and c_w is the specific heat of the water. From the problem statement above, we have

$$\dot{q}_{Water} = 64 \ \frac{lb}{ft^3} \left(0.5\frac{gal}{min}\right) \left(\frac{ft^3}{7.48 \ gal}\right) \left(\frac{60 \ min}{hr}\right) \left(1\frac{BTU}{lb-°F}\right)(T_{in}-100) \ °F$$

$$\dot{q}_{Water} = 256.64 \ (T_{in}-100) \ \frac{BTU}{hr} \qquad (7\text{-}43)$$

Equating Equations (7-40) and (7-43) gives

$$29.2 \left[\frac{T_{in}-100}{\ln\left(\frac{T_{in}-29}{71}\right)} \right] = 256.64 \ (T_{in}-100)$$

$$\ln\left(\frac{T_{in}-29}{71}\right) = 0.1138$$

or

$$\frac{T_{in} - 29}{71} = e^{.1138} = 1.1205$$

This gives

$$T_{in} = 108.6\,°F$$

The heat loss from the warm water to the surrounding seawater can now be calculated from Equation (7-43) as

$$\dot{q}_{Water} = \rho_w\, \dot{V}_w\, c_w\, \left(T_{in} - T_{out}\right)$$

or

$$\dot{q}_{Water} = 64\,\frac{lb}{ft^3}\left(0.5\,\frac{gal}{min}\right)\left(\frac{ft^3}{7.48\,gal}\right)\left(\frac{60\,min}{hr}\right)\left(1\,\frac{BTU}{lb-°F}\right)(108.6 - 100)\,°F$$

$$\dot{q}_{Water} = 256.64\,(108.6 - 100)\,\frac{BTU}{hr}$$

$$\dot{q}_{Water} = 2207\,\frac{BTU}{hr} \qquad [647.2\ watts]$$

7.8   Design of Divers' Garments--Passive Thermal Protection

In the following discussion we will investigate the basic components of heat loss from wet and dry diving suits, and show the changes in effectiveness of these garments with variations in the diver's environment. Since engineers and physiologists often express the same physical parameters with different terminology, thermal resistance or insulation in this discussion will be expressed in the unit of "Clo". A widely accepted unit today, one Clo is defined as the thermal insulation required to maintain the "average" resting man in thermal equilibrium while exposed to a comfortable 70°F atmosphere (Gagge *et al*, 1969), with conversion factors given as

$$1\ Clo = 0.18\,\frac{m^2-hr-°C}{kcal} = 0.88\,\frac{ft^2-hr-°F}{Btu} \qquad (7\text{-}44)$$

When thermal protection was called for in pre-World War II diving operations, multiple pairs of thermal underwear (long johns) were used in conjunction with the dry diver's dress until sufficient warmth could be achieved. This bulky suit satisfied, and continues to satisfy even today, the diver's needs for all but extremely cold missions. Unfortunately, as the diver goes deeper the trapped gas inside the suit is compressed (called *suit squeeze*), causing the suit material to buckle around the diver's skin, causing discomfort unless additional gas can be added.

With the advent of open-circuit SCUBA, the limitations in diver mobility resulting from the bulky suit became evident and improvements were sought. These efforts often resulted in the achievement of less suit bulk while sacrificing insulation qualities and waterproof integrity. Even when operationally acceptable for short duration missions, the susceptibility of these lightweight "dry" outfits to leaks from defects, tears, and wear caused frequent annoyances.

In the early 1950's, a new approach was found to address the difficult problem of diver thermal protection. Tight-fitting, closed-cell, foam rubber suits were designed to permit a thin film of water to exist between the suit and the diver's skin. When wearing these "wet" suits, the initial heat loss from the diver's body serves to heat this small quantity of water, at which time the thermal gradient at the skin and further heat loss is reduced. While usually inferior with regard to thermal protection, these wet suits eliminate the problems of suit leakage and squeeze associated with the dry suits.

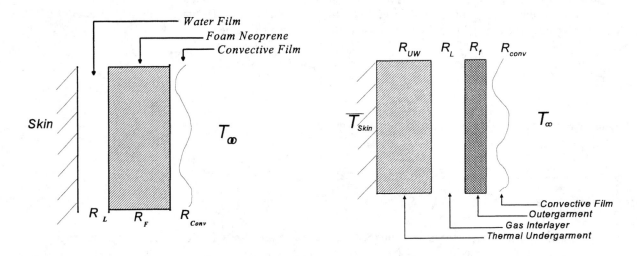

Figure 7-9: Thermal resistance elements of a wet suit.

Figure 7-10: Thermal resistance elements of a dry suit.

The heat loss from a good fitting, passive diver's suit occurs primarily by conduction through the suit and undergarments, and by convection between the surface of the suit and its surroundings. Usually, radiation plays an extremely small part in sub-surface diver heat losses; this is so, since the outside surface temperatures of a diver's suit is generally within 1° -2° F of the ambient water temperature (see radiation heat transfer). The net heat transfer through the diver's suit can be determined by using the method described previously in Equation (7-27), where the overall heat transfer coefficient, U, (or *suit conductance*) is found as the inverse of the sum of the resistances for each suit layer, or

For Wetsuits, U_w

$$U_W = \frac{1}{R_L + R_f + R_{conv}}$$

(7-45)

where R_L is the resistance to heat flow through the thin film of water, R_f is the resistance to heat flow through the foam neoprene, and R_{conv} is the convective heat transfer coefficient between the diver's suit and the surroundings.

For Drysuits, U_D

$$U_D = \frac{1}{R_{UW} + R_L + R_f + R_{conv}}$$

(7-46)

where the resistances are similar to those for a wetsuit above, except that there is an additional resistance to heat flow offered by the thermal underwear, R_{UW}, and R_L is due to a gas layer rather than water. Additionally, the resistance of the outergarment, R_f, in some cases is derived from a thin, rubber-coated nylon layer rather than foam neoprene.

Note that in most cases, the suit surface can be treated as a flat plate when calculating the heat loss. This can be confirmed by computing the thermal resistance offered by a foam neoprene thickness covering a cylinder using cylindrical coordinates, Equations (7-29) or (7-32), when compared with flat plate analysis, Equation (7-27). In cylindrical coordinates, the inherent thermal resistance of the foam can be represented by

$$R_f = \frac{r_1}{K} \ln\left(\frac{r_2}{r_1}\right) \qquad [\textit{ cylindrical coordinates }]$$

(7-47)

When approximated as a flat plate, the foam resistance will be

$$R_f = \frac{r_2 - r_1}{K} = \frac{L}{K} \qquad [\textit{ flat plate }]$$

(7-48)

Comparing the computed resistances for cylindrical and flat plate analyses will give an estimate of the magnitude of the error seen by a flat plate assumption. It can be shown that a flat plate assumption, with $L = r_2 - r_1$, gives a good approximation for the thermal resistance of the covered cylinder if

$$\frac{L}{r_1 \ln\left(\frac{L + r_1}{r_1}\right)} \approx 1$$

(7-49)

For instance, a material thickness of 1 cm that covers a 30 cm diameter cylinder gives the quantity

$$\frac{1}{15 \ln\left(\frac{1 + 15}{15}\right)} = 1.03$$

indicating that the error from a flat plate assumption is approximately 3%. The same material thickness covering a 15 cm cylinder will give a 6.5% error. As a general rule, the error from a flat plate assumption will decrease sharply as the relative magnitude of the material thickness decreases when compared to the cylinder diameter (less than 1% error will occur when computing the thermal resistance of a 1cm material thickness covering a 120 cm cylinder, as in the case of an insulated recompression chamber).

Thus reasonable accuracy can be obtained when estimating the heat loss from a diver's suit by assuming that the suit insulation can be modeled as a flat plate with a body surface area given by a correlation of diver anthropometry data (Dubois, 1916) as

$$A = 0.108 \ W^{0.425} \ H^{0.725} \tag{7-50}$$

where A is the diver's body surface area, given in ft^2; W is the diver weight, lb; and H is the diver height, inch.

7.8.1 Outer Garment Insulation, R_f

The outer garments of most dry suits, and all wet suits are fabricated from closed-cell, foam neoprene. Good fitting, foam rubber wet suits give excellent thermal protection for short duration, shallow water dives, even in polar regions. In fact, the wet suit is still preferred by many commercial, military, and sport divers today. However, the effectiveness of the foam rubber wet suit to retain diver body heat diminishes rapidly as depth increases. The compression of the closed-cell foam caused by increased hydrostatic pressures at depth acts to simultaneously decrease the material's thickness as the cells collapse, and increase the thermal conductivity of the foam, both contributing to a decrease in the thermal resistance. This compound degradation in insulation value with depth causes a 0.25-inch thick closed cell foam to become as ineffective as a thin layer of 0.125-inch thick solid rubber in keeping a diver warm when environmental pressures increase beyond approximately 8 atmospheres (230 ft or 70 m).

The effectiveness of any material as a thermal insulator is primarily dependent upon its ability to entrap gases (usually air). Thus, porous materials such as foam rubber, with a high volume of entrapped air, or nitrogen, serve as excellent insulators in an uncompressed state. Jacob (1949) described an expression for calculating the apparent thermal conductivity, K_a, of porous insulating materials, showing its dependency on the void fraction of the entrapped gas, as

$$K_a = K_s \left[\frac{1 - \left(1 - a \ \dfrac{K_p}{K_s}\right) b}{1 + (a - 1) \ b} \right] \tag{7-51}$$

with

$$a = \frac{3 \ K_s}{2 \ K_s + K_p} \qquad and \qquad b = \frac{V_p}{V_s + V_p} \tag{7-52}$$

where b is defined as the void fraction, V_s is the total solid volume, V_p is the total entrapped gas volume, K_s is the thermal conductivity of the solid, and K_p is the thermal conductivity of the entrapped gas.

Butler (1972) showed that these expressions can be modified to predict the apparent thermal conductivity of foam neoprene at depth by assuming that the solid material is incompressible, and that the entrapped gas compresses as an ideal gas; i.e., the entrapped gas volume can be replaced with

$$V_p = V_{p_0} \left(\frac{P_0}{P} \right) \tag{7-53}$$

where V_{P_0} is the total gas volume at the surface, P_0 is the atmospheric pressure at the surface (i.e., 1 Ata), and P is the atmospheric pressure at depth (Ata).

Figure 7-11 shows the predicted degradation in thermal conductivity for difference grades of foam neoprene with densities variations from 10 lbm/ft³ to 20 lbm/ft³ (this covers the acceptable foam densities prescribed by MIL-W-82400, the military specification for neoprene used in wetsuits). This figure indicates that such density variations have a significant effect on the material thermal conductivity at the surface, and even more so at depth.

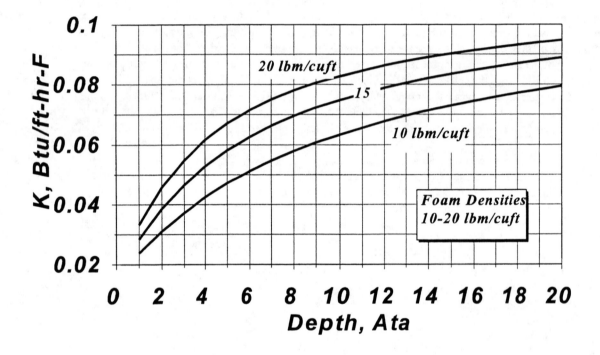

Figure 7-11: Effect of neoprene foam density on its thermal conductivity at hyperbaric conditions. (Densities cover the range prescribed by MIL-M-82400)

Assuming that the foam thickness also decreases in a manner predictable by the ideal gas law, we can derive this thickness as depth increases as

$$L = L_0 \left[\frac{1}{1 + b'\left(\frac{P}{P_0} - 1\right)} \right]$$

(7-54)

where b' is the compressed gas void fraction at depth, given by

$$b' = \cfrac{1}{1 + \cfrac{V_s}{V_{P_0}\left(\dfrac{P_0}{P}\right)}} \tag{7-55}$$

With the approximations given in Equations (7-51) and (7-54), the foam conductance, h_f, defined as the thermal conductivity divided by thickness, can be calculated as depth increases as

$$h_f = \frac{K_a}{L} = \left(\frac{K_s}{L_0}\right) \cdot \left[\frac{1 - \left(1 - a\,\dfrac{K_p}{K_s}\right)b'}{1 + (a - 1)\,b'}\right] \cdot \left[1 + b'\left(\frac{P}{P_0} - 1\right)\right] \tag{7-56}$$

or the thermal resistances (i.e., Clo values) can be found as depth increases by using the definitions for Clo in Equation (7-44), giving:

$$Clo_f = \frac{5.547}{h_f\left(\dfrac{kcal}{m^2\text{-}hr\text{-}°C}\right)} \qquad or \qquad \frac{1.136}{h_f\left(\dfrac{Btu}{ft^2\text{-}hr\text{-}°F}\right)} \tag{7-57}$$

These expressions were used to calculate the effects of pressure on the thermal resistance of foam neoprene, as shown in Figure 7-12.

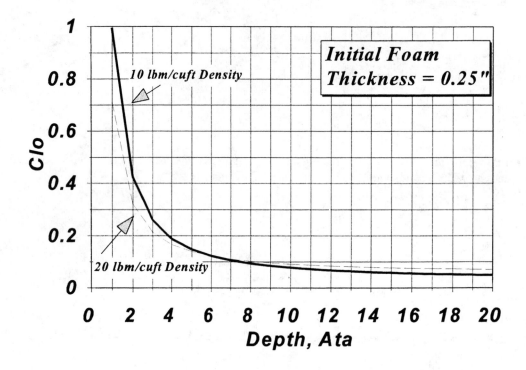

Figure 7-12: Insulation afforded by 1 cm foam neoprene at hyperbaric conditions.

7.8.2 Insulation Due to Surface Convection, R_{conv}

The thermal resistance component derived from the suit's convective film between its surface and the environment (recall that the surface resistance is the reciprocal of this convective film coefficient) can be approximated as flow over cylinders (Witherspoon *et al*, 1970). These convective film coefficients can be approximated using the convective heat transfer correlations given previously in Tables 7-1 and 7-2. However, a more empirical approach was proposed by McAdams (1942), who showed that the average convective coefficient can be calculated using the equation

$$\overline{h_{conv}} = \left(0.35 + 0.56 \, Re_D^{0.5} \right) Pr^{0.31} \frac{K}{D} \tag{7-58}$$

where $\overline{h_{conv}}$ is the average convective coefficient for the cylinder, kcal/m²-hr-°C; Re_D is the Reynolds number based on the cylinder diameter (see Equation (7-19)), Pr is the Prandtl number of the fluid adjacent to the suit surface (Equation (7-20)), K is the thermal conductivity of this fluid, kcal/m-hr-°C; and D is the cylinder diameter, m.

Equation (7-44) can be applied to convert this film conductance into an equivalent insulation value as

$$Clo_{conv} = \frac{5.547}{h_{conv}} = \frac{5.547}{\left(0.35 + 0.56 \, Re_D^{0.5}\right) Pr^{0.31} \dfrac{K}{D}} \qquad (7\text{-}59)$$

When the fluid adjacent to the suit happens to be water, as in diving applications, only minor effects are seen in the average film coefficient over the range of pressures and temperatures normally encountered. Thus, the cylinder diameter and fluid velocity are the major parameters of concern in the determination of this insulation component. Figure 7-13 shows that in the case of water flowing over cylinders approximating various segments of the human body, the insulation value of this film is quite small--in all cases less than 0.02 clo. However, prior to diver entry into the water, the insulating value of the film can be quite significant, contributing in excess of 1 Clo to the garment as indicated in Figure 7-13 with low air flow rates. This illustrates the reason that a waterproof suit which provides good passive insulation for temperature extremes in water requires a very different design from a suit for land use.

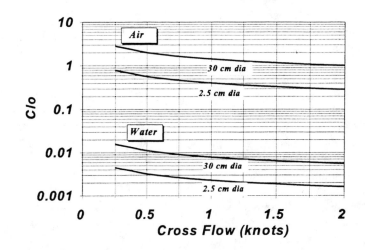

Figure 7-13: Thermal resistances of surface films in air and water.

7.8.3 Insulation Due to Thermal Undergarments

Most drysuits rely on the insulation value of the thermal undergarment to retain body heat in cold environments. Rubberized fabric outergarments, and closed-cell foam neoprene garments at depth, offer only minimal thermal resistance. Thus, proper design of the thermal undergarment is essential to gaining adequate protection for cold water exposures.

As was noted above for closed-cell foam, the thermal efficiency of a diver's underwear is dependent upon its ability to entrap and retain gases, in particular, air. An ideal drysuit underwear material would be composed of small gas pockets to minimize both natural and forced convective currents between the diver's body and the outergarment. In addition, the ideal underwear would minimize thermal paths by conduction through the material substrate by using materials with low thermal conductivity. Due to the high probability of water infiltrating even the best drysuit designs, selected materials should also retain most of their insulation properties when in contact with water. (I.e., materials that are hydrophobic in nature, such as Thinsulate, have been shown to retain much of their insulation capability when wet; see Table 7-6.)

Although the interiors of most drysuits on the market today are pressure equalized with surrounding water pressures by way of an inflation gas (drysuits having inflation and exhaust valves to vary the volume of trapped gas inside the suit are called *variable volume drysuits*), there still exists small pressures variations between the diver's chest and lower extremities (approximately 1 - 2 psi). The material should offer low compression properties to retain the entrapped gases in the lower extremities due to this normal suit "squeeze". Yet, the inherent material stiffness to resist compression should not significantly affect the diver's mobility. In effect, the underwear would furnish an optimum tradeoff between low compression for gas retention with sufficiently low stiffness for good diver mobility.

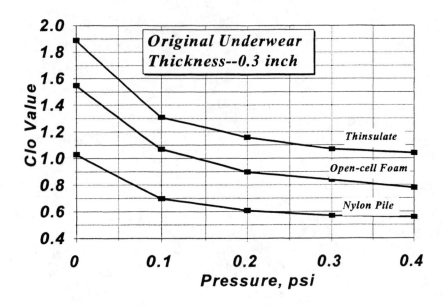

Figure 7-14: Effect of suit squeeze on undergarment insulation.

Most conventional underwear materials used in conjunction with dry suits fall into one of three major categories: open-cell urethane foam, nylon pipe (sometimes referred to as "Wooly Bear"), cotton waffle, or micro-fiber batts (similar to Thinsulate[8]).   Refer to Table 7-6 for a summary of the thermal properties of typical materials used in diving undergarments. While all of these materials offer varying degrees of insulation, they all have low resistance to compression from even small levels of suit squeeze, see Figure 7-14. Note the rapid decay in the insulation values of typical divers' underwear with squeeze of less than 0.5 psi. This explains the difficulty of maintaining adequate thermal protection in the legs and feet unless the suit is over-pressurized in upper chest to eliminate the lower suit squeeze. Such a suit would be overly inflated in the chest, resulting in excessive suit buoyancy.

7.8.4 Predicting the Thermal Insulation From Wetsuits and Drysuits

The thermal characteristics established above for the various components of wetsuits and drysuits can be used to predict the insulation values of sample composite suits by rewriting Equations (7-45) and (7-46) in terms of total Clo values, such that

For Drysuits

$$Clo_D = Clo_{UW} + Clo_L + Clo_f + Clo_{conv}$$

---

[8]Thinsulate is a registered tradename of 3M Corporation

where the subscripts *D, UW, L, f* and *conv* indicate the thermal resistances of the total drysuit ensemble, the thermal underwear, trapped gas layer, outergarment (either foam or rubberized fabric) and the convective film, respectively.

For Wetsuits

$$Clo_W = Clo_L + Clo_f + Clo_{conv}$$

where the subscripts *W* and *L* indicate the thermal resistances of the total wetsuit ensemble and the trapped liquid film, respectively.

Figures 7-15 and 7-16 shows the calculated thermal insulation values for sample drysuits using the above analysis. These results were verified with experimental manikin test data at depths up to 16 Ata (Wattenbarger and Breckinridge, 1978). Note the rapid drop-off in Clo values in the first 4 Ata for the wetsuits and drysuits having foam neoprene outergarments. This drop-off in insulation is likewise accompanied by a reduction in suit buoyancy as the closed-cell foam compresses. Beyond this depth, the compression of the closed-cell foam neoprene is essentially completed, giving the diver approximately the same thermal protection as he would have derived from a rubberized fabric suit.

Table 7-5: Typical Insulation Values of Wetsuits and Drysuits at Various Ambient Pressures

Suit	Insulation Values, Clo	
	Surface	4 Ata
Nude Manikin	0.8 (in air) 0.1 (in water)	---
0.25" Wetsuit	0.77	0.25
0.25" Foam Drysuit	1.90 (in air) 0.94 (in water)	---
0.25" Foam Drysuit w/nylon pile underwear	2.33 (in air) 1.20 (in water)	0.60
0.4" Rubberized Fabric Drysuit w/ 0.3" urethane foam underwear	2.10 (in air) 0.87 (in water)	0.87
0.4" Rubberized Fabric Drysuit w/ 0.3" Thinsulate underwear	2.40 (in air) 1.20 (in water)	1.20

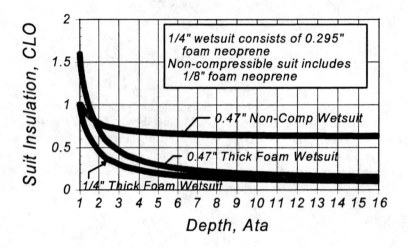

Figure 7-15: Predictions of the insulation values of various wetsuits at hyperbaric conditions.

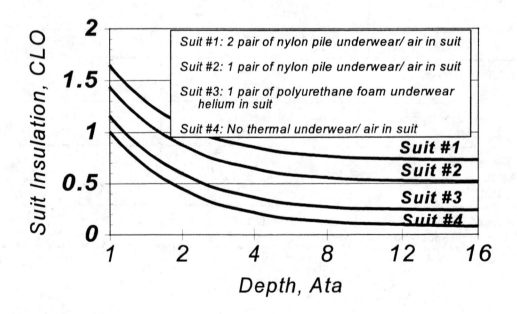

Figure 7-16: Predictions of the insulation values of various drysuit combinations at hyperbaric conditions.

TABLE 7-6: APPROXIMATELY THERMAL CONDUCTIVITY OF SELECTED MATERIALS

Material	Temperature °F	Density lbm/ft³	Thermal Conductivity Btu/ft-hr-°F	Thermal Conductivity W/m-°C	Clo/inch
Foam, polyurethane, open cell	70	8.0 (dry)	0.021 (dry) 0.121 (wet)	0.036 (dry) 0.209 (wet)	4.51 (dry) 0.78 (wet)
Foam, neoprene, closed cell	70	14.5	0.030	0.052	3.16
Nylon pile (Wooly bear)	70		0.028	0.048	3.38
M400 Thinsulate[1]	70	3.3 (dry)	0.019 (dry) 0.027 (wet)	0.033 (dry) 0.047 (wet)	4.98 (dry) 3.51 (wet)
Neoprene rubber coated nylon	70	81.0	0.120	0.208	0.79
Cotton, fabric	70		0.046	0.080	2.06
Cork board	70	10	0.025	0.043	3.79

[1]Thinsulate is a registered tradename of 3M Corporation

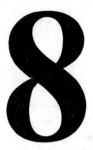

Humidity Control

Objectives

The objectives of this chapter are to:
- understand the thermodynamic relationships as they apply to hyperbaric psychrometrics
- derive equations for use in developing psychrometric charts for applications of mixed gases under pressure
- predict heating and cooling loads required to maintain acceptable levels of comfort
- provide analysis techniques for designing gas conditioning in hyperbaric life support systems
- predict respiratory heat losses due to breathing gas mixtures in hyperbaric environments.

8.1   Introduction

Normal air-conditioning processes at sea level with atmospheric air are well understood. In an enclosed room, temperature and humidity levels can easily be predicted and manipulated using a standard psychrometric chart and a sling psychrometer. In hyperbaric chambers, however, the breathing gas is often a mixture of gases which differs from normal air in composition and partial pressures.

The U.S. Navy Diving Gas Manual presents humidity charts for use with breathing gas mixtures. There are three charts to cover the range of pressures encountered in diving. Interpolation is necessary for depths not specified on the charts. The units given are not standard for psychrometric calculations and therefore ordinary psychrometric charts can not be used for predicting humidity levels at various depths and gas mixtures.

In this chapter we examine the thermodynamic equations necessary to construct new charts for specific depths and gas mixtures. As we will learn, the introduction of gas mixtures (i.e. helium) into the hyperbaric environment make ordinary instruments such as the sling psychrometer unreliable for psychrometric measurements. Also, construction of new charts for every different depth or gas mixture is a cumbersome process at best. We will examine the Universal Humidity Chart (Sexton, 1972) to specifically address this problem.

8.2   Psychrometrics

8.2.1 Basic Relationships

In a previous chapter, it was shown that carbon dioxide removal from breathing gases is based on maintaining a simple maximum partial pressure in the breathable medium. Gas circulation equipment can be designed based on assumed human production rates of CO_2. However, in addition to CO_2, the human respiration process also produces water vapor. No absolute limit can be set for humidity, particularly under higher pressures where multiple gas mixtures are used. For underwater habitats, diving bells and Deck Decompression Chambers (DDC), a design value of 50% relative humidity is usually the goal to maintain a level of comfort for the divers. However, whenever there is an opening to the sea, high humidity becomes more difficult to control. Also, as will become evident in this chapter, humidity in a hyperbaric, mixed gas environment becomes difficult to measure and control.

In order to work with hyperbaric psychrometrics, the perfect gas assumption is used in gas mixtures. Also, for gas-vapor mixtures, the following definitions apply.

8.2.1.1   Dew Point Temperature

If a vapor-gas mixture is cooled at a constant pressure, the temperature at which condensation of the vapor begins is the dew point temperature (T_{dp}).

8.2.1.2   Dry Bulb Temperature

Dry bulb temperature is the temperature or habitat room temperature as obtained by a normal thermometer (T).

8.2.1.3   Wet Bulb Temperature

Wet bulb temperature (T_{wb}) is defined as the temperature at which water, by evaporating into moist gas at a given dry-bulb temperature and humidity ratio can bring the gas to saturation adiabatically. In practice, wet bulb temperature is measured by passing an unsaturated air-vapor mixture over a wetted surface until a condition of dynamic equilibrium has been attained. When this condition has been reached, the heat transferred from the air-vapor stream to the liquid film to evaporate part of it is equal to the energy carried from the liquid film to the air-vapor stream by the diffusing vapor. When this equilibrium condition is obtained, the resulting temperature of the air-vapor mixture is the wet bulb temperature.

8.2.1.4   Relative Humidity

Relative humidity (RH) refers to the ratio of the actual amount of water vapor in the atmosphere compared to the maximum possible amount of water vapor that the atmosphere could hold at the existing dry bulb temperature. When relative humidity is 100%, the dry bulb temperature and wet bulb temperature will be identical. At these relative humidities, the body's thermoregulatory mechanisms will be inhibited since evaporation will cease from the surface of the skin, negating the normal cooling effect due to the latent heat of evaporation, and all perspiration will be lost as liquid water. At 100% relative humidity the atmosphere is completely saturated with water vapor and any slight temperature decrease or pressure increase will cause condensation, fog or rain in a closed environment.

Relative humidity is defined as

$$\phi = \frac{\rho_V}{\rho_s}$$

(8-1)

where ρ_V is the density of the vapor in the mixture of gas and vapor, and ρ_S is the density the vapor would have at the mixture temperature (T) if it were saturated. This latter density can be found in the steam tables as the density of saturated vapor at T. In all psychrometric problems, the amount of water vapor is small and its partial pressure is very low. Consequently, ideal or perfect gas behavior (see Chapter 2) works well under these conditions so that

$$\rho_v = \frac{P_v}{RT} \quad and \quad \rho_s = \frac{P_s}{RT}$$

(8-2)

where P_v is the water vapor partial pressure and P_s is the saturated water vapor partial pressure. Equations 8-1 and 8-2 are combined to give

$$\phi = \frac{P_v}{P_s}$$

(8-3)

8.2.1.5   *Absolute Humidity Ratio*

The absolute humidity ratio (w), also known as the humidity ratio, is defined as the mass of water vapor in a gas-vapor mixture (m_v) divided by the mass of *dry* gas (m_{gas}). Using dry gas as a basis makes psychrometric computation simpler since for a given volume of dry gas, we can write

$$w = \frac{m_v}{m_{gas}} = \frac{\rho_v}{\rho_{gas}}$$

(8-4)

Again, by assuming that ideal gas behavior can be applied to both the water vapor and the dry gas, we can write

$$w = \frac{\frac{R_{gas}T}{P_{gas}}}{\frac{R_v T}{P_v}}$$

Noting that the partial pressure of the dry gas is the total pressure minus the partial pressure of the water vapor, allows us to write

$$w = \frac{P_v \frac{R_{gas}}{R_v}}{P_{total} - P_v}$$

(8-5)

We saw in Chapter 2 that R_{gas} for a mixture of gases can be found by a mole-fraction average. For two gases, gas a and gas b, the average molecular weight of the mixture is

$$M_{mix} = \frac{n_a}{n_t} M_a + \frac{n_b}{n_t} M_b = X_a M_a + X_b M_b \tag{8-6}$$

where n_a and n_b are the number of moles in each constituent gas, n_t is the total number of moles, and X_a and X_b are the volume fractions for each constituent gas. The number of moles in any substance is

$$n = \frac{m}{M} \tag{8-7}$$

where m is the mass of the gas and M is its molecular weight. Knowing M_{mix}, R_{gas} is found from

$$R_{gas} = \frac{R_u}{M_{mix}} \tag{8-8}$$

where R_u is the universal gas constant.

The reader should be cautioned that an ideal gas assumption is not always appropriate for cool dense gas mixtures. Since hyperbaric atmospheres tend to produce these conditions at higher pressures, we must examine the validity of our perfect gas assumptions for deeper dives. Deeper dives require the inert carrier gas helium in high concentrations. Since helium is monatomic, it shows only minor deviation from perfect gas behavior, making our assumption still valid. However, the deepest dives reintroduce nitrogen to the gas mixture to offset High Pressure Nervous Syndrome (HPNS). In these extreme hyperbaric conditions, depending upon the concentration of nitrogen, a more accurate psychrometric prediction using Van Der Waal's equation (see Chapter 2) should be considered. We will not deal with Van Der Waal's equation in this chapter. However, the serious student is encouraged to run analyses to evaluate the change in psychrometric predictions at elevated pressures using Van Der Waal's equation.

8.2.2 Adiabatic Humidification

In sea level air conditioning, the adiabatic humidification process is an important one for two reasons: It can be carried out by spray chambers, and it is approximated by the *constant wet bulb line*, an important chart process that allows a simple wet bulb temperature to assist in finding the actual humidity of the air.

In a hyperbaric mixed-gas situation, the slope of the lines of constant wet bulb temperature is dependent upon pressure--the higher the pressure, the more nearly vertical the lines. This means that extremely accurate measurements of wet bulb temperature would be required at greater depths. Furthermore, with the introduction of helium as the main constituent of the habitat atmosphere, there is no reason to believe that a wet bulb line and a line of adiabatic humidification are the same under eight or ten atmospheres of mostly helium pressure.

However, it is apparent that the lines on the psychrometric chart are still important to life support considerations. The development of the equations relating to adiabatic humidification provide us with other very important equations that predict heating and cooling loads on life support or unmanned gas-vapor systems.

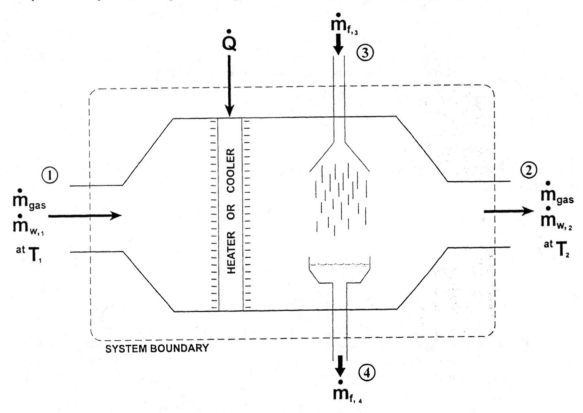

Figure 8-1: Vapor and heat exchange to a flowing stream

Figure 8-1 shows a generalized process in which both heat and vapor may be added to, or taken from, a flowing stream. A mixture of gas and water vapor enter at ①, and gain (or lose) heat in the heater/cooler and vapor from the sprayed water entering at ③. The heated (or cooled) and humidified air leaves at ②. Note that $\dot{m}_{gas,1} = \dot{m}_{gas,2}$, but that $\dot{m}_{w,1} \neq \dot{m}_{w,2}$ providing $\dot{m}_{f,3} \neq \dot{m}_{f,4}$, where $\dot{m}_{gas}$, $\dot{m}_{w}$, and $\dot{m}_{f}$ refer to the mass flow rates of the dry gas, water vapor, and liquid water, respectively. The general conservation of energy equation describing this process, assuming no work is done, no frictional effects are present, and no significant velocity changes occur is

$$\dot{Q} = \sum \dot{m} h_{out} - \sum \dot{m} h_{in} \qquad \text{(8-9)}$$

where $\dot{Q}$ is the heat addition/removal rate, $\dot{m}$ is mass flow rate and h is enthalpy. Then (from Figure 8-1)

$$\dot{Q} = \dot{m}_{gas}(h_{gas,2} - h_{gas,1}) + (\dot{m}_{w,2}h_{w,2} - \dot{m}_{w,1}h_{w,1}) + (\dot{m}_{f,4}h_{f,4} - \dot{m}_{f,3}h_{f,3}) \qquad \text{(8-10)}$$

↑   ↑   ↑

(dry gas)   (water vapor term)   (liquid water term)

Dividing this equation through by $\dot{m}_{gas}$ and applying Equation 8-4, we obtain

$$Q' = (h_{gas,2} - h_{gas,1}) + (w_2 h_{w,2} - w_1 h_{w,1}) + (\dot{m}_{f,4}h_{f,4} - \dot{m}_{f,3}h_{f,3})/\dot{m}_{gas} \qquad \text{(8-11)}$$

where Q' is heat per mass of gas and w is the humidity ratio. Note that the amount of liquid water flowing in at ③ and leaving at ④ is not necessarily the same since humidification may occur. Therefore, a mass flow balance on the water gives

$$w_2 - w_1 = (\dot{m}_{f,3} - \dot{m}_{f,4}) / \dot{m}_{gas} \qquad \text{(8-12)}$$

Also, we can define a mixture enthalpy, H, as the total enthalpy of the dry gas and the contained water vapor (per mass of dry gas) as

$$H = h_{gas} + w h_w \qquad \text{(8-13)}$$

Combining these last three equations yields

$$Q' = H_2 - H_1 + (\dot{m}_{f,4}h_{f,4} - \dot{m}_{f,3}h_{f,3}) / \dot{m}_{gas} \qquad \text{(8-14)}$$

Equation 8-14 can be used for general design purposes when humidification plus heating and cooling is desired. In the special case of a habitat chamber open to the sea from which water is evaporating into the chamber, $\dot{m}_{f,4}$ can be considered equal to zero, and

$$Q' = H_2 - H_1 - (w_2 - w_1) h_{f,3} \qquad \text{(8-15)}$$

since Equation 8-12 becomes $\dot{m}_{gas}(w_2 - w_1) = \dot{m}_{f,3}$.

Figure 8-2 shows the final simplification of this system and the one of major interest--the adiabatic humidification process. In this situation, moist air passes over an insulated water supply. In time the water and the exit air assume the same temperature--the *temperature of adiabatic saturation*. Since no heat is being added during this process, Q' will be zero, and since the temperature of the water source equals the exit temperature we can write $h_{f,3} =$

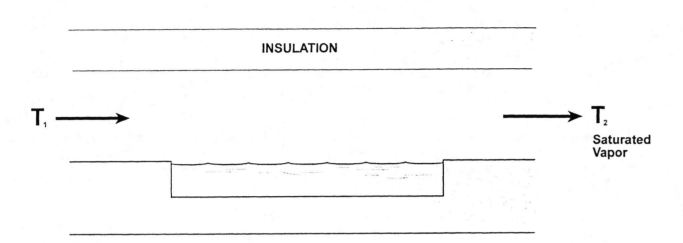

Figure 8-2 Adiabatic humidification process

$h_{f,2}$. Thus, under these conditions Equation 8-15 becomes

$$H_1 + (w_2 - w_1) h_{f,2} = H_2 \qquad (8\text{-}16)$$

In the case of normal air-water vapor mixtures the process illustrated in Figure 8-2 is well approximated by the sling psychrometer in which a wet bulb thermometer (this is essentially a thermometer whose bulb is covered with gauze soaked in clean water) is whirled in moist air and reads the *wet bulb temperature*. At high pressures, when the environment consists mostly of helium gas, we will assume that the wet bulb temperature can be measured using an instrument similar in concept to Figure 8-2, with a thermocouple at the exit to measure T_2 in our habitat. We will use this use this measurement to construct a special psychrometric chart below, examine its use, and finally, examine a special Universal Humidity Chart.

8.2.3 Psychrometric Chart Construction

During the construction of this psychrometric chart for high pressure applications, we will assume that the vapor is water, but the breathing gas may be a combination of oxygen, helium, and possibly nitrogen. The gas mixture will have a specific heat ($C_{p,gas}$) as defined in Chapter 2 (Equation 2-39) and an average gas constant, as defined in Equation 8-8.

The X-axis of a psychrometric chart is the dry bulb temperature T. The Y-axis is w, the absolute humidity ratio, expressed in mass of water vapor per mass of dry gas. The first line to identify on this chart is the saturated water vapor line, or line of 100% relative humidity. This can be accomplished by using our definition of humidity ratio expressed in Equation 8-5, with P_v equal to the saturated vapor pressure, P_s. We will also make the assumption that in deep water, $P_{total} >> P_v$. Under these conditions, Equation 8-5 is approximately

$$w = \frac{R_{gas}}{R_v} \cdot \frac{P_v}{P_{total}}$$

(8-17)

Example: What will be the humidity ratio at 100% relative humidity for a 10% oxygen and 90% helium mixture when the ambient pressure is 100 psia and the temperature is 80°F.

Solution: The gas constant for this gas mixture was previously found in Section 2.10.3 as 227.1 ft-lbf/lbm-°R. The gas constant for water vapor can likewise be found by dividing the Universal Gas Constant by the molecular weight of water (18.01 lbm/mol), giving

$$R_v = \frac{1544 \; \frac{ft-lbf}{mol-°R}}{18.01 \; \frac{lbm}{mol}} = 85.7 \; \frac{ft-lbf}{lbm-°R}$$

Table 8-1 lists the saturated pressures for water vapor taken from the steam tables. Note that at 80 °F the pressure of saturated vapor is approximately 0.5 psia. Applying Equation 8-17, we find the absolute humidity ratio for this heliox gas mixture at 100 psia, 100% relative humidity as

$$w = \frac{227.1 \; \frac{ft-lbf}{lbm-°R}}{85.7 \; \frac{ft-lbf}{lbm-°R}} \cdot \frac{0.5 \; psia}{100 \; psia} = 0.0132 \; lbm \; water \; vapor \; per \; lbm \; gas$$

Table 8-1: Properties of Saturated Vapor Versus Temperature
(taken from <u>Steam Tables</u> by Keenan *et al*, 1969)

Temp, °F	P_s, Sat Vapor Press, psia	ρ_s, Density of Sat Vapor lbm/cuft	h_{fg}, Latent Heat of Evap Btu/lbm	Temp, °F	P_s, Sat Vapor Press, psia	ρ_s, Density of Sat Vapor lbm/cuft	h_{fg}, Latent Heat of Evap Btu/lbm
32	0.08854	0.000302	1075.8	110	1.2748	0.003768	1031.6
35	0.09995	0.000339	1074.1	120	1.6924	0.004919	1025.8
40	0.12170	0.000409	1071.3	130	2.2225	0.006356	1020.0
45	0.14752	0.000491	1068.4	140	2.8886	0.008130	1014.1
50	0.17811	0.000587	1065.6	150	3.718	0.010302	1008.2
60	0.2563	0.000829	1059.9	160	4.741	0.012938	1002.3
70	0.3631	0.001152	1054.3	170	5.992	0.016113	996.3
80	0.5069	0.001579	1048.6	180	7.510	0.019908	990.2
90	0.6982	0.002137	1042.9	200	11.526	0.029727	977.9
100	0.9492	0.002854	1037.2	212	14.696	0.037313	970.3

Humidity ratios for other dry bulb temperatures can similarly be found for this gas environment. The line defined by these humidity ratios across a range of dry bulb temperatures will be the upper boundary (100% relative humidity) for our psychrometric chart. Above this line, droplets of water exist in the gas.

Lines of constant relative humidity below 100% are easily found from Equations 8-3 and 8-17. For example, at 50% relative humidity and 80°F, the water vapor pressure will be

$$P_v = \phi \cdot P_s = 0.5 \cdot 0.5 \; psia = 0.25 \; psia$$

and it is easy to show that the humidity ratio at 50% relative humidity and 80°F is 0.0066 lbm of water vapor per lbm of dry heliox. These lines of constant relative humidity can be directly related to the saturated vapor line using proportional dividers on the *w* versus *T* plot.

Two important lines typically shown on these psychrometric charts are the lines of adiabatic saturation and total constant enthalpy (*H*). To generate these lines, we first define h_{gas} as

$$h_{gas} = C_{p,gas} T \qquad (8\text{-}18)$$

which references h_{gas} to a convenient zero enthalpy datum of 0°F.

We can approximate the enthalpy of water vapor, h_w , with the equation

$$h_w = 1076 + 0.44\,(T,^\circ F - 32) \qquad \frac{Btu}{lbm} \qquad (8\text{-}19)$$

where 1076 is the enthalpy in Btu per pound mass needed to change one pound of water at 32°F to one pound of vapor (see *latent heat of evaporation* in Table 8-1), and 0.44 is the specific heat of the vapor (expressed in Btu/lbm-°F) in the low temperature regime. Note that the enthalpy datum for the vapor is then 32°F. This difference in datums is not important since we will never use these quantities except in difference computations.

Equation 8-16 for the case of adiabatic humidification is

$$H_2 - H_1 = (w_2 - w_1)\,h_{f,2} \qquad (8\text{-}20)$$

where *H* is found from Equation 8-13. Expanding 8-20 gives (with signs changed throughout)

$$-h_{gas,2} - w_2 h_{w,2} + h_{gas,1} + w_1 h_{w,1} = -w_2 h_{f,2} + w_1 h_{f,2}$$

We now add the term $w_1 h_{w,2}$ to both sides and collect terms to get

$$h_{gas,1} + w_1 h_{w,1} - (h_{gas,2} + w_1 h_{w,2}) = w_2(h_{w,2} - h_{f,2}) - w_1(h_{w,2} - h_{f,2})$$

Notice that $(h_{w,2} - h_{f,2})$ is simply the difference between the vapor and liquid enthalpies at condition 2, which is $h_{fg,2}$, the latent heat of evaporation (see Table 8-1). Substituting this definition for the latent heat, the right side of the above equation then becomes

$$h_{fg}(w_2 - w_1)$$

The left side of the equation can be simplified by substituting Equations 8-18 and 8-19 and canceling terms to give

$$(T_2 - T_1)(C_{p,gas} + 0.44\,w_1)$$

In a typical hyperbaric situation,

$$C_{P,gas} \gg 0.44 w_1$$

This was confirmed in our previous example above, in which the maximum humidity ratio (at 100% relative humidity) for a 90/10 heliox mixture at 100 psia, 80 °F was 0.0132 lbm water vapor per lbm of dry gas. The specific heat for this same gas mixture was shown in Section 2.10.2 to equal 0.76 Btu/lbm-°F, or 130 times larger that 0.44 w_1.

With the above simplifications, the adiabatic heating process shown in Figure 8-2, originally described in

Equation 8-20, reduces to

$$C_{P,gas}(T_1 - T_2) = h_{fg,2}(w_2 - w_1) \tag{8-21}$$

For computational applications, it is helpful to express a relationship for $h_{fg,2}$ as a function of T_2 (°F) as

$$h_{fg,2} = 1091.6 - 0.56T_2 \tag{8-22}$$

which simply expresses the *T-h* vapor line on the steam table in equation form. To draw a line of adiabatic humidification on our psychrometric chart, we first select a temperature T_2 and a humidity ratio w_2 on the saturation line (100% RH). Then choose a T_1 such that $T_1 > T_2$ and compute w_1 from Equation 8-21. This gives a new point on the same line of adiabatic saturation. If these lines are curved, we need several points to define each curve. Lines of constant adiabatic humidification can best be found by writing Equation 8-21 in the form

$$\frac{\Delta w}{\Delta T} = -\frac{C_{p,gas}}{h_{fg,2}} \tag{8-23}$$

For any line, the two terms on the right side of Equation 8-23 are constant. Thus, the slope of the adiabatic humidification line on our *w-T* coordinate system will be constant for all values of *w* and *T*. In addition, we note that this slope value only changes from line to line as $h_{fg,2}$ changes. Equation 8-22 predicts changes in h_{fg} of only about 25 Btu/lbm (out of over 1000 Btu/lbm) over a human comfort range of perhaps 40°F. This causes negligible change to the slope of the *w-T* lines of adiabatic humidification. Thus, if we obtain a single line, all other lines can be drawn parallel with the first line with reasonable accuracy.

Example: In all heating and cooling situations, we must work with *H*, the total enthalpy based on the mass of dry gas. Consider for example Equation 8-20 derived for adiabatic humidification. Assume that pure helium gas is being saturated with water vapor at 100 psia total pressure at a temperature of 100°F. Is adiabatic humidification a fair assumption for this process?

Solution: We can use Equation 8-17 to calculate a maximum humidity ratio for this saturated helium as w_2 = 0.0428 lbm vapor/lbm helium. We will assume that the humidification process started with dry gas (w_1 = 0). The enthalpy of liquid water at an exit temperature of 100°F, $h_{f,2}$, can be found in steam tables to be 68 BTU/lbm water. Applying Equation 8-20 for this process gives

$$\Delta H = (w_2 - w_1)h_{f,2} = \left(0.0428 \ \frac{lbm \ vapor}{lbm \ helium} \cdot 68 \ \frac{Btu}{lbm \ vapor} \right) = 2.94 \ \frac{Btu}{lbm \ helium}$$

This shows that the usual assumption made about Equation 8-20, namely that $H_1 = H_2$, is somewhat in error for our special conditions, at least at higher temperatures and with large humidity changes. For normal air conditioning calculations, it is usually assumed that lines of constant adiabatic humidification and lines of constant *H* are identical. Equation 8-17 shows that since helium has such a high gas constant, the effective *w* for any pressure is much greater with helium than in the case of air.

To compute lines of constant *H* on our chart, it is necessary to first obtain H_2 at a given point on the 100% RH line. This is done by reading T_2 and w_2 from the chart and then solving Equations 8-18 and 8-19 for the separate enthalpies of the dry gas and water vapor. These are combined in Equation 8-13 to get H_2. Since the total enthalpy is constant, $H_2 = H_1$. Substituting Equations 8-18 and 8-19 into Equation 8-13 gives the general equation for constant H as

$$T_2 C_{P_{gas}} + 1076 w_2 + 0.44 w_2 T_2 = T_1 C_{P_{gas}} + 1076 w_1 + 0.44 w_1 T_1 \qquad \textbf{(8-24)}$$

An easily obtained second point on our constant H curve occurs at the point where the initial humidity ratio w_1 is zero. Setting w_1 at zero in Equation 8-24 allows us to solve for T_1

$$T_1 = T_2 + \frac{1076 w_2 + 0.44 w_2 T_2}{C_{P_{gas}}} \qquad \textbf{(8-25)}$$

A third point on a line of constant H should be found by choosing an intermediate value of w_1 and solving Equation 8-24 for T_1. This is only necessary if the Equation 8-25 calculation indicates that the constant H line has deviated from the line of adiabatic saturation passing though the $w_2 - T_2$ point.

Thus, the major parameters in any psychrometric problem can be expressed in graphical form. Of course, the equations given here can be used for computer or hand computation when a chart is not needed.

8.2.4 Universal Humidity Chart

Since most deep diving involves heliox mixtures, it is desirable to construct a humidity chart which is independent of pressure and gas mixture by choosing the appropriate units for the ordinate of the psychrometric chart. Instead of expressing the humidity ratio in pounds of water vapor / pound of dry gas, Sexton (1972) suggested that we express it in terms of pounds of water vapor per cubic foot of dry gas. Sexton showed that by restating the definition of relative humidity as

$$\rho_v = \phi \rho_s \qquad \textbf{(8-26)}$$

(this results from Equation 8-3 by assuming that water vapor behaves as an ideal gas), lines of constant relative humidity can be drawn by selecting a value for ϕ and using tabulated values of ρ_s versus T from the <u>Steam Tables</u> (Table 8-1) to plot ρ_V as a function of T. The resulting humidity chart shown in Figure 8-3, referred to as the Universal Humidity Chart, is suitable for use with gas mixtures of various compositions and for various pressures.

Constant Dew Point Lines   Lines of constant dew point temperature on the Universal Humidity Chart are also lines of constant partial pressure of water vapor since the partial pressure of water vapor is unchanged until condensation occurs. In addition, water vapor partial pressure corresponds to the saturation pressure at the dew point temperature of the mixture. Therefore, for a constant dew point temperature,

$$P_v = \phi = P_s \quad at \quad T_{dp}$$

Employing the ideal gas relations, Equation 8-2 gives

$$P_s @ T_{dp} = (\rho_s @ T_{dp}) R_v T_{dp} \qquad \textbf{(8-27)}$$

and

$$\rho_v R_v T_v = (\rho_s @ T_{dp}) R_v T_{dp}$$

or

$$\rho_v = (\rho_s @ T_{dp}) \frac{T_{dp}(absolute)}{T(absolute)} \tag{8-28}$$

Equation 8-28 shows that lines of constant dew point temperature on the Universal Humidity Chart (Figure 8-3) are not horizontal as on a standard psychrometric chart, but slope slightly downward with increasing temperature.

Energy Calculations   Unlike conventional psychrometric charts, the Universal Humidity Chart does not include lines of constant mixture enthalpy for use in energy calculations. Therefore, the equations developed below and shown on the chart must be used. These equations were derived based on the assumption that most gases used in diving applications are diatomic (nitrogen or oxygen) or monatomic (helium) gases. Although other non-simple gases can be encountered in diving mixtures, carbon dioxide for instance, the percentages of these gases will be small in life support applications and can be ignored.

Each gas in a mixture of gases behaves as if it occupies the total volume at the mixture temperature, so that the equation of state for each gas constituent is

$$P_i V = m_i R_i T$$

The constant pressure specific heat of a diatomic gas or mixture thereof over temperature ranges consistent with life support applications can be approximated by

$$C_{p_a} = 0.0045 R_a \quad (Btu/lbm - {}^\circ R) \tag{8-29}$$

where the subscript "a" denotes the diatomic gas. Similarly for a monatomic gas (or mixture thereof)

$$C_{p_b} = 0.00324 R_b \tag{8-30}$$

where the subscript b denotes the monatomic gas.

A gas that is being heated or cooled at constant pressure requires energy given by

$$Q = H_2 - H_1$$

Consider a constant pressure heating of the mixture of monatomic and diatomic gases from T_1 to T_2. The amount of energy that must go into this mixture of monatomic and diatomic gases can be calculated as

$$Q = H_2 - H_1 = m_a C_{p_a}(T_2 - T_1) + m_b C_{p_b}(T_2 - T_1)$$

Collecting terms and applying Equations 8-29 and 8-30

$$Q = \left(\frac{T_2}{T_1} - 1\right)(0.0045 m_a R_a T_1 + 0.00324 m_b R_b T_1)$$

Substituting the equation of state for these gas constituents, the total energy per unit of the original volume becomes

$$\frac{Q}{V_1} = \left(\frac{T_2}{T_1} - 1\right)(0.0045 P_a + 0.00324 P_b)$$

Now, dividing the above equation with the total mixture pressure P, and replacing the pressure ratios by the corresponding volume fractions X_i (note that $X_a = P_a / P$ and $X_b = P_b / P)$ we obtain

$$\frac{Q}{PV_1} = \left(\frac{T_2}{T_1} - 1\right)(0.0045 X_a + 0.00324 X_b)$$

For this two gas mixture

$$X_a + X_b = 1$$

Therefore, we can write

$$\frac{Q}{PV_1} = \left(\frac{T_2}{T_1} - 1\right)(0.0045 - 0.00126 X_b)$$

The Universal Humidity Chart was generated with pressure expressed in atmospheres. Thus, converting the above equation with total pressure from lbf/ft^2 to atmospheres (1 Ata equals 2116 lbf/ft^2) gives:

$$\frac{Q}{\overline{P}V_1} = \left(\frac{T_2}{T_1} - 1\right)(9.52 - 2.72 X_b) \qquad (8\text{-}31)$$

where X_b is the volume fraction of the monatomic gas component; Q is the energy that must be added to the mixture to go from T_1 to T_2, given in Btu; $\overline{P}$ is the total pressure, given in Ata, V_1 is the gas volume, in ft^3, and T is in °R.

Sexton (1972) demonstrated that Equation 8-31 is sufficient for calculating energies required for even humid gas mixtures over the temperature range of the Universal Humidity Chart with little error. Therefore, with the monatomic gas assumed to be helium and an arbitrary gas enthalpy (H_{gas}) defined for the chart as

$$H_{gas} = 9.52 - 2.72 X_{He} \qquad (Btu) \qquad (8\text{-}32)$$

allows us to write Equation 8-31 as

$$\frac{Q}{V_1} = \bar{P} \cdot \frac{H_{gas}}{T_1} (T_2 - T_1)$$ (8-33)

Equation 8-33 gives an expression for the amount of heat that must be added per unit volume to the dry gas mixture during the heating/cooling process. The energy per unit volume for the water vapor can be found by again assuming that the water vapor behaves as an ideal gas (this is not a bad assumption over the relatively small temperature range and at the low partial pressures seen in most life supporting environments). Under these conditions, we can write

$$Q_v = m_v C_{p_v}(T_2 - T_1)$$

where m_v is the mass of the water vapor added during the process, and C_{pv} is an average specific heat for the added water vapor over the temperatures occurring in the heating/humidification process. If we assume an average specific heat for the water vapor over the temperature range of interest to be 0.445 Btu/lbm-°F, we can calculate the amount of heat added to the water vapor per unit volume as

$$\frac{Q_v}{V_1} = 0.445 \; \rho_{vl} \; (T_2 - T_1)$$

where ρ_{vl} is the density of the water vapor at the initial temperature T_l (°R). Adding this energy to the energy for the dry gas, given in Equation 8-33, gives the total energy addition for the moist gas mixture as

$$\frac{Q + Q_v}{V_1} = \left[\bar{P} \cdot \frac{H_{gas}}{T_1} + 0.445 \; \rho_{vl} \right] (T_2 - T_1)$$ (8-34)

Example: At what rate must energy be added to heat and humidify air that is flowing at 1 ft³/min with initial conditions of 32 °F, 50% RH, 1 Ata to final conditions of 84.2 °F, 100% RH, 1 Ata?

Solution: --First, the gas enthalpy can be calculated from Equation 8-32 as $H_{gas} = 9.52 + 2.72 \,(\, 0 \,) = 9.52$.

-- Next, ρ_{vl} at 32 °F, 50% RH is estimated from Figure 8-3 as 0.00015 lb vapor/ft³ gas. (Note: this could also be derived by taking 50% of the density of saturated water vapor at 32 °F from Table 8-1.)

-- Applying Equation 8-34 to calculate the energy required to heat the original moist gas, we get

$$Energy = \left(1 \; x \; \frac{9.52}{492} + 0.445 \; x \; 0.00015 \right) (544.2 - 492) = 1.0135 \; \frac{Btu}{ft^3 \; mix}$$

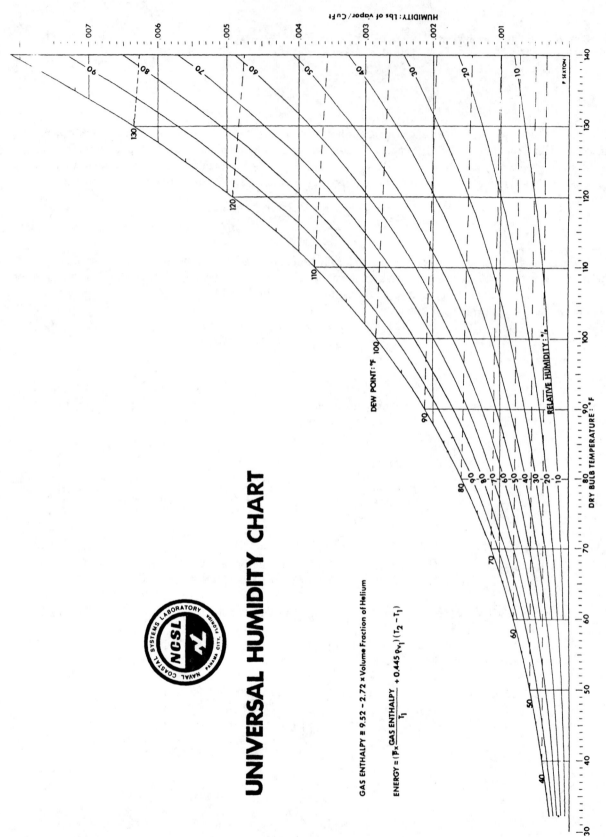

Figure 8-3 Universal Humidity Chart (Taken from Sexton, 1972)

Additional energy will required to evaporate extra vapor to increase the vapor content to 84.2 °F, 100% RH (this can be estimated from Figure 8-3 to result in a $\rho_{v2} = 0.00175$ lb vapor/ft³ gas). Thus, the added mass of water vapor to reach the final condition is

$$Added\ vapor = \rho_{v2} - \rho_{v1} = 0.00175 - 0.00015 = 0.0016\ \frac{lb\ vapor}{ft^3\ mix}$$

--The latent heat required to evaporate this added mass of water from a liquid to a vapor at 84.2 °F can be found as (h_{fg} at 84.2 °F is estimated from Table 8-1 as 1046 Btu/lbm)

$$Added\ Latent\ Energy = h_{fg}\ (\rho_{v2} - \rho_{v1}) = 1046\ \frac{Btu}{lbm\ vapor}\ x\ 0.0016\ \frac{lbm\ vapor}{ft^3\ mix} = 1.6736\ \frac{Btu}{ft^3\ mix}$$

-- The total rate of energy addition to complete this heating/humidification process can now be calculated as

$$Total\ Energy\ Rate = 1\ \frac{ft^3}{min}\ x\ (1.013 + 1.674)\ \frac{Btu}{ft^3\ mix} = 2.687\ \frac{Btu}{min}$$

8.2.5 Mixtures

One of the main applications of a chart is in systems where a mixture of two different gas-vapor streams occur. In a hyperbaric chamber, for example, one stream is the respired, humid air leaving the lungs of the chamber personnel, and the other might be the gas-vapor flow through some sort of dehumidifier. Such mixing situations are computed using a mass balance on the water vapor. Mixing streams 1 and 2 to give a resulting stream 3 gives

$$w_1 m_{gas,1} + w_2 m_{gas,2} = w_3 (m_{gas,1} + m_{gas,2}) \qquad \text{(8-35)}$$

where the unknown mixed humidity; w_3 can be computed if the individual dry gas flows $m_{gas,1}$ and $m_{gas,2}$ are known. Equation 8-26 allows the computation of one parameter of the mixed state (w_3). The other parameter needed to fix the mixed flow is the mixed enthalpy which can be obtained from an energy balance

$$H_1 m_{gas,1} + H_2 m_{gas,2} = H_3 (m_{gas,1} + m_{gas,2}) \qquad \text{(8-36)}$$

Since lines of H and w cross each other, they fix a specific location on the chart. In many cases, the third point lies on, or very close to, the straight line connecting points 1 and 2. Clearly, this third point defines the steady state of the air-vapor mixture in the chamber. If it is close to 100% RH, discomfort, corrosion and electronic problems can be anticipated.

8.2.6 Engineering Processes

There are five basic processes that are done with most standard heating/cooling equipment: *simple heating, simple cooling, dehumidification by simple cooling, adiabatic humidification and chemical dehumidification*. These processes are shown in Figure 8-4. Since high humidity, and/or cold temperatures, are the most common situations in life-support systems under water, we are mainly concerned with chemical or cooling dehumidification and simple heating. Humidification by cooling can often utilize the surrounding water as a cold sink. If a counterflow heat exchanger is used, some of the initial cooling can occur there and the heat removed can be added to the counter current stream of gas and vapor, thus reducing the heating load. Such a system requires a gas-to-gas countercurrent unit, a gas-to-water cooler, and a gas heater (depending on how the heating is done). If the habitat is well insulated, it might be possible to eliminate the heater. In any case, the heating and cooling loads can be computed by reading the total enthalpy at each state, taking the difference and multiplying by the gas flow.

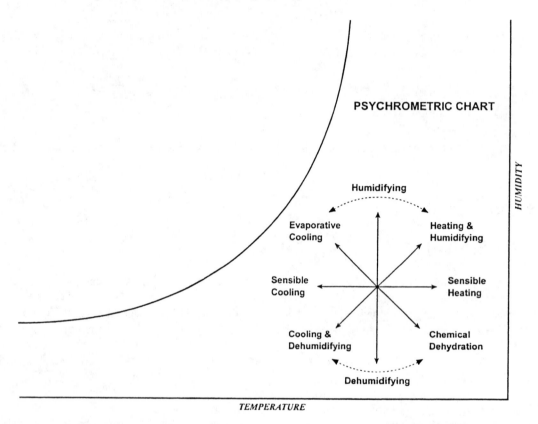

Figure 8-4 Gas conditioning process on the psychrometric chart

Example: A large underwater lab is to be fitted for operation in 200 feet of seawater such that the workers can live in the habitat for days or weeks. The breathing gas in the lab is 60% helium, 30% nitrogen, and 10% nitrogen, and the lab atmosphere is continuously circulated through an absorbent to remove CO_2.

There are 10 men in the lab. Assume each man requires 1 cubic foot of gas per minute. The gas is exhaled at 98°F and is saturated with moisture. At the same time, lab gas is circulated through a seawater cooler that cools the gas to 40°F, then through a heater that brings the temperature back to 80°F. Assume the lab is insulated and no heat is lost through the walls. The cooler flow and the exhaled gas flow mix continuously. Find the equilibrium lab conditions when the cooler-heater flow is the same as, twice, and then four times the lung-gas flow. (Note that the heat loss problem is covered in Chapter 7.)

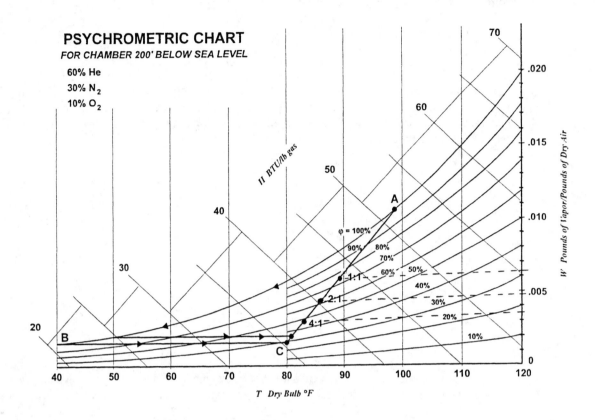

Figure 8-5 Psychrometric chart for example

Solution: Figure 8-5 is a psychrometric chart constructed from the equations in section 8-3 using the conditions for this problem. Path A→B→C indicates the process of gas conditioning. Connecting points A and C;

(1) for 1:1 flow; the equilibrium lab conditions are found half way between A and C ∴

T_{mix} = 89°F   73% RH w = 0.0063 lb vapor / lb gas

(2) for 2:1 flow, the equilibrium lab conditions are found 2/3 of the distance along the line AC

T_{mix} = 86°F   62% RH w = 0.0047 lb vapor / lb gas

(3) for 4:1 flow, the equilibrium lab conditions are found 4/5 of the distance along the line AC

T_{mix} = 84°F   49% RH w = 0.0035 lb vapor / lb gas

Alternative Solution using the Universal Humidity Chart

(1) for 1:1 flow   (applying Equation 8-35 to get the humidity ratio of the mixture)

$$T_{mix} = 89°F \qquad 73\% \text{ RH} \qquad w = 0.0014 \text{ lb vapor / ft}^3$$

Note: Caution should be taken when comparing the humidity ratios derived with the Universal Humidity Chart and those found in the previous method since the first method is based on mass of vapor per mass of gas, while the Universal Chart is based on mass of vapor per volume of gas. The humidity ratio found from the Universal Chart can be converted by dividing it by the density of the gas.

(2) for 2:1 flow

$$T_{mix} = 86°F \qquad 62\% \text{ RH} \qquad w = 0.0011$$

(3) for 4:1 flow

$$T_{mix} = 84°F \qquad 50\% \text{ RH} \qquad w = 0.00075$$

Example: For the three mixing designs given in the previous example, find the daily cooling loads (in Btu's) that you would give to the heat exchanger designer. How much water is removed per day in each of these cases?

Solution: First, we will find the basic mass flow rate of dry gas

$$\dot{m}_{gas} = \rho_{gas} \dot{V} ; \quad \rho_{gas} = \frac{P}{R_{gas}T} ; \quad P = 104 \, psia ; \quad R_{gas} = \frac{R_u}{M_{gas}(14.0)}$$

$$\therefore \quad \rho_{gas} = \frac{(104)(144)(14)}{1545 \ T}$$

$$\dot{V} = 10 \ men \left(1\frac{ft^3}{min} \right) (60 \ \frac{min}{hr}) = 600 \frac{ft^3}{hr}$$

assume $T \sim 86°F = 546°R$

$$\dot{m} = \frac{(104)(144)(14)}{(1545)(546)}(600) = 149 \frac{lb_{gas}}{hr}$$

(1) from Figure 8-5, for 1:1 flow

$$H_{in\ cooler} = 42.8 \ \frac{Btu}{lb_{gas}}$$

$$H_{out} = 21$$

$$\dot{Q} = (42.8 - 21) \ \frac{Btu}{lbm} \ (149 \ \frac{lbm}{hr}) = 3248 \ \frac{Btu}{hr}$$

$$\dot{m}_{water} = \dot{m}_{gas} \ (w_{in} - w_{out}) = (0.0063 - 0.0015)(149)(24) = 17.2 \frac{lb}{day}$$

(2)   For 2:1 flow

$$\dot{Q} = (41.0 - 21)(149)(2) = 5960 \frac{Btu}{hr}$$

$$\dot{m}_{water} = (0.0047 - 0.0015)(149)(24)(2) = 22.7 \frac{lb}{day}$$

(3)   For 4:1 flow

$$\dot{Q} = (38 - 21)(149)(4) = 10132 \frac{Btu}{day}$$

$$\dot{m}_{water} = (0.0034 - 0.0015)(149)(24)(4) = 26.8 \frac{lb}{day}$$

Using the Universal Chart: For 1:1 flow

$$\dot{V} = 600 \ \frac{ft^3}{hr}$$

$$Gas\ enthalpy = 9.52 - (2.72)(0.60) = 7.89$$

$$Energy = \left(7.05 \cdot \frac{7.89}{558} + 0.445(0.00033) \right)(500 - 558) = -5.79 \frac{Btu}{ft^3}$$

$$\dot{Q} = (-5.79 \ \frac{Btu}{ft^3})(600 \ \frac{ft^3}{hr}) = 3474 \frac{Btu}{hr}$$

$$\dot{m}_{water} = w_{in} - w_{out} = (0.0014 - 0.00033)(600)(24) = 15.4 \frac{lb}{day}$$

Example: Suppose the water temperature in the previous example rose to a point where the cooler could only get the water temperature down to 50°F (instead of 40°F as before). What flow in the cooler-heater would be required to obtain the same lab gas moisture content as with the cooler flow at twice that of the lung flow? To what temperature should the cooler-heater flow be heated, in this case, to make the mixed temperature identical to that when the cooled temperature was 40°F? In other words, the mixed condition is to be identical to that in (a) with the cooler-heater flow at twice the lung flow, but now can it only be cooled to 50°F. To what must the cooler flow be increased and at what temperature must heating be terminated to do this?

Solution: From Figure 8-5: lung flow $w = 0.0117$ (fixed)

Following line at 50° back to line A-C, terminate heating at 82°F ∴ new flow

$w = 0.002$ for every lb m lung

$$(1) \qquad (0.117) + \dot{m}_{cool}(0.002) = (1 + \dot{m}_{cool})(0.0047)$$

$$\dot{m} = 2.6 \qquad \therefore \text{ new flow increases to } 2.6\text{:}1$$

Or using the Universal Humidity Chart, Lung flow $w = 0.0025 \dfrac{lb}{ft^3}$

following line back at 50°F cooling
terminate heat at 82°F

∴ new w for flow = .0005

for every 1 ft³ m lung

$$(1)(0.0025) + v_{cool}(0.0005) = (1 + v_{cool})(0.0011)$$

$$\dot{v} = \frac{0.0014}{0.0006} = 2.3\text{:}1 \quad \textit{volume flow}$$

8.2.7 Respiratory Heat Loss

For conditioning the environment in the previous problem, our main concerns were simple heating and dehumidification. The heating and cooling loads of interest did not address the energy required to humidify or dehumidify the gas since that energy was dumped as waste heat into the seawater.

Cooling dehumidification and chemical dehumidification will generate heat, and some waste heat may be recovered to reduce energy requirements, making waste heat loads a design consideration. However, as we saw in Chapter 3, a critical concern in life support is respiratory heat loss.

Refer again to Figure 8-4. When gas is inspired to the lung at temperatures below 98°F and RH below 100%, the body is required to heat and humidify the gas. This process on the chart is indicated on the upper right path. Notice that the path can be broken into components of sensible heating (horizontal line; w = constant) and humidifying (vertical line; T = constant). With a standard psychrometric chart or a chart constructed similar to the previous problem, the lines of constant enthalpy allow us to find the total energy required in a process and also to break this into the components of sensible and latent heat directly from the chart.

The Universal Humidity Chart allows us to find the sensible heating energy requirement from Equation 8-34. To calculate the latent heat energy and obtain the total heating requirement, we need to refer to Section 8-2 and recall the evaporation or "boiling enthalpy" as the energy required in latent heat of vaporization. We can then compute heat loss due to humidification from $Q = m\, h_{fg2}$ on the Universal Humidity Chart.

Example: A jogger inhales cold air with a dry bulb temperature of 32°F at 50% RH. Air pressure is 1 atmosphere. His exhalation is 100% RH at 84°F. The jogger's respiratory minute volume (see Chapter 3) is 48 LPM. At what rate is the jogger losing water vapor and heat?

Solution: Using the *Universal Humidity Chart*:

At the initial condition (inhaling) the humidity of the air is found from the Universal Humidity Chart to be $0.0002\, lb/ft^3$

The final condition is $0.00175\, lb/ft^3$.

The amount of water vapor lost from the joggers body is found by taking the difference of these amounts and multiplying by the RMV.

$$water\ loss = (final\ humidity - initial\ humidity)\ RMV$$

$$48\,\frac{liters}{min} = 1.7\,\frac{ft^3}{min}$$

$$\therefore\ water\ loss = \left(0.00175\,\frac{lb}{ft^3} - 0.0002\,\frac{lb}{ft^3}\right)\left(1.7\,\frac{ft^3}{min}\right)\left(60\,\frac{min}{hr}\right) = 0.158\,\frac{lb}{hr}$$

Alternate Solution: Using a *standard psychrometric chart*:

$$water\ loss = \dot{m}_{air}(w_2 - w_1)$$

$$since\ \dot{m}_{air} = \rho_{air}\,\dot{V},\quad for\quad \rho_{air} = 0.071\, lb/ft^3$$

$$\dot{m}_{air} = (0.071\, lb/ft^3)(1.7\, ft^3/min)(60\,min/hr) = 7.24\ lb/hr$$

From any *standard psychrometric* chart

w_1 @ 32°F, 50% RH = 0.00186 lb vapor/lb gas
w_2 @ 84°F, 100% RH = 0.0255 lb vapor/lb gas

$\therefore$ water loss = (7.24 lb gas/hr)(0.0255 - 0.00186) lb vapor/lb gas = 0.17 lb/hr   (~ 1/3 cup)
This alternate solution compares within 10% of the solution found above using the Universal Humidity Chart.

Heat Loss Solution using the Universal Humidity Chart: First, compute Gas Enthalpy

Using Equation 8-32, $H_{gas} = 9.52 - 2.72(0) = 9.52$

Then the energy/volume can be found using Equation 8-34

$$= [1\,\text{ata}\,(9.52/492) + .445\,(.0002)]\,(544 - 492) = 1.011 \text{ Btu/ft}^3$$

Finally, multiplying this energy per gas volume by the RMV gives the rate at which sensible heating is added

$$= [1.011 \text{ Btu/ft}^3][1.7 \text{ ft}^3/\text{min}][60 \text{ min/hr}] = 103 \text{ Btu/hr}   \text{ (Sensible heat addition)}$$

This is the sensible heat required to raise the gas temperature in the lung from 32°F to 84°F.

Now, calculate the latent heat required to increase the humidity of the lung gas to 100% RH @ 84°F.

From the steam table (Table 8-1) h_{fg} @ 84°F = 1046 Btu/lbm

∴ latent heat = (1046 Btu/lbm of water) (0.17 lb water per hour) = 178 Btu/hr

So the total heat loss becomes

Total Heat Loss = Sensible Heat + Latent Heat = 103 + 178 = 281 Btu/hr

This rate of heat loss is approximately 12% of the jogger's metabolic heat output of 2285 Btu/hr. (See Chapter 3 for review of metabolic heat production rates.)

Alternate Heat Loss Calculation: Using a standard psychrometric chart

$$Total\,Heat\,Loss = \dot{m}\,(H_2 - H_1)$$

$$= (7.24 \text{ lb/hr})(48.3 - 9.7) = 279.5 \text{ Btu/hr}$$

The sensible heat loss $(T_1 \rightarrow T_2,\ w = 0)$

H_1 @ 34°F, 50% RH = 9.7

H_2 @ 84°F, ~ 17% RH = 24.7

$\dot{Q} = \dot{m}\,(H_2 - H_1)$

$$= 7.24\,(24.4 - 9.7) = 106.4 \text{ Btu/hr}$$

The latent heat loss $(w_1 \rightarrow w_2,\ T = 0)$

$H_1 = 24.7$

$H_2 = 48.3$

$Q = (7.24)(48.3 - 24.4) = 173 \text{ Btu/hr}$

8.3   Closure

Psychrometric predictions for hyperbaric, mixed-gas situations are important in life support considerations. The significance of these predictions ranges from sustaining an acceptable level of human comfort, to maintaining electronic systems at operationally acceptable humidity levels, and finally, the crucial issue of human respiratory heat loss. Proper application of the concepts developed in this chapter will result in the analysis required to design comfortable, safe habitats which function at an optimum level of maintenance.

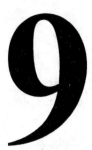

Applied Fluid Mechanics to Dive Systems

Objectives

The objectives of this chapter are to
● review some of the physical principles which relate to the transport of fluids from one point to another through a piping system
● understand the concepts of compressible and incompressible flow in a piping system
● be able to evaluate the pressure drops in pipes and umbilical, or be able to evaluate the fluid flow rate based on known inlet and exit pipe pressures
● present evaluation methods to predict the power requirements for pumps and compressors

9.1   Introduction

The most commonly employed method of transporting gases and liquids from one point to another is to force the gas or fluid to flow through a piping system. For instance, the gas ventilation requirements for a surface-supplied diver or underwater habitat (discussed in Chapter 6) is often satisfied by piping compressible fluids (gases) through a pipe or hose between the surface and the diver/habitat. Likewise, the thermal protection requirements of a diver discussed in Chapter 7 are often achieved by pumping an incompressible fluid (warm water) from the surface to a diver's hot water suit and respiratory gas heater. In so doing, the diver's body can be surrounded with a warm micro-climate, even in extremely cold environments, and respiratory heat losses can be minimized.

So extensive are the applications of hydraulics and fluid mechanics to life support systems design that it is essential that the life support engineer familiarize himself /herself with at least the elementary laws of fluid flow. This chapter will attempt to review these elementary laws and show their applications to typical underwater missions.

9.2   Incompressible Flow

Because of the great variety of fluids being delivered to underwater systems, a single equation which can be used for the flow of any fluid in pipes or hoses offers obvious advantages. Such an equation is the Darcy[9] formula, expressed in Equation (9-1). For steady flow of liquids in pipes or hoses, the Darcy formula can be used to calculate the pressure drop in that pipe or hose using the expression

$$H_L = f \cdot \frac{L}{D} \cdot \frac{V^2}{2g}$$ (9-1)

where H_L is the head loss resulting from the flow of a viscous liquid, ft; f is an experimentally determined friction factor; L is the hose length, ft; D is the hose diameter, ft; ρ is the density of the liquid, lb/ft³; V is the flow velocity, ft/sec; and g is the local acceleration of gravity at sea level (32.2 ft/sec²). Although the Darcy formula can be derived by means of dimensional analysis, the friction factor f has been determined experimentally----the most useful and widely accepted data of friction factor for use with the Darcy equation have been presented by L. F. Moody (Moody, 1944) shown in Figure 9-1.

As can be seen in this graphical display, often called the Moody diagram, the friction factor f is a function of the dimensionless Reynolds number Re and the relative roughness of the hose interior e/D, where

$$Re = \frac{\rho \, V \, D}{\mu}$$

consisting of the fluid density ρ, lbm/ft³; fluid velocity V, ft/sec; pipe diameter D, ft; and liquid viscosity μ, lbm/ft-sec; the absolute hose roughness e, ft can be found in Table 9.1.

In lieu of Figure 9-1, friction factors can also be determined during laminar flow (i.e., $Re < 2000$) as

$$f = \frac{64}{Re} \qquad for \;\; Re \; < \; 2000$$ (9-2)

---

[9]The Darcy formula is also known as the Weisbach formula or the Darcy-Weisbach formula; also, as the Fanning formula, sometimes modified so that the friction factor is one-fourth the Darcy friction factor.

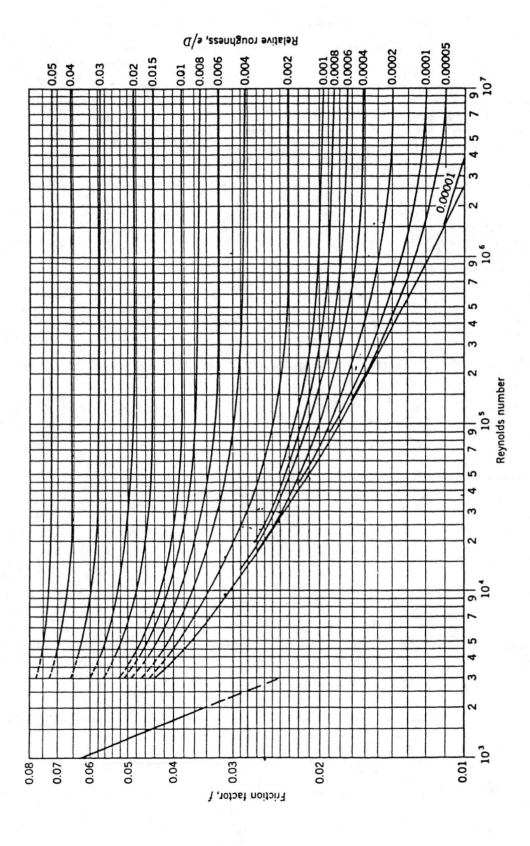

Figure 9-1: Friction factors for flow in pipes.

Table 9-1: Absolute Roughness of Various Pipe Materials

Material	Roughness, e (ft)
Glass, plastic	Smooth
Drawn tubing	0.000005
Wrought iron, steel	0.00015
Asphalted cast iron	0.0004
Galvanized iron	0.0005
Cast iron	0.00085
Wood stave	6×10^{-4} to 3×10^{-3}
Concrete	10^{-3} to 10^{-2}
Riveted steel	3×10^{-3} to 3×10^{-2}

For turbulent flow (i.e., $Re > 4000$), the Colebrook formula can be used to derive friction factors as

$$\frac{1}{\sqrt{f}} = -2 \log_{10}\left[\frac{\frac{e}{D}}{3.7} + \frac{2.51}{Re \sqrt{f}} \right] \qquad for \ Re > 4000 \qquad (9\text{-}3)$$

Note that flows having Reynolds numbers in the transition region between laminar and turbulent (Re between 2000 and 4000) will give vastly different values of f when using the relationships for either laminar or turbulent flow. In this narrow region, the reliability of friction factors derived from either the Moody diagram or Equations (9-2) or (9-3) must be used with caution.

9.2.1 Minor Losses.

Most umbilical systems will have additional pressure losses due to bends, elbows, valves, connectors, etc which will be in addition to the pressure drop of the hose. Typically, it will be necessary to resort to experimental results to characterize these losses. Such information is generally given in the form

$$H_{L_M} = K \frac{V^2}{2g} \qquad (9\text{-}4)$$

where K is called the *minor loss coefficient* (values of this loss coefficient for some typical valves and fittings is shown in Table 9.2), and H_{L_M} is the head loss associated with viscous flow in these various components.

Table 9-2: Minor Loss Coefficients for Various Valves and Fittings

Valve or Fitting	*K*
90° Elbow, std sweep	0.3-0.7
90° Elbow, long sweep	0.2-0.5
Tee, flow through run	0.15-0.5
Tee, flow through 90° branch	0.6-1.6
Gate valve, open	0.1-0.2
Swing check valve, open	2.0-10.0
Globe valve, open	5.0-16.0
Ball check valve	50.-90.0
Lift check valve	8.0-15.0
Square edge entry	0.4-0.6

The total head loss in a hose or pipe in which an incompressible, viscous liquid is flowing can be found by combining the hose loss with the minor losses to give

$$H_L = \left[f \cdot \frac{L}{D} + \sum K \right] \frac{V^2}{2g} \qquad \text{(9-5)}$$

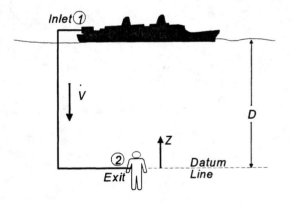

This total head loss for a liquid flowing between any two locations in a piping system, designated here as positions #1 and #2, can be related to the corresponding pressure differential between those two positions by using the steady-flow energy equation for an incompressible fluid; i.e.,

$$Z_1 + \frac{V_1^2}{2g} + \frac{P_1}{\gamma} = Z_2 + \frac{V_2^2}{2g} + \frac{P_2}{\gamma} + wk_{12}\frac{g_c}{g} + H_{L_{12}} \qquad \text{(9-6)}$$

Figure 9-2: Pipe system used to supply a liquid flow to a diver.

where Z is the elevation of the pipe locations relative to some arbitrary datum line, ft; V is the flow velocity at each position, ft/sec; P is the absolute pressure at each location, lbf/ft²; γ is the specific weight of the fluid, lbf/ft³; g is the local acceleration of gravity, ft/sec²; g_c is the dimensional constant, 32.2 lbm-ft/lbf-sec²; wk_{12} is the mechanical work done on the fluid between positions #1 and #2 (i.e., external work added by some type of pump).

In the special case of a piping system with a constant diameter hose or umbilical, and which has no external work being added between positions #1 and #2, we have

$$V_1 = V_2 \qquad and \qquad wk_{12} = 0$$

By substituting these observations in the steady-flow energy equation gives

$$P_1 = P_2 + \gamma \left[\left(Z_2 - Z_1 \right) + H_{L_{12}} \right] \qquad (9\text{-}7)$$

The application of Equation (9-7) to find the pressure drop in a typical piping system used to deliver incompressible fluids can best be demonstrated in the following example.

Example: Warm water (100° F) is being supplied to a diver's hot water suit at the rate of 3 gallons per minute through a 300 foot long smooth plastic hose having an internal diameter of 0.5 inches. The sum of all minor loss coefficients in elbows, valves, and connectors in this circuit is estimated to be 10.0. At what pressure must the water be supplied at the surface to reach a diver located at a depth of 250 FSW? Assume that the density and viscosity of the water are 62.0 lb/ft³ and 0.458 x 10⁻³ lbm/ft-sec, respectively.

Solution: We can first find the flow velocity from the volumetric flow rate specified in the problem by dividing this flow rate by the cross-sectional area of the hose

$$V = \frac{\dot{V}}{A_{cs}} = \frac{\left(3 \; \frac{gal}{min} \right) \cdot \left(\frac{min}{60 \; sec} \right) \cdot \left(\frac{ft^3}{7.48 \; gal} \right)}{\frac{\pi}{4} \left(\frac{0.5 \; inch}{12 \; \frac{inch}{ft}} \right)^2} = 4.9 \; \frac{ft}{sec}$$

The Reynold's number for this flow velocity is calculated as

$$Re = \frac{\rho \cdot V \cdot D}{\mu} = \frac{\left(62 \; \frac{lbm}{ft^3} \right) \left(4.9 \; \frac{ft}{sec} \right) \left(\frac{0.5 \; inch}{12 \; \frac{inch}{ft}} \right)}{0.458 \; x \; 10^{-3} \; \frac{lbm}{ft\text{-}sec}} = 27,638$$

Entering the Moody diagram with $Re = 27,638$ on the "smooth" pipe curve, we can obtain a friction factor f equal to 0.023.

The Colebrook formula, Equation (9-3), could also be used to obtain f using an iterative approach. The use of the Colebrook formula is particularly beneficial when computing pressure drops with a computer, where graphical displays for the friction factor are not available. In the above application, starting with any arbitrary value for f (we will use the value of f found graphically above) and assuming an e/D ratio equal to zero. This gives

$$\frac{1}{\sqrt{f}} = -2 \, \log_{10}\left[\frac{0}{3.7} + \frac{2.51}{27{,}638 \, \sqrt{0.023}} \right] = 6.445 \qquad \Rightarrow \quad f = 0.024$$

We could have just as easily started with a different initial value for the friction factor, and calculated a new value using the method described above. If necessary, this new friction factor value can be refined further by substituting this new value of *f* back into the Colebrook equation and again solving for a *f* in an iterative manner until the desired accuracy is obtained. Generally, only two to three iterations are sufficient to obtain accuracies to four decimal places.

The total head loss in the piping system can now be found from Equation (9-5) as

$$H_{L_{12}} = \left[f \cdot \frac{L}{D} + \sum K \right] \frac{V^2}{2g}$$

$$H_{L_{12}} = \left[0.023 \cdot \frac{300 \, ft}{\frac{0.5}{12} ft} + 10.0 \right] \frac{\left(4.9 \frac{ft}{sec} \right)^2}{2 \left(32.2 \frac{ft}{sec^2} \right)} = 65.5 \, ft$$

Referring to the piping system illustrated in Figure 9-2, we can arbitrarily establish a datum line at a depth of 250 FSW such that at a depth of 250 FSW (location #2), Z_2 is 0 ft; and at the surface (location #1), Z_1 is 250 ft. We could have just as easily established the zero datum line at the surface, making $Z_1 = 0$ and $Z_2 = -250$ ft, giving the same result when we subtract these two elevations in Equation (9-7).

Also, we know that the pressure at the exit of the umbilical is equal to the hydrostatic pressure at a depth of 250 FSW, such that

$$P_2 = \frac{250 + 33}{33} \, Ata \cdot 14.7 \, \frac{psia}{Ata} = 126.1 \, psia$$

Applying the steady-flow energy equation for an incompressible fluid to this piping system (Equation 9-7) with the total head loss calculated above, we are able to find the required inlet pressure to the umbilical to maintain the water flow to the diver as

$$P_1 = P_2 + \gamma \left[\left(Z_2 - Z_1 \right) + H_{L_{12}} \right]$$

Rearranging the above equation, we can solve for P_1

$$P_1 = 126.1 \; psia + \frac{62 \; \frac{lbf}{ft^3} \left[(0 - 250) \; ft + 65.5 \; ft \right]}{144 \; \frac{in^2}{ft^2}}$$

$$P_1 = 126.1 \; psia - 79.4 \; psi = 46.7 \; psia$$

A similar approach could be taken to calculate fluid delivery pressures at the diver's location when the surface supply pressure is known. An iterative approach will be necessary to calculate flow rates in these piping systems with known supply and delivery pressures. A description of this iterative approach will be given in the following discussion of compressible flow systems.

9.3   Compressible Flow

In the above discussion of pressure drops with incompressible fluids we used the Darcy formula, which uses a constant fluid density ρ and fluid velocity V. By definition, the density of compressible fluids will decrease as the gas travels from the inlet to the exit of a pipe due to a reduction in gas pressure. Additionally, this decreased density will necessarily result in an increase in gas velocity to satisfy a conservation of mass flow rate in the piping system

$$\dot{m} = \rho_1 \; V_1 \; A_1 = \rho_2 \; V_2 \; A_2 \tag{9-8}$$

where A is the cross sectional area of the pipe, ρ is the gas density, V is the gas velocity, and the subscripts 1 and 2 indicate the conditions at the hose inlet and outlet, respectively.

9.3.1 Approximating Pressure Drops Using the Darcy Formula

For very small pressure drops relative to the absolute pressures involved, the pressure drops for compressible fluids can be closely approximated by the results for incompressible flow using the Darcy equation, Equation 9-1. When dealing with compressible fluids, such as air or other gases, the following restrictions have been proposed in applying the Darcy formula for making pressure drop approximations (Crane Co, 1980):

a) If the calculated pressure drop $(P_1 - P_2)$ is less than about 10% of the inlet pressure P_1, reasonable accuracy will be obtained if the density used in the Darcy formula is based upon either the upstream or downstream conditions, whichever may be known.

b) If the calculated pressure drop $(P_1 - P_2)$ is greater than about 10%, but less than about 40% of the inlet pressure P_1, the Darcy equation may be used with reasonable accuracy by using a gas density based upon the average of upstream and downstream conditions.

c) For greater pressure drops, such as are often encountered in long pipe lines, such as gas supply umbilical, the method given below should be used.

9.3.2 Hose Pressure Drops With Steady, Isothermal Flow of Ideal Gases

The steady flow of gases in pipes or hoses will be treated in the following discussion as isothermal flow of an ideal gas. The solutions for pressure drop under isothermal conditions will, in most cases, vary little with those from an adiabatic flow with friction. The major issue that must be addressed when considering compressible flow is that the flow will always remain subsonic (i.e., Mach number must be less than 1.0). Friction tends to decrease the pressure along a pipe for subsonic flow, but causes a pressure rise for supersonic velocities. Thus, continuous transitions from subsonic to supersonic are impossible. The following expression relates pressure drop and friction for steady, isothermal flow in a hose

$$\frac{P_1^2 - P_2^2}{P_1^2} = k \, M_1^2 \left[2 \, \ln\!\left(\frac{P_1}{P_2}\right) + f \, \frac{L}{D} \right] \tag{9-9}$$

where P_1 is the upstream pressure (*absolute*), lbf/in^2; P_2 is the downstream pressure (*absolute*), lbf/in^2; k is the ratio of gas specific heats, c_p/c_v; M_1 is the upstream flow Mach number , given by

$$M_1 = \frac{V_1}{\sqrt{g_c \, k \, R \, T}} \tag{9-10}$$

where V_1 is the flow velocity at the inlet to the hose, ft/sec; g_c is the dimensional constant = 32.2 lbm-ft/lbf-sec^2; R is the gas constant, ft-lbf/lbm-°R; T is the gas temperature, °R; f is the friction coefficient discussed previously (Note: the Re used to find f is based on flow conditions at the inlet to the hose); L and D are the pipe length and diameter, respectively, given in feet.

The rather awkward expression given in Equation (9-9), with variables for pressure found on both sides, can be simplified for long pipes, where

$$f \, \frac{L}{D} \gg 2 \, \ln\!\left(\frac{P_1}{P_2}\right) \tag{9-11}$$

In these applications we can approximate the pressure drop in a "long" pipe as

$$\frac{P_1^2 - P_2^2}{P_1^2} = k \, M_1^2 \, f \, \frac{L}{D} \tag{9-12}$$

This can best be demonstrated in the following example.

Example: A 1500 foot long umbilical, constructed from ½-inch diameter (ID) drawn tubing (roughness, e, is 0.000005 ft) supplies 1000 SCFM of a heliox mixture containing 99% helium and 1% oxygen to a personnel transfer capsule (PTC) at a depth of 1200 FSW. The entrance pressure to the hose is 2500 psia. What will be the pressure drop in this hose assuming isothermal flow at 40 F? (Assume the ratio of specific heats, k=1.66).

Solution: Given

$P_1 = 2500$ psia $\qquad\qquad$ $T = 40\ °F = 500\ °R$

$L = 1500$ feet $\qquad\qquad$ $D = 0.5$ inch $= 0.04167$ feet

We can find the gas properties for the 99% helium/1% oxygen mixture using the methods described in Chapter 2 to give

Viscosity: $\qquad\qquad$ $\mu = 1.28 \times 10^{-5}$ lbm/ft-sec

Gas Density: $\qquad\qquad$ ρ @ 70° F, 1 Ata (SCFM)= 0.01107 lbm/ft^3

$\qquad\qquad\qquad\qquad\qquad$ ρ @ 40° F, 2500 psia= 1.8376 lbm/ft^3

Gas constant: $\qquad\qquad$ $R = 360.7$ ft-lbf/lbm-°R

The mass flow rate through the hose can be found as

$$\dot{m} = \dot{V}_{SCFM} \cdot \rho_{SCFM} = 1000\ \frac{ft^3}{\min} \cdot 0.01107\ \frac{lbm}{ft^3} = 11.07\ \frac{lbm}{\min} = 0.1845\ \frac{lbm}{\sec}$$

With this flow rate and the gas density at 2500 psia, the velocity of the gas at the inlet to the hose can be found by application of Equation (9-8) to give

$$V_1 = \frac{\dot{m}}{\rho_1 A_1} = \frac{0.1845\ \frac{lbm}{\sec}}{1.8376\ \frac{lbm}{ft^3} \cdot \frac{\pi}{4}\left(\frac{0.5}{12}ft\right)^2} = 73.6\ \frac{ft}{\sec}$$

This flow velocity corresponds to a flow Mach number at the hose inlet of

$$M_1 = \frac{V_1}{\sqrt{g_c\,k\,R\,T}} = \frac{73.6\ \frac{ft}{\sec}}{\sqrt{32.2\ \frac{ft\text{-}lbm}{lbf\text{-}sec^2}\,(1.66)\left(360.7\ \frac{ft\text{-}lbf}{lbm\text{-}°R}\right)(500\,°R)}}$$

or

$$M_1 = 0.0237$$

Also, the Reynolds number corresponding to this flow at inlet conditions is

$$Re_1 = \frac{\rho_1 V_1 D}{\mu_1} = \frac{1.8376\,(73.6)\left(\frac{0.5}{12}\right)}{1.28 \times 10^{-5}} = 4.4 \times 10^5$$

Referring to Figure 9-1, with a Reynolds number of 4.4 x 10^5, and

$$\frac{e}{D} = \frac{0.000005 \; ft}{\frac{0.5}{12} \; ft} = 0.00012$$

we find a friction factor f of 0.0145. Again, the Colebrook formula could have also been solved iteratively to find this friction factor.

Now, assuming isothermal flow in a "long hose", we can apply Equation (9-12) to obtain the following:

$$\frac{P_1^2 - P_2^2}{P_1^2} = k \; M_1^2 \; f \; \frac{L}{D} = 1.66 \; (0.0237)^2 \; (0.0145) \left(\frac{1500}{\frac{0.5}{12}} \right) = 0.4867$$

or

$$\frac{2500^2 - P_2^2}{2500^2} = 0.4867 \qquad \Rightarrow \qquad P_2^2 = 3,208,125 \left(\frac{lbf}{in^2} \right)^2$$

giving P_2 = 1791 psia, or a pressure drop in the hose of

$$P_1 - P_2 = 2500 - 1791 = 709 \; psi$$

Note: We should now check our previous assumptions in using Equation (9-11), which was only valid for subsonic flow conditions and for long hoses. In making the "long hose" assumption, recall that we assumed that

$$f \; \frac{L}{D} \gg 2 \; \ln \left(\frac{P_1}{P_2} \right)$$

Checking this assumption, we find

$$f \; \frac{L}{D} = 0.0145 \left(\frac{1500}{\frac{0.5}{12}} \right) = 522 \qquad and \qquad 2 \; \ln \left(\frac{P_1}{P_2} \right) = 0.67 \qquad [VALID]$$

Also, checking the Mach number at the end of the hose (1791 psia and 40°F)

$$\rho_2 = \frac{144 \; P}{R \; T} = \frac{144 \cdot 1791}{360.7 \cdot 500} = 1.35 \; \frac{lbm}{ft^3}$$

Applying Equation (9-8), this gives a gas velocity at the hose exhaust of

$$V_2 = \frac{\dot{m}}{\rho_2 \, A_2} = \frac{0.1845 \, \frac{lbm}{sec}}{1.35 \, \frac{lbm}{ft^3} \cdot \frac{\pi}{4} \left(\frac{0.5}{12} ft \right)^2} = 100.2 \, \frac{ft}{sec}$$

which results in a flow Mach number at the hose exit of

$$M_2 = \frac{V_2}{\sqrt{g_c \, k \, R \, T}} = \frac{100.2 \, \frac{ft}{sec}}{\sqrt{32.2 \, \frac{ft\text{-}lbm}{lbf\text{-}sec^2} \, (1.66) \left(360.7 \, \frac{ft\text{-}lbf}{lbm - {}^\circ R} \right) (500\,{}^\circ R)}}$$

or

$$M_2 = 0.032 \qquad [WELL \; BELOW \; 1.0]$$

In some applications, dealing with compressible or incompressible flows in a piping systems, the flow rate may be unknown but known pressures exist at the inlet and exit of the piping system. Under these conditions, it may be necessary to calculate the gas flow rate within the piping system with these fixed pressures. Since the flow rate is unknown in this type of problem, straight forward determinations of the friction factors and Mach numbers are not possible. An iterative approach will be necessary as described by the following example.

Example: A 1200 foot long umbilical supplies a heliox mixture containing 99% helium and 1% oxygen to a personnel transfer capsule (PTC) at a depth of 1000 FSW. The pressure at the PTC is set to be 100 psi over bottom pressure, and the manifold pressure regulator on the surface is set at 600 psig. Determine the maximum rate of gas flow in a 0.25 inch diameter hose assuming that there is sufficient heat transfer through the hose to maintain the gas at 70F. (Gas constant = 360.7 ft-lbf/lbm-R; k = 1.66, viscosity = 1.34 x 10^{-5} lbm/ft-sec)

Solution: In this example, pressures on each end of the umbilical are known, but the mass flow rate is not known. Thus, we have two unknowns--- Mach number and friction factor--- in our compressible flow equation (Equation 9-12). These two unknowns will necessitate an iterative approach in solving this problem. One method of solution is to assume a value of f to solve for the Mach number, followed by a check of this assumption. This process will allow an iterative improvement in the value of f until no further refinements are required. The following procedure could be used for this iterative method:

Since, for long pipes

$$\frac{P_1^2 - P_2^2}{P_1^2} = k \, M_1^2 \, f \, \frac{L}{D} \tag{9-13}$$

we can rearrange Equation (9-13) to solve for the unknown Mach number as

$$M_1 = \sqrt{\frac{\dfrac{P_1^2 - P_2^2}{P_1^2}}{k f \dfrac{L}{D}}}$$ (9-14)

with

$$P_1 = 600 \; psig = 614.7 \; psia = 88,516.8 \; \frac{lbf}{ft^2}$$

$$P_2 = \frac{D + 33}{33} (14.7) + 100 = 560.2 \; psia = 80,662.2 \; \frac{lbf}{ft^2}$$

These known pressures, gas properties and hose geometries can be substituted into Equation (9-14) to give an expression for the Mach number as only a function of the unknown friction factor

$$M_1 = \sqrt{\frac{\dfrac{88,516.8^2 - 80,662.2^2}{88,516.8^2}}{1.66 \; f \; \dfrac{1200}{\dfrac{0.5}{12}}}} = \sqrt{\frac{1.771 \times 10^{-6}}{f}}$$ (9-15)

This expression can be solved iteratively until the correct friction factor is found which corresponds to the calculated gas stream velocity. For instance, if we start by arbitrarily assuming a friction factor $f = 0.01$, then

$$M_1 = \sqrt{\frac{1.771 \times 10^{-6}}{0.01}} = 0.0133 = \frac{V_1}{\sqrt{g_c \; k \; R \; T}}$$

Rearranging the above expression to solve for the gas velocity at the inlet of the umbilical, we have

$$V_1 = 0.0133 \sqrt{32.2 \; \frac{ft\text{-}lbm}{lbf\text{-}sec^2} \; (1.66) \left(360.7 \; \frac{ft\text{-}lbf}{lbm\text{-}°R} \right) (530°R)} = 42.5 \; \frac{ft}{sec}$$ (9-16)

We can now calculate the Reynolds number based on this flow velocity at the inlet, with

$$\rho_1 = \frac{144 \cdot 614.7}{360.7 \cdot 530} = 0.443 \; \frac{lbm}{ft^3}$$

giving

$$Re_1 = \frac{\rho_1 \, V_1 \, D}{\mu_1} = \frac{0.443 \, \frac{lbm}{ft^3} \left(42.5 \, \frac{ft}{sec} \right) (0.0208 \, ft)}{1.34 \, x \, 10^{-5} \, \frac{lbm}{ft-sec}} = 2.92 \, x \, 10^4 \qquad \text{(9-17)}$$

Referring to the Moody diagram, Figure 9-1, with this Reynolds number of 2.92×10^4 and a roughness factor e/D for drawn tubing of

$$\frac{e}{D} = \frac{0.000005 \, ft}{\frac{0.5}{12} \, ft} = 0.00012$$

we obtain a friction factor $f = 0.024$. This differs significantly from our original assumption for f of 0.01. Thus, we will repeat the sequence of solutions for Equations (9-15), (9-16), and (9-17) with this new friction factor, $f = 0.024$, giving

$$M_1 = 0.0086 \quad \Rightarrow \quad V_1 = 27.5 \quad \Rightarrow \quad Re_1 = 1.89 \, x \, 10^4 \quad \Rightarrow \quad f = 0.026$$

A second iteration, now using the refined value for the friction factor, $f = 0.026$, gives

$$M_1 = 0.0083 \quad \Rightarrow \quad V_1 = 26.5 \quad \Rightarrow \quad Re_1 = 1.82 \, x \, 10^4 \quad \Rightarrow \quad f = 0.026$$

This stabilized solution for the friction factor indicates that the maximum rate of gas flow through the umbilical with the conditions described above will have an inlet velocity of 26.5 ft/sec, giving a volumetric flow rate at inlet conditions of the following:

$$\dot{V}_1 = V_1 \, A_1 = 26.5 \, \frac{ft}{sec} \cdot \frac{\pi}{4} (0.0208 \, ft)^2 = 9 \, x \, 10^{-3} \frac{ft^3}{sec} \qquad [0.54 \, CFM]$$

and the mass flow rate will be

$$\dot{m} = \rho_1 \, \dot{V}_1 = 0.443 \, \frac{lbm}{ft^3} \cdot 9 \, x \, 10^{-3} \, \frac{ft^3}{sec} = 3.99 \, x \, 10^{-3} \, \frac{lbm}{sec}$$

It is left for the reader to confirm the validity of our "long hose" assumption, and also confirm that the Mach number remains below 1.0 throughout the umbilical.

9.4   Pumps and Compressors

It is often necessary to estimate the power requirements needed to supply the required flow rates of liquids or gases in a life support system loop or umbilical. To arrive at these estimates, it will first be necessary to determine the amount of mechanical work involved in propelling the gases or liquids through the circuit. Again, we will look at liquids as incompressible, viscous fluids and gases as compressible, ideal fluids.

9.4.1 Requirements for Pumping Liquids

In a typical hydraulic system, as shown in Figure 9-3, the fluid is being pumped down to a diver or hydraulic tool. The liquid will be pumped from a supply at surface pressure and delivered through a hose (including connectors, valves, bends, etc) to an elevated pressure at the diver site.

The steady flow energy equation for this incompressible, viscous flow system was given previously as

$$Z_1 + \frac{V_1^2}{2g} + \frac{P_1}{\gamma} = Z_2 + \frac{V_2^2}{2g} + \frac{P_2}{\gamma} + wk_{12}\frac{g_c}{g} + H_{L_{12}} \qquad (9\text{-}18)$$

where 1 and 2 identifies any two locations in the circuit, and wk_{12} is the mechanical work done on the fluid by a pump between these two locations. Notice that by sign convention, the value of wk_{12} in this equation will be negative when work is done on the fluid by the pump.

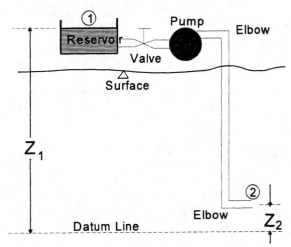

Once this value of work is found, the power requirement to run the pump can be found by

$$WHP = \frac{\dot{m}\ |wk_P|}{550\ \dfrac{ft\text{-}lbf}{Hp\text{-}sec}} \qquad (9\text{-}19)$$

where *WHP* is the required *water horsepower*, i.e., the power delivered to the fluid; and $\dot{m}$ is the mass flow rate of the fluid, lbm/sec. The *brake horsepower, BHP*, or the power which must be delivered to the pump from an external motor, can be related to the pump efficiency as

Figure 9-3: Pumping liquids to a location beneath the surface.

$$BHP = \frac{WHP}{\eta_P} \qquad (9\text{-}20)$$

where η_P is defined as the *pump efficiency* which accounts for the frictional losses in the pump. A typical pumping application will best illustrate the power requirements to deliver a flow of liquids to a location beneath the surface.

Example: Water is being pumped at a rate of 3 gallons per minute from a surface reservoir to a depth of 250 FSW. The water is being supplied through 300 feet of smooth plastic pipe having an internal diameter of 0.5 inches. The umbilical entry pressure required to maintain this flow rate was shown previously to be 46.7 psi (see earlier example at beginning of this chapter). What power must be supplied to the pump to maintain this flow if the pump efficiency is 60%? (The density of the water being pumped is 62.4 lbm/ft³; local acceleration of gravity is 32.2 ft/sec²)

Solution: Since the locations identified in Equation (9-18) can be arbitrary, we will assume location #1 is the inlet to the pump, and location #2 is the pump exit as shown in Figure 9-4; the elevations (i.e., Z locations) and cross-sectional areas of the pump inlet and exit are assumed to be equal. Water from the surface reservoir is assumed to enter the pump at 14.7 psia and exit the pump at 46.7 psia.

Rearranging Equation (9-18) to solve for pump work, we have

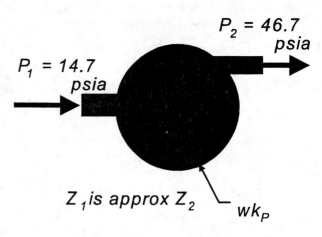

Figure 9-4: Pump requirements to deliver water to a diver at 250 FSW..

$$wk_P \left(\frac{g_c}{g} \right) = (Z_1 - Z_2) + \frac{V_1^2 - V_2^2}{2g} + \frac{P_1 - P_2}{\gamma} - H_{L_{12}}$$

Continuity of flow across the pump requires that

$$\dot{m}_1 = \dot{m}_2$$

or

$$(\rho \, V \, A)_1 = (\rho \, V \, A)_2$$

where ρ is the fluid density (ρ_1 and ρ_2 are constant for incompressible flow); V is the flow velocity and A is the cross-sectional area of the pump inlet and exit. However, since the pump inlet and exit areas are equal, then

$$V_1 = V_2$$

and approximately equal elevations of the inlet and exit give

$$Z_1 \approx Z_2$$

Also, the head loss across the pump will be assumed to equal zero in the above analysis and later accounted for using the pump efficiency. Making the above substitutions above gives

$$wk_P\left(\frac{g_c}{g}\right) = 0 + 0 + \frac{\left(14.7\ \frac{lbf}{in^2} - 46.7\ \frac{lbf}{in^2}\right)144\frac{in^2}{ft^2}}{\gamma\ \frac{lbf}{ft^3}}$$

where

$$\gamma = \rho\left(\frac{g}{g_c}\right) = 62.4\ \frac{lbm}{ft^3} \cdot \frac{32.2\ \frac{ft}{sec^2}}{32.2\ \frac{lbm\text{-}ft}{lbf\text{-}sec^2}} = 62.4\ \frac{lbf}{ft^3}$$

Thus,

$$wk_P\left(\frac{g_c}{g}\right) = \frac{(14.7 - 46.7)\cdot 144}{62.4} = -73.8\ ft$$

or

$$wk_P = -73.8\ ft \cdot \frac{32.2\ \frac{ft}{sec^2}}{32.2\ \frac{lbm\text{-}ft}{lbf\text{-}sec^2}} = -73.8\ \frac{ft\text{-}lbf}{lbm}$$

This mechanical work can now be substituted into Equation (9-19) to give the power delivered to the water from the pump as

$$WHP = \frac{\dot{m}\ |wk_P|}{550\ \frac{ft\text{-}lbf}{Hp\text{-}sec}}$$

$$WHP = \frac{3\ \frac{gal}{min} \cdot \frac{ft^3}{7.48\ gal} \cdot \frac{1\ min}{60\ sec} \cdot 62.4\ \frac{lbm}{ft^3} \cdot |-73.8|\ \frac{ft\text{-}lbf}{lbm}}{550\ \frac{ft\text{-}lbf}{Hp\text{-}sec}} = 0.055\ Hp$$

Applying Equation (9-20), the brake horsepower can now be found as

$$BHP = \frac{WHP}{\eta_P} = \frac{0.055}{0.6} = 0.092 \; Hp$$

9.4.2 Compressor Requirements

The work, and consequently the power, required to compress gases can be approximated by assuming that the fluid behaves as an ideal gas while undergoing a polytropic process. A polytropic process is defined as any process in which the relationship between pressure and specific volume for the gas can be described as

$$P \, v^n = C \tag{9-21}$$

where C is a constant, P is pressure, v is the gas specific volume and n is the polytropic exponent, with

$$0 < n < \infty$$

Note: The polytropic exponent for a constant temperature process can be shown to have a value of 1, giving Equation (9-21) the form

$$P \, v = Constant$$

which was shown in Chapter 2 to be an expression of Boyles Law. Similarly, a constant pressure process will have a polytropic exponent n equal to zero, giving

$$P \, v^0 = Constant \qquad or \qquad P = Constant$$

During a compression process involving an idea gas, a reversible, adiabatic (isentropic) process will be assumed where the polytropic exponent n is equal to the ratio of the gas specific heats k. I.e.,

$$n = k = \frac{c_p}{c_v}$$

If we define the condition of an ideal gas at the beginning of this isentropic compression process as state point #1, and the condition of the gas at the completion of the compression process as state point #2, this polytropic process can be described as

$$P_1 \, v_1^k = P_2 \, v_2^k \tag{9-22}$$

or

$$\frac{P_2}{P_1} = \left(\frac{v_1}{v_2}\right)^k = \left(\frac{v_2}{v_1}\right)^{-k} \tag{9-23}$$

Therefore,

$$\frac{v_2}{v_1} = \left(\frac{P_1}{P_2}\right)^{\frac{1}{k}} = \left(\frac{P_2}{P_1}\right)^{-\frac{1}{k}} \tag{9-24}$$

We can also write the equation of state for the ideal gas as

$$\frac{P_1 v_1}{T_1} = \frac{P_2 v_2}{T_2} \tag{9-25}$$

or

$$\frac{T_2}{T_1} = \left(\frac{P_2}{P_1}\right)\left(\frac{v_2}{v_1}\right) \tag{9-26}$$

Substituting the polytropic relationships given in Equations (9-23) and (9-24) into the equation of state for an ideal gas , Equation (9-26), we can show that

$$\frac{T_2}{T_1} = \left(\frac{v_1}{v_2}\right)^{k-1} = \left(\frac{P_2}{P_1}\right)^{\frac{k-1}{k}} \tag{9-27}$$

Now, for any reversible, non-flow process (i.e., a piston-cylinder arrangement as seen in a reciprocating-type compressor) the work involved in that process can be expressed as

$$wk_c = \int_1^2 P \, dv \tag{9-28}$$

where again, if the process is isentropic, we can write

$$P = \frac{C}{v^k} \tag{9-29}$$

Substituting Equation (9-29) into Equation (9-28) and integrating, the amount of work supplied by the compressor to this gas can be found as

$$wk_c = C \int_1^2 \frac{dv}{v^k} = C \left[\frac{v^{1-k}}{1-k}\right]_1^2 = C \left[\frac{v_2 v_2^{-k} - v_1 v_1^{-k}}{1-k}\right] \tag{9-30}$$

But, since

$$C = P_1 v_1^k = P_2 v_2^k \qquad (9\text{-}31)$$

then

$$wk_c = \frac{P_2 v_2^k v_2^{-k} - P_1 v_1^k v_1^{-k}}{1-k} \qquad (9\text{-}32)$$

or

$$wk_c \ (isentropic) = \frac{P_2 v_2 - P_1 v_1}{1-k} \qquad (9\text{-}34)$$

and since ideal gases can be described as $P \ v = R \ T$, we can also write

$$wk_c \ (isentropic) = \frac{R \ (T_2 - T_1)}{1-k} \qquad (9\text{-}35)$$

The deviation from isentropic behavior for the real compression process can be accounted for by defining an *isentropic compressor efficiency*

$$\eta_c = \frac{wk_c \ (isentropic)}{wk_c \ (real)} \qquad (9\text{-}36)$$

such that

$$wk_c \ (real) = \frac{P_2 v_2 - P_1 v_1}{\eta_c \ (1-k)} = \frac{R \ (T_2 - T_1)}{\eta_c \ (1-k)} \qquad (9\text{-}37)$$

The power requirements for the real compression process can then be determined in a manner similar to that which was used previously to find the pumping requirements for incompressible liquids; i.e.,

$$HP_c = \frac{\dot{m} \ |wk_c \ (real)|}{550 \ \dfrac{ft\text{-}lbf}{Hp\text{-}sec}} \qquad (9\text{-}38)$$

The following example will demonstrate the application of these principles to find the power requirements for gas compressors.

Example: A single-stage air compressor delivers air from inlet conditions of 14.7 psia to outlet conditions of 200 psia at the rate of 1000 SCFM. The isentropic compressor efficiency is 60% and the mechanical efficiency of the compressor is 75%. What size motor is required to run this compressor? (The ratio of specific heats for air is 1.4; the gas constant for air is 53.3 ft-lbf/lbm-°R; inlet temperature of the air is 70°F.)

Solution: At state point #1, the density of the air is (standard conditions of 70°F, 14.7 psia)

$$\rho_1 = \frac{144 \, P_1}{R \, T} = \frac{144 \, \frac{in^2}{ft^2} \cdot 14.7 \, \frac{lbf}{in^2}}{53.3 \, \frac{ft-lbf}{lbm-°R} \cdot 530°R} = 0.075 \, \frac{lbm}{ft^3}$$

and

$$v_1 = \frac{1}{\rho_1} = 13.35 \, \frac{ft^3}{lbm}$$

Assuming an isentropic compression process, we can write

$$P_1 \, v_1^{\,k} = P_2 \, v_2^{\,k} \qquad or \qquad v_2 = v_1 \left(\frac{P_1}{P_2} \right)^{\frac{1}{k}}$$

or

$$v_2 = 13.35 \left(\frac{14.7}{200} \right)^{\frac{1}{1.4}} = 2.07 \, \frac{ft^3}{lbm}$$

and

$$wk_c \, (isentropic) = \frac{200 \, \frac{lbf}{in^2} \left(144 \, \frac{in^2}{ft^2} \right) \left(2.07 \, \frac{ft^3}{lbm} \right) - 14.7 \, \frac{lbf}{in^2} \left(144 \, \frac{in^2}{ft^2} \right) \left(13.35 \, \frac{ft^3}{lbm} \right)}{1-1.4}$$

$$wk_c \, (isentropic) = -78,294 \, \frac{ft-lbf}{lbm}$$

The actual work involved in this compression process is found by applying the definition of the isentropic efficiency given in Equation (9-36)

$$wk_c \, (real) = \frac{-78,294}{\eta_c} = \frac{-78,294}{0.6} = -130,490 \, \frac{ft-lbf}{lbm}$$

(Note: The negative sign confirms that work is being done on the working fluid.)

The power requirement is now found using Equation (9-38) with an air mass flow rate given by

$$\dot{m} = \rho_{SCFM} \cdot \dot{V}_{SCFM} = 0.075 \, \frac{lbm}{ft^3} \left(1000 \frac{ft^3}{min} \right) \left(\frac{min}{60 \, sec} \right) = 1.25 \, \frac{lbm}{sec}$$

This gives

$$HP_c = \frac{1.25 \; \dfrac{lbm}{sec} \; \left| \; -130{,}490 \; \dfrac{ft-lbf}{lbm} \; \right|}{550 \; \dfrac{ft-lbf}{Hp-sec}} = 296.6 \; Hp$$

A motor used to drive this compressor would have to deliver a brake horsepower of

$$BHP = \frac{HP_c}{\eta_{Mech}} = \frac{296.6}{0.75} = 395.4 \; Hp$$

9.5   Closure

Pumps and compressors are essential components of any underwater or hyperbaric diving system. Proper sizing of these components to deliver the correct flow rates of gases and liquids is critically important to achieve adequate ventilation and thermal protection. The laws and principles discussed in this chapter should provide the basic tools to satisfy these requirements.

10

UBA Design

Objectives

The objectives of this chapter are to
● introduce the student to various types of underwater breathing apparatus and present an overview of critical engineering concerns which must be considered when designing these breathing circuits
● assess the gas supply requirements for different classes of underwater breathing apparatus
● give a description of lung volumes and circuit volume requirements
● give an assessment of the critical breathing characteristics of an apparatus, including static lung loading, peak inhalation and exhalation pressures, circuit work-of-breathing and dynamic elastance
● conduct an analysis of circuit weight and buoyancy including the importance of component placement
● discuss the hydrodynamic resistance of various breathing apparatus.

10.1 Introduction

Underwater breathing apparatus (UBA's) can be categorized according to the manner in which breathing gases are delivered to the diver. This differentiation of UBA designs conventionally fits into one of three classes as depicted in Figure 10-1; open-circuit, semi-closed circuit, or closed circuit. While this broad classification covers the manner in which gas is utilized in the UBA, it does not fully differentiate the specific manner in which gases are delivered for sub-categories of each. The U. S. Navy (U.S. NEDU, 1994) has established a useful classification system for UBA's which will be used here to identify performance goals for 5 different UBA categories, including

- Category 1. Open-circuit, demand systems
- Category 2. Open-circuit, umbilical supplied, demand systems
- Category 3. Open-circuit, umbilical supplied, steady-flow systems
- Category 4. Closed and semi-closed, lung powered systems
- Category 5. Semi-closed, ejector or pump driven systems

A general description of UBA categories will follow in the order of the quantity of gas that is required to operate these systems.

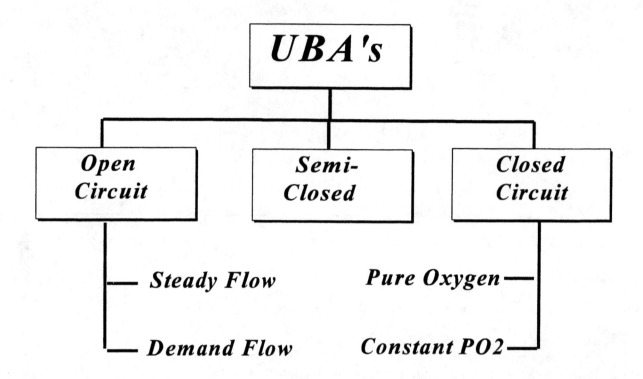

Figure 10-1: Classifications of underwater breathing apparatus.

10.1.1   Open-Circuit Systems, Categories 1, 2 and 3

The least complex of these categories are the UBA's which operate in an open circuit mode, whereby a fresh breathing gas supply is continually delivered to the diver via a surface-supplied umbilical or a diver-carried gas source. While simple in design, these systems are extremely wasteful of gas and find practical applications only in relatively shallow diving operations.

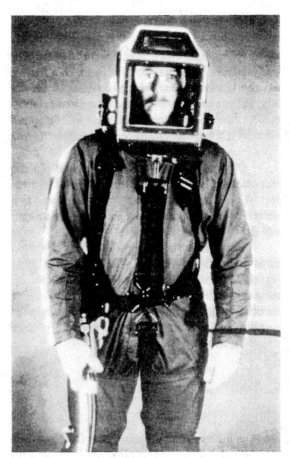

Figure 10-2: MK 12 Surface Supplied Diving System--open-circuit, steady-flow UBA. (U.S. Navy photo)

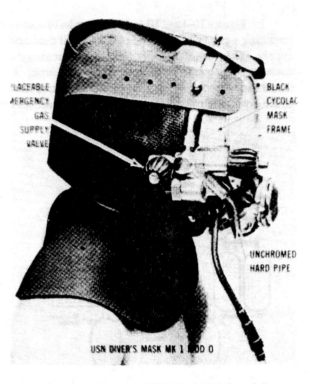

Figure 10-3: U.S. Navy MK 1 Mod 0 Lightweight Diving System--open-circuit, demand flow UBA. (U.S. Navy photo.)

Figures 10-2 and 10-3 show two different versions of an open-circuit system. The first type, very similar in design to the early diving helmets developed by Augustus Siebe (ca 1840) and typified today by the U. S. Navy's MK 12 Surface Supplied Diving System, uses a steady stream of gas to ventilate the diver's helmet or face mask. The rate at which gas is supplied to these systems is generally established to ensure that metabolically-produced carbon dioxide from the diver is adequately flushed from the helmet or mask. Although the diver uses only a small portion of the oxygen content from the respiratory gases in these systems, the carbon dioxide-enriched exhaust gases are purged to the surrounding seawater, making the remaining oxygen in this exhaust gas unavailable to the diver.

The second type of open-circuit system shown in Figure 10-3, typified by the presence of a demand regulator similar to that used in the "Aqua Lung" developed by Jacques Cousteau and Emile Gagnan during the mid-1940's, has become the system of choice for sport divers today and most shallow, surface-supplied operations. These systems supply a fresh stream of breathing gas at ambient water pressure upon demand during the diver's inspiration phase. During the exhalation phase the demand regulator closes and the fresh supply of gas ceases until the diver's inhalation triggers the demand valve to re-open. Gas consumption when using these systems is directly linked to the diver's activity level and is quantified by the respiratory minute volume (RMV), seen previously in Chapter 3. While more gas conservative than the steady flow systems, the exhaust gases from such open-circuit, demand systems contain approximately 17% oxygen when air is the supply gas--unused oxygen which is lost to the surrounding seawater. There is also a considerable volume of inert gas (typically nitrogen or helium) that will be lost along with the oxygen.

10.1.2   Semi-Closed Circuit Systems, Categories 4 and 5

Figures 10-4 and 10-5 show examples of underwater breathing apparatuses which recirculate most of the diver's breathing gases, while injecting only a small percentage (nominally 10%) of the total circuit flow with a fresh gas supply. The fresh gas supply delivers the necessary make-up oxygen to compensate for the oxygen that the diver consumes during each pass through the diver's lungs. Consequently, approximately 10% of the total circuit flow will be exhausted from the circuit to maintain a constant circuit volume. The remainder of the circuit flow will be recycled to the diver after passing through a chemical scrubber to remove the diver's metabolically-produced carbon dioxide.

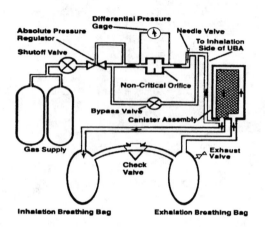

Figure 10-4: MK 6 Semi-closed circuit UBA; self-contained (U.S. Navy photo).

Obviously, semi-closed systems are far more conservative of the breathing gas supply as shown in Table 10.1. This makes their utility for deep diving applications more practical than either open-circuit steady flow, or demand systems.

The injection of fresh gas into these systems can occur in two different methods. The MK 6 UBA, Figure 10-4, utilized a simple metering valve (sonic orifice) to inject a constant mass flow rate into the circuit. These sonic orifices are based on the principle that as long as the ratio of downstream-to-upstream pressures surrounding these orifices is

$$\frac{P_2}{P_1} \leq \left(\frac{2}{k+1} \right)^{\frac{k}{k-1}} \qquad \textbf{(10-1)}$$

where P_1 is the upstream pressure, P_2 is the downstream pressure, and k is the ratio of specific heats for the

injected gas, the flow through the orifice will be sonic (choked flow), and the mass of the gas passing through these orifices will remain constant. For air or oxygen, where k = 1.4, this ratio is 0.528 (the ratio is 0.488 when injecting helium). This implies that as long as the downstream pressure on these injectors remains less than 52.8% of the upstream pressure, the injected mass flow rate will be constant. The injection flow rate, controlled only by the diameter of the orifice, must be carefully determined to ensure that sufficient oxygen will be added to the circuit in the makeup gas to maintain a safe oxygen level within the circuit over a wide range of diver oxygen consumption rates.

For deep diving applications, the injection of fresh gas can be used to assist in the movement of gas flow around the semi-closed circuit. The

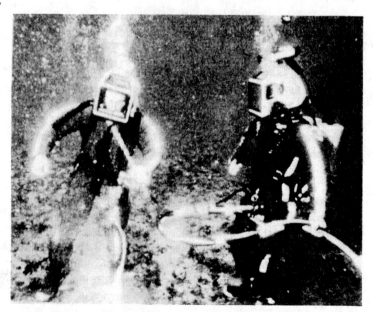

Figure 10-5: MK12 Mixed-Gas Diving System; surface-supplied, semi-closed circuit. (U.S. Navy photo.)

MK12 Mixed-Gas Surface Supported Diving System, shown in Figure 10-5, includes a small gas ejector, or jet pump. A small, high pressure stream (primary flow or makeup gas) is injected through this gas ejector into the breathing circuit to drive the gas circulation (secondary flow). This resulting pumping action assists the diver in propelling dense gases around the breathing circuit, thereby offsetting the added flow resistance of these dense gases which would otherwise lead to diver fatigue. A proper selection of the ejector nozzle has been shown to maximize the efficiency of this pumping action (Nuckols and Sexton, 1987).

10.1.3 Closed-Circuit Systems, Category 4

The most conservative type of breathing apparatuses with regard to minimizing gas requirements are the closed-circuit UBA's. These systems can be categorizes as either pure *oxygen rebreathers*, like the Draeger LAR V shown in Figure 10-6, or *mixed-gas systems* which maintain a constant partial pressure of oxygen, represented by the U.S. Navy's MK 16 shown in Figure 10-7. Both systems use the diver's lung power to recirculate the breathing gases through a carbon dioxide scrubber during the diver's exhalation, followed by these gases residing in some type of counterlung within the circuit (the counterlung could consist of one or more breathing bags, a diaphragm or bellows) until the diver is ready to start his inhalation phase. Since no gases are exhausted to the surrounding seawater, the oxygen consumed by the diver is the only gas volume that needs to be replenished within the circuit, except when the circuit gases are compressed as the diver increases depth. The absence of exhaust gases also means no tell tale bubbles are left in the diver's track, making these systems desirable where covertness is important.

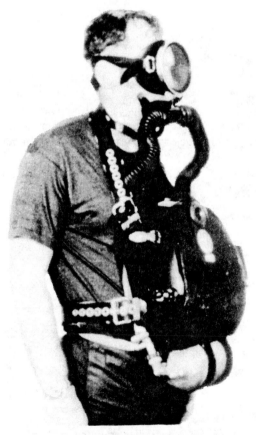

Figure 10-6: Draeger LAR V closed-circuit pure oxygen rebreather. (U.S. Navy photo.)

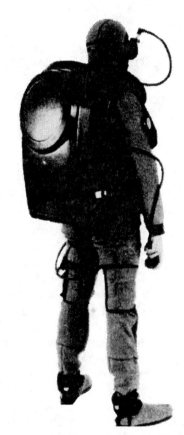

Figure 10-7: MK 16 closed-circuit, constant oxygen partial pressure UBA. (U.S. Navy photo.)

The first pure oxygen rebreather was designed in 1879 by Henry Fleuss, an English merchant seaman. His system, utilizing caustic potash for carbon dioxide absorption and an oxygen source pressurized to only 450 psig -- the state-of-the-art in pressure vessel technology at that time, allowed Alexander Lambert in 1880 to swim back into a flooded tunnel being built under the Severn River in England to close a jammed door and make necessary repairs. Simple in design and operation, pure oxygen rebreathers are limited to shallow operations due to the possibility of oxygen toxicity (see discussion of oxygen toxicity in Chapter 3).

When closed-circuit operations are required at depths beyond approximately 25 feet of seawater, dilution of the oxygen content in the breathing circuit is necessary. Generally, this dilution is accomplished with some inert gas such as nitrogen or helium. However, since the diver will consume the oxygen within the circuit, it is necessary to accurately monitor the breathing atmosphere to ensure that the oxygen level will not drop too low to cause hypoxia nor become to high to cause oxygen toxicity. For the breathing apparatus shown in Figure 10-7, similar in design to the U.S. Navy's MK15 and MK16 UBA's, oxygen is mixed with a *diluent gas* to maintain a preset oxygen partial pressure (PO_2) which is within the physiologically acceptable limits for the diver--generally in the neighborhood of 0.7 ATA. *Oxygen sensors* continually monitor the oxygen level in the circuit, and electrically signal either solenoid or piezo-electric valves to add oxygen when these sensors detect that the level of oxygen has dropped below the preset value. While such systems are able to provide gas-efficient operations to depths in excess of 200 FSW, the additional complexity of these electronic systems makes their cost significantly higher than pure oxygen rebreathers.

10.2 Engineering Design Considerations

When designing an underwater breathing apparatus, whether open, semi-closed or closed-circuit, it is critically important that the breathing circuit provides a gas environment which is adequate for the mission. Additionally, the physical characteristics of the system should not place undue limitations on the diver's ability to breathe normally and work productively. The following engineering concerns must be carefully evaluated to minimize restrictions on the diver:

Engineering Design Concerns For UBA's

- Provide adequate gas source
- Provide adequate carbon dioxide removal/adsorption
- Provide provisions for condensation
- Minimize external dead space
- Provide sufficient counter-lung volume
- Minimize static lung loading
- Minimize peak inhalation/exhalation pressures
- Minimize work-of-breathing (resistive breathing effort)
- Minimize system weight (air) and buoyancy
- Match center-of-gravity with center-of-buoyancy
- Minimize hydrodynamic resistance

Carbon dioxide removal and the removal of condensation from breathing apparatuses were previously discussed in Chapter 5 and will not be repeated here. The reader should review Chapter 5 when addressing this critical design concern for underwater breathing apparatuses.

10.3 Gas Requirements

The primary advantage of closed and semi-closed breathing apparatus when compared to open-circuit systems is the savings in respiratory gases, particularly as the mission depth increases. These gas savings with closed and semi-closed systems are usually offset with added design complexity, as discussed above, and increased operational maintenance; i.e., scrubbers, breathing bags, oxygen sensors, etc. The following example compares the gas requirements for different categories of UBA's for a typical dive mission to demonstrate their gas consumptions relative to open-circuit, demand systems.

Example: Calculate the gas requirements for a moderately hard working diver at 200 FSW in 50°F water. Compare the relative consumption rates for different categories of UBA circuits.

Solution: We saw earlier (Figure 3-5) that a moderately hard working diver can be expected to have a respiratory minute volume (RMV) of approximately 18-35 liters per minute (BTPS)[10]; i.e., at conditions of body temperature (98.6°F), ambient pressure (in this example 7.06 ATA, and saturated with water vapor. Let's assume that the diver RMV is 30 LPM with a corresponding oxygen consumption rate, given by Equation (3-2), of

$$\dot{V}_{O_2} , SLPM = \frac{RMV\ (BTPS)}{24} = 1.25$$

Delivery of this quantity of oxygen to meet the metabolic requirements of the diver can be met in different ways depending on the type of circuit design, as the following analyses will show.

10.3.1   Open-circuit, steady flow

The ventilation requirements for a diver's helmet or full face mask was given earlier in Equation (6-22) as

$$\dot{V}_{gas}, SCFM = \frac{P_T * \dot{V}_{O_2} * RQ * F}{26.3\ [P_{CO_2}\ (design\ point) - P_{CO_2}\ (input)]}$$

If we assume a typical respiratory quotient (RQ) of 0.85 (defined by Equation (3-3)) and a mixing effectiveness factor **F** of 1.0 (i.e., complete mixing within the helmet as defined by Equation (6-21)), the required ventilation rate when using surface air (containing 0.035% carbon dioxide) to maintain a carbon dioxide level of 1.0% SEV (0.01 ATA) within the helmet is

$$\dot{V}_{gas}, SCFM = \frac{7.06 * 1.25 * 0.85 * 1}{26.3\ [\ 0.01 - 0.00035\ (7.06)]} = 37.9\ SCFM$$

---

[10]Specified conditions as follows:
BTPS--98.6 °F, surrounding seawater pressure
Standard liters (SL) or standard liters per minute (SLPM)--32 °F, 1.0 ATA
Standard cubic feet (SCF) or standard cubic feet per minute (SCFM)--70 °F, 1.0 ATA

Noting the conditions for SCFM are 1.0 ATA and 70°F, the actual ventilation rate (ACFM[11]) at bottom conditions can be found using Equation 10-2 below to give

$$\dot{V}_{gas}, \, ACFM = \dot{V}_{gas}, \, SCFM \; * \; \left(\frac{1.0 \; ATA}{7.06 \; ATA} \right) \; * \; \left(\frac{50 \; + \; 460° \; R}{530° \; R} \right) = 5.2 \; ACFM$$

The results given in the above example are not unlike those for most open-circuit, steady flow systems where ventilation rates are typically set at 4 - 6 ACFM to flush metabolically-produced carbon dioxide from the helmet or mask.

10.3.2   Open-Circuit, Demand Flow

Since respiratory gases will be exhausted to the surrounding environment only during exhalation with an open-circuit, demand system, the gas consumption rate for these systems is exactly equal to the diver's respiratory minute volume (RMV). Thus, in this comparison example the diver is consuming gas a 30 liters per minute, BTPS (98.6°F, 7.06 ATA). At standard conditions, the equivalent consumption rate is

$$\dot{V}_{gas}, \, SCFM = \frac{\dot{V}_{gas}, \, BTPS}{28.3 \; liters/ft^3} \left(\frac{7.06 \; ATA}{1.0 \; ATA} \right) \left(\frac{530° \; R}{98.6 \; + \; 460° \; R} \right) = 7.1 \; SCFM$$

In this example, the gas consumption requirements for the demand flow system are seen to be less than 20% of that for the steady-flow system shown above.

10.3.3   Semi-Closed Circuit, Lung Driven

For lung-driven systems, similar to that shown in Figure 10-4, the rate at which gas is circulated around the circuit is equal to the diver's respiratory minute volume. As discussed in section 10.1.2 above, fresh makeup gas is generally injected through a small metering valve at a rate equivalent to approximately 10% of this circuit flow rate. We can easily see that this injection rate will be 10% of the gas consumption shown above for the open-circuit, demand system, or

$$\dot{V}_{gas} = 0.7 \; SCFM$$

This recycling of approximately 90% of the circuit flow represents a considerable gas savings.

---

[11]Actual cubic feet per minute (ACFM) can be found as follows

$$\dot{V}_{gas}, \, ACFM = \dot{V}_{gas}, \, SCFM \; * \; \left(\frac{1.0 \; ATA}{P_{Depth} \; ATA} \right) \; * \; \left(\frac{T^o_{Depth} \; R}{530° \; R} \right) \qquad \text{(10-2)}$$

10.3.4   Semi-Closed Circuit, Ejector Driven

Semi-closed systems used in deep diving, such as the system shown in Figure 10-5, will maintain a helmet ventilation rate of 4-6 ACFM to keep the carbon dioxide levels in the helmet manageable; similar to the helmet ventilation rates shown above for open, steady flow systems. However, during these applications a jet pump is used to drive the circulation through the diver's helmet and carbon dioxide scrubber. While the design of this jet pump must be optimized for the specific mission, the primary flow to drive these jet pumps can be estimated as 10% of the circuit flow, or 0.52 ACFM for this example. At standard conditions, the equivalent consumption rate in this example will be

$$\dot{V}_{gas}, SCFM = 0.52\ ACFM \left(\frac{7.06\ ATA}{1.0\ ATA} \right) \left(\frac{530^o\ R}{50\ +\ 460^o\ R} \right) = 3.8\ SCFM$$

10.3.5   Closed-Circuit, Pure Oxygen

Closed-circuit systems provide the maximum level of gas conservation. Since the only gas leaving the circuit is the oxygen being consumed by the diver, $\dot{V}_{O_2}$, the gas consumption rate for an oxygen rebreather in this example would be 1.25 SLPM. For comparison purposes, this consumption rate is converted into equivalent units as

$$\dot{V}_{gas}, SCFM = \frac{\dot{V}_{O_2},\ SLPM}{28.3\ liters/ft^3} \left(\frac{530^o\ R}{492^o\ R} \right) = 0.048\ SCFM$$

Note that as the diver increases depth the compression of the circuit gas volume must be compensated by the injection of additional oxygen into the circuit. However, since this oxygen is still available to the diver it is not considered as a consumable in this comparison.

10.3.6   Closed-Circuit, Constant PO$_2$

The oxygen consumption calculated above for the oxygen rebreather will be the same for this circuit. However, a second gas source is necessary to dilute the oxygen, as necessary to maintain a constant oxygen partial pressure. The *diluent gas*, consisting of a breathable mixture of oxygen and inert gas, is injected through a demand valve located in the breathing bag to compensate for the compression of the circuit volume as the diver goes to depth. However, after the diver reaches his maximum depth, further injection of the diluent gas should not be necessary. The bottle capacity for this diluent gas is generally rated the same as the oxygen bottle.

10.3.7   Comparison of Gas Requirements

Table 10.1 compares the gas supply requirements for a moderately hard working diver at 200 FSW with the different breathing apparatus circuits discussed above. The relative consumption rate is based on the consumption rate of the familiar open-circuit, demand systems being used by most sport divers. The duration calculations give the times for a diver to consume the gas in a bottle which is rated at 80 SCF when pressurized to 3000 psig (205 ATA) at 70°F.

It should be noted that not all of the gas contained in the bottle will be available to the diver since some of the gas volume will continue to reside in the bottle after the bottle pressure comes into equilibrium with the surrounding seawater pressure. This *residual volume* for a bottle, expressed in standard cubic feet (SCF), can be calculated using the formula

$$V_{Residual}, \ SCF = V_{Rated}, \ SCF \left(\frac{P_{Depth}, \ ATA}{P_{Rated}, \ ATA} \right) \left(\frac{530^\circ \ R}{T^{\ o}_{Depth} \ R} \right) \tag{10-3}$$

where V_{Rated} is the rated capacity of the bottle in SCF, P_{Depth} is the surrounding seawater pressure, P_{Rated} is the bottle pressure when filled to rated capacity, and T_{Depth} is the surrounding seawater temperature. Equation 10-3 can be used to determine the available volume of gas left in this 80 SCF bottle after pressure equalizes with the ambient pressure at 200 FSW (7.06 ATA) at 50°F as

$$V_{avail}, \ SCF = 80 \left[1 - \left(\frac{7.06 \ ATA}{205 \ ATA} \right) \left(\frac{530^\circ \ R}{50 + 460^\circ \ R} \right) \right] = 77.1 \ SCF$$

Table 10.1 compares the time that it will take a diver to consume this available volume when using the different UBA circuit designs discussed above. Note that the extremely long duration shown for the closed-circuit design would be excessive for most dive missions; a smaller bottle capacity would generally be used.

Table 10-1: Comparison of Gas Consumption Rates For Different UBA Circuit Modes
(Moderately hard working diver at 200 FSW)

Circuit Mode	Gas Consumption, SCFM	Relative Consumption[3]	Duration of 80 SCF Bottle, minutes
Open, Steady Flow	37.9	5.33	2.03
Open, Demand Flow	7.1	1.0	10.9
Semi-Closed, Lung Driven	0.71	0.1	108.6
Semi-Closed, Ejector Driven	3.8	0.54	20.3
Closed Circuit	0.048	0.0068	1606 (26.8 hrs)

[3] Gas consumption rates are compared with open-circuit, demand flow systems.

10.4 Static Lung Loading

Breathing gases enter the lungs whenever the pressure inside the lungs drops below the pressure of the gas source that we are breathing. This reduction in lung pressure is created when our diaphragm and the muscles surrounding the ribcage cause the lung volume to expand. The inverse relationship between the pressure and volume of gases dictates that this lung volume expansion will result in a drop in pressure, resulting in inhalation. The reverse sequence, diaphragm relaxation followed by a reduction in lung volume, will occur during the exhalation phase. During normal respiration at surface conditions, the amplitudes of these pressure variations in the lungs will be extremely small, generally varying from atmospheric pressure by less than 1 mmHg (Guyton, 1976, pg 517). While an average adult can develop lung pressures in excess of 100 mmHg during a single forced expiration against a large external resistance, and a negative lung pressure of approximately -80 mmHg during a forced inhalation, such pressure extremes could not be maintained during normal respiration. Indeed, during surface air breathing the lung pressure will vary only minimally with the gas source pressure.

In the case of a diver, the weight of water pressing around a diver's ribcage can make it difficult for him to breathe unless the gas source from which the diver is breathing is at a pressure sufficient to counterbalance these inward forces. A gas source that is pressurized higher than the water pressure surrounding the ribcage will create a positive hydrostatic imbalance (NEDU, 1994) which will tend to force-feed the diver with gas during inspiration, but make it difficult for the diver to exhale. Conversely, a gas source that is at a lower pressure than the water pressure surrounding the lungs will create a negative hydrostatic imbalance which will make it more difficult for the diver to inhale, but facilitate expiration. Since the hydrostatic pressure being exerted on the ribcage varies approximately linearly with depth, it is necessary to define a reference position on the ribcage when talking about the relative hydrostatic pressures. The position of the *suprasternal notch (SN)*, the v-shaped notch at the top of the sternum, has become the accepted reference point for describing positions around the diver's lungs. In an upright man, the suprasternal notch lies approximately 17 cm below the mouth (Knafelc, 1988).

The schematics shown in Figure 10-8 demonstrate how these hydrostatic imbalances (often called *static lung loadings*) between the surrounding water pressure at the level of the suprasternal notch and the breathing gas source are established in a UBA design, and the importance of the compliant volume locations (ie, breathing bags locations) in a breathing circuit. Imagine in the first schematic, Figure 10-8a, that the diver's source of breathing gas is the gas which has been captured in an inverted bucket having an open bottom. When breathing air on the surface through a hose connected to this inverted bucket, the air source pressure within the bucket will not vary from the air pressure exerted against the outside of the ribcage. Small cyclic variations in lung pressure, above and below atmospheric, will occur as the diver breathes from this source.

Next, submerge the diver and his breathing source as shown in Figure 10-8b. As the bucket is lowered in the water column, the air/water interface inside the bucket will gradually move upward until the pressure of the gas trapped in the bucket equals the hydrostatic pressure at the depth of this interface. Note in this condition that the vertical position of this air/water interface is at the same depth as the diver's suprasternal notch. Similar to the breathing characteristics seen in Figure 10-8a, small cyclic variations in lung pressure will occur above and below the suprasternal notch reference pressure during respiration. The same breathing characteristics could be established with a closed-circuit UBA having a breathing bag that is positioned at the same vertical position as the suprasternal notch provided that the collapse plane of the bag, the vertical plane separating the full and empty portions of the bag, is at the same vertical position as the SN.

In Figure 10-8c, the inverted bucket has been lowered in the water column such that the position of the air/water interface is at a greater depth than the SN reference plane. Under these circumstances, the pressure of the breathing source inside the bucket will be higher than the water pressure surrounding the ribcage at the level of the SN reference; i.e., a *positive static lung loading* will be established. To exhale, the diver's respiratory muscles will have to contract forcefully to expel gas back into the bucket, or similarly into a breathing bag. However, during inhalation this positive source pressure will tend to force-feed the diver.

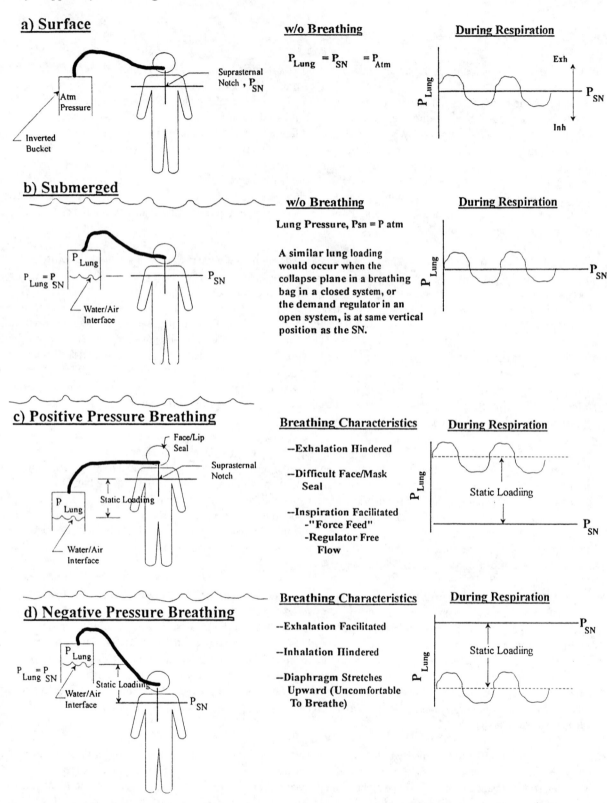

Figure 10-8: Effects of breathing bag positions and collapse plane locations on static lung loadings.

In Figure 10-8d, the inverted bucket has been elevated in the water column such that the position of the air/water interface in the bucket is at a shallower depth than the SN reference plane. Under these circumstances, the pressure of the breathing source will be lower than the water pressure surrounding the diver ribcage at the level of the SN reference plane; i.e., a *negative static lung loading* will be seen. Exhalation will be facilitated in this configuration. However, to inhale the diver will have to create a high negative pressure to pull the gas source from the bucket or a breathing bag.

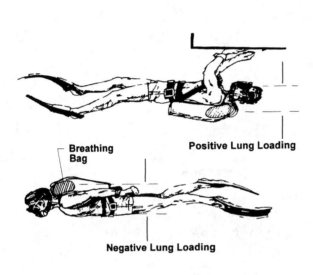

Figure 10-9: Sensitivity of diver orientation to static lung loading. (From NOAA Dive Manual, 1991)

Excessively high static lung loadings, either positive or negative, can result in diver fatigue after prolonged respiration with this hydrostatic imbalance. What then are the optimal source pressures to counterbalance the inward forces on the ribcage? What is the ideal position for breathing bag placement? Unfortunately, there is no single answer to this important design question. This uncertainty occurs since the position of the collapse plane in any breathing bag is sensitive to the orientation of the diver within the water column, as shown in Figure 10-9. A breathing circuit that has the breathing bag positioned in a backpack, similar to the U. S. Navy's MK 15 or MK16, creates a neutral-to-positive lung loading when the diver is vertical in the water column, but results in a negative lung loading when the diver is swimming in a horizontal, face down (supine) position. Positioning the breathing bag in a chest pack, similar to the LAR V, creates a near neutral lung loading when the diver is vertical, but a positive lung loading when the diver is in a supine swimming posture.

A placement of the breathing bag which will result in a static source pressure equivalent to the hydrostatic pressure that exists at the lung centroid P_{LC} appears to be the optimum pressure for diver comfort during immersion (Taylor, Morrison, 1989). Unfortunately, maintaining the breathing bag collapse plane at the lung centroid, defined as 13.6 cm below the suprasternal notch in an upright diver, and 7 cm above the plane of the sternal notch in a horizontal, face down diver, would be impractical. Short of a chest implant, this location is impossible, meaning that this optimum pressure for diver comfort cannot be obtained for all diver orientations. However, the U. S. Navy has established an allowable hydrostatic imbalance which ranges ±10 cmH$_2$O in any direction from the lung centroid pressure. For helmeted diving, the U.S. Navy Experimental Diving Unit (NEDU) recommends maintaining helmet pressures between lung centroid pressure and 10 cmH$_2$O above lung centroid pressure. For non-helmeted diving, NEDU recommends pressures ranging from lung centroid to 10 cmH$_2$O below lung centroid; see Figure 10-10.

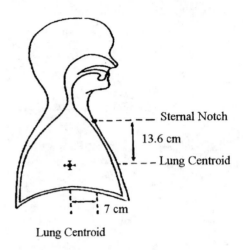

Figure 10-10: Location of lung centroid relative to the suprasternal notch (taken from NEDU Manual 1-94, 1994)

10.5 Peak Pressures and Work-of-Breathing

As the respiratory muscles expand and contract lung volume during normal breathing on the surface, energy is expended to overcome the nonelastic tissue and airway resistances in the lungs. During normal quiet breathing with healthy lungs, this energy is minimal, only 2 to 3 per cent of the total energy expended by the body (Guyton, 1976, pg 520).

However, during submerged respiration additional energy must be expended to overcome the hydrostatic imbalances discussed above, as well as, the added flow resistances in the diver's breathing apparatus. These added flow resistances, ever increasing as the breathing medium becomes more dense with increasing depth, make the diver's breathing more difficult and can result in diver fatigue. A UBA designer must minimize the expenditure of the diver's energy which will be required to overcome the external resistances in the breathing apparatus.

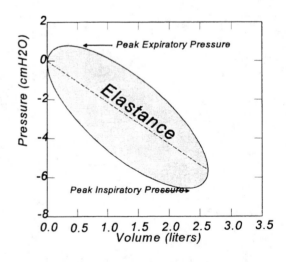

Figure 10-11: Pressure-volume loop for a closed-circuit UBA (taken from NEDU Manual 1-94, 1994).

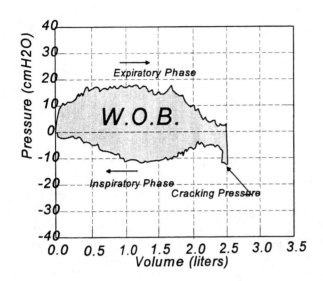

Figure 10-12: Typical pressure-volume characterization for an open-circuit, demand regulator.

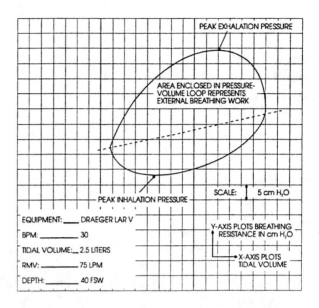

Figure 10-13: Pressure-volume characterization for the Draeger Lar V closed-circuit UBA.

The breathing characteristics of a UBA are analyzed by plotting the variations of mouth pressure seen during a complete breathing cycle against lung volume, as shown in Figure 10-11. As the diver inhales, negative pressures are recorded in the diver's mouth, reaching a *peak inspiratory pressure* (minimum circuit pressure relative to the initial mouth pressure) prior to the end of the inhalation phase. As the diver begins exhaling, the mouth pressure rises, reaching a *peak expiratory pressure* (maximum circuit pressure) prior to the completion of the respiration cycle. The resulting P-V loops will appear quite different depending on the design of the UBA; indeed each UBA category will show its own unique characteristic. The breathing characteristics of two different UBA categories are demonstrated in Figures 10-12 and 10-13, each giving important information about its own breathing characteristics. For instance, a fundamental thermodynamic principle says that the area enclosed within a P-V cycle can be equated to the work involved in completing that cycle; i.e.

$$W = \oint P \ dV \qquad \qquad (10\text{-}4)$$

The work derived from these P-V loops, referred to as the *work-of-breathing (WOB)* or *resistive effort*, quantifies the energy that the diver will have to expend to overcome the resistances in the breathing apparatus. Historically, measurements of *WOB* are normalized with the tidal volume to yield an indication of the work per unit volume, given in kg-m/l or joules/l. With pressure recordings given in cmH_2O and lung volume measured in liters, *WOB* calculations for a typical breathing apparatus can be made as follows:

$$WOB = \frac{W}{Lung\ Vol} = \frac{\oint P\ dV}{Lung\ Vol}$$

$$WOB\left(\frac{kg-m}{\ell}\right) = \frac{Loop\ Area\ (cmH_2O\ *\ \ell)}{100\ *\ Tidal\ Vol\ (\ell)} \qquad (10\text{-}5)$$

$$WOB\left(\frac{joule}{\ell}\right) = 9.807\ *\ WOB\left(\frac{kg-m}{\ell}\right)$$

Design goals for peak respiratory pressures and work-of-breathing (resistive effort) have been established by the U. S. Navy according to the UBA category and diver activity level; see Table 10-2. Efforts to minimize peak pressures and *WOB* should concentrate on eliminating the need for the diver to use his own lung power to force peak flows through highly restrictive components such as carbon dioxide scrubbers or check valves. A successful technique used to reduce peak pressures and *WOB* in the design of some closed-circuit UBA's incorporates dual breathing bags, one located on each side of the carbon dioxide scrubber. By doing this, the diver's breathing cycle is now isolated from the highly resistive components, making peak gas flows through the scrubber no longer a requirement.

Table 10-2: Performance Goals For The Design of Underwater Breathing Apparatus
(taken from NEDU Manual 01-94, June 1994)

$\dot{V}O_2$ (L/min)	RMV (L/min)	V_T (L)	f (BPM)	PEAK FLOW RATE (L/sec)	CATEGORY 1 DEPTH 0 to 198 fsw AIR RESISTIVE EFFORT kg·m/L	CATEGORY 1 kPa (J/L)	CATEGORY 2 0 to 198 fsw AIR 0 to 1000 fsw HeO$_2$ RESISTIVE EFFORT kg·m/L	CATEGORY 2 kPa (J/L)	CATEGORIES 3 & 5 0 to 200 fsw AIR 0 to 1500 fsw HeO$_2$ $\Delta P^{(3)}$ (kPa)	RESISTIVE EFFORT kg·m/L	kPa (J/L)	CATEGORY 4 0 to 150 fsw AIR $\Delta P^{(3)}$ (kPa)	RESISTIVE EFFORT kg·m/L	kPa (J/L)	CATEGORY 4 0 to 1500 fsw HeO$_2$ $\Delta P^{(3)}$ (kPa)	RESISTIVE EFFORT kg·m/L	kPa (J/L)
0.90	22.5	1.5	15	1.18	0.14[1]	1.37[1]	0.18[1]	1.76[1]	0.147	0.024	0.231	0.108	0.017	0.170	0.147	0.024	0.231
1.60	40.0	2.0	20	2.09	0.14[1]	1.37[1]	0.18[1]	1.76[1]	0.393	0.063	0.617	0.324	0.052	0.509	0.393	0.063	0.617
2.50	62.5	2.5	25	3.27	0.14[1]	1.37[1]	0.18[1]	1.76[1]	0.982	0.157	1.542	0.746	0.120	1.172	0.982	0.157	1.542
3.00	75.0	2.5	30	3.93	(2)	(2)	(2)	(2)	1.375	0.220	2.159	1.080	0.173	1.696	1.375	0.220	2.159
3.60	90.0	3.0	30	4.71	(2)	(2)	(2)	(2)	1.964[4]	0.315	3.085	1.610[4]	0.258	2.529	1.964[4]	0.315	3.085

Notes: [1] Categories 1 and 2 are not always capable of making the 75 L/min performance requirements at their maximum operating depths. State-of-the-art in open-circuit demand UBA is such that 62.5 L/min is the limit for reasonable breathing work values.
[2] No work of breathing goal is established for Category 1 and 2 RMVs greater than 62.5 L/Min, however UBAs may be evaluated at 75 and 90 L/Min if capable of performing at these higher work rates.
[3] ΔP max is measured from neutral (no flow) to full inhalation or exhalation.
[4] An RMV of 90 L/min is of interest to verify system performance but 75 L/min is the actual performance goal.

10.6 Dynamic Elastance

When using open-circuit systems, a diver experiences constant source pressure during a respiratory cycle unless the diver changes his orientation in the water during the breathing cycle. This is a result of the fixed delivery pressure for open, steady flow systems and the fixed surrounding pressures acting on the regulator in open, demand systems. The reference from which the resistive pressures are plotted on their P-V loops will thus remain constant for these systems, as shown in Figure 10-12.

On the other hand, closed and semi-closed circuit UBA's have a variable system pressure due to the vertical motion of the collapse plane in the breathing bag, or neckdam, as they empty and fill during the respiratory cycle. Consequently, the P-V loop for closed-circuit systems will have a sloping system pressure, typical of the sloping loop shown in Figure 10-13. This slope is identified as the *UBA elastance* (Joye, Clarke, Carlson, Thalmann, 1994), given in cmH$_2$O/l or kPa/l, which can be derived from the P-V plot by dividing the peak-to-peak pressures ΔP that are recorded in the breathing cycle by the tidal volume ΔV, i.e.

$$Elastance = \frac{\Delta P}{\Delta V} \qquad (10-6)$$

Unless other design constraints dictate otherwise, UBA's should be designed to minimize elastance. This is most easily achieved by designing the breathing bag, neckdam or diaphragm such that the vertical motion of the collapse plane will be minimized during the breathing cycle.

Although definitive goals have not yet been established for UBA elastance, existing closed-circuit UBA's being used by the U.S. Navy have elastances which are typically less than 0.7 kPa/l when their breathing bags are properly inflated (Clarke, 1995). However, the elastance of some emergency bail-out systems for diving helmets have been measured as high as 2.0 kPa/l, levels which would be tolerable for only short intervals during an emergency.

10.7 Weight/Buoyancy -- Subsystem Placement

Although it is always desirable to make the entire UBA assembly as near to neutrally buoyant as possible, ie

$$\sum UBA\ subsystem\ weights = \sum UBA\ subsystem\ buoyant\ forces \qquad (10-7)$$

individual components are rarely neutrally buoyant. The breathing bags and hoses are almost always positively buoyant, while the gas bottle, UBA frame and cover, and CO$_2$ scrubber are frequently negative. The positioning of subsystem components in an underwater breathing apparatus can have a significant impact on the swimmability of that apparatus. This is true since the relative positions of the UBA center-of-gravity (CG) and center-of-buoyancy (CB) determine the existence and magnitude of a righting moment inherent with the UBA that will be exerted on the diver. If the CG and CB are co-located as shown in Figure 10-14a, no righting moment will be observed as the diver swims in any orientation relative to the water column. However, when the negative components are centrally located near one end of the UBA and the positive components are centrally located near the opposite end, an undesirable righting moment will be acted upon the diver, as seen in Figure 10-14b. All things being equal, the UBA designer should make every effort to minimize this righting moment **unless** the mission calls for the diver to be in a single orientation throughout the dive. In that case the righting moment could be used to the diver's advantage by helping the diver remain in the desired orientation.

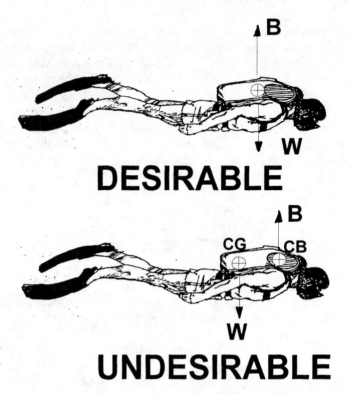

Figure 10-14: Effect of UBA center-of-gravity (CG) and center-of-buoyancy (CB) on diver righting moment.

The relative positions of the individual UBA subsystems, along with their known weights (in air) and volume displacements can be used to locate the positions of the CG and CB relative to some arbitrary set of axes as

$$CG_X = \frac{\sum X_i * W_i}{\sum W_i} \qquad\qquad CG_Y = \frac{\sum Y_i * W_i}{\sum W_i} \qquad\qquad \textbf{(10-8)}$$

and

$$CB_X = \frac{\sum X_i * B_i}{\sum B_i} \qquad\qquad CB_Y = \frac{\sum Y_i * B_i}{\sum B_i} \qquad\qquad \textbf{(10-9)}$$

where W_i is the weight (in air) of the ith component in the UBA; B is the buoyant force due to the displacement of seawater by the ith component; X_i and Y_i are the positions of the centroid of the ith component from some arbitrary origin. The following example demonstrates how the righting moment can be characterized for a UBA design.

Example: The primary components for an experimental, closed-circuit breathing apparatus, designed to be worn on the diver's chest, are tabulated in Table 10-3 along with the component weights, locations and displacement volumes for each. Calculate the net buoyant force and inherent righting moment that this UBA will exert on a diver swimming in a prone, face-down posture.

Table 10-3: CG/CB Analysis For An Experimental UBA Design

Component	Weight, LB	Buoyancy, LB	X, in	Y, in	X * W	Y * W	X * B	Y * B
Bottle	-8.00	3.84	15.25	2.25	-122.00	-18.00	58.56	8.64
Canister	-9.50	8.00	9.50	4.30	-90.25	-40.85	76.00	34.40
Bag	-0.50	7.81	5.00	3.00	-2.50	-1.50	39.04	23.42
Hoses	-1.50	2.37	-4.00	0.00	6.00	0.00	-9.47	0.00
Shell	-4.70	2.24	6.50	4.00	-30.55	-18.80	14.56	8.96
Total	-24.20	24.26			-239.30	-79.15	178.69	75.42

Net Buoyant Force, LB =	0.06			CG_x =	9.89		CB_x =	7.37
				CG_y =	3.27		CB_y =	3.11

Net Righting Moment, in-lb =   -61.02

Note: X and Y are measured from the inside, top of UBA

Although the sum of all component weights (in air) approximately equals the sum of all component buoyant forces (24.2 pounds), the horizontal locations of the CG and CB, relative to an arbitrary coordinate system shown in the sketch in Table 10-3, are separated by approximately 2.5 inches (CG_x = 9.9 inches, CB_x = 7.4 inches). This separation establishes a righting moment equal to the product of this separation distance times the total system weight, ie

$$Righting\ Moment = (\ CG_X - CB_X\ ) * \sum UBA\ Subsystem\ Weights \qquad (10\text{-}10)$$

This separation of CB and CG establishes a righting moment of approximately 61 in-lbs (5.1 ft-lbs) which will be transferred to the swimming diver. This moment will tend to right the diver into a vertical posture unless the diver exerts an additional effort to remain horizontal.

Table 10-4: CG/CB Analysis For a Modified Experimental UBA Design

Component	Weight, LB	Buoyancy, LB	X, in	Y, in	X * W	Y * W	X * B	Y * B
Bottle	-8.00	3.84	15.25	2.25	-122.00	-18.00	58.56	8.64
Canister	-5.20	8.00	9.50	4.30	-49.40	-22.36	76.00	34.40
Bag	-0.50	7.81	5.00	3.00	-2.50	-1.50	39.04	23.42
Hoses	-1.50	2.37	-4.00	0.00	6.00	0.00	-9.47	0.00
Shell	-4.70	2.24	6.50	4.00	-30.55	-18.80	14.56	8.96
Lead Weight	-4.80	0.44	-4.50	3.10	21.60	-14.88	-1.98	1.36
Total	-24.70	24.70			-176.85	-75.54	176.71	76.79

Net Buoyant Force, LB =	-0.00			CG_x =	7.16		CB_x =	7.16
				CG_y =	3.06		CB_y =	3.11

Net Righting Moment, in-lb =   -0.11   (Placing the lead weights at the top of the UBA effectively cancels the righting moment on the diver.)

This moment can be effectively eliminated, if so desired, by modifying the individual component weights and displacements, or by re-positioning the existing components. For example, in Table 10-4, the CO_2 scrubber canister has been redesigned using more lightweight materials. The weight savings from the canister redesign (approximately 4 pounds) were re-positioned in the form of a lead weight toward the UBA top (toward the diver's head), causing the CG and CB to be near-identically positioned. Similar benefits in CG/CB matchup could be seen by reconfiguring the existing components within physical and physiological constraints.

10.8 Hydrodynamic Resistance

Minimizing the hydrodynamic drag of a UBA becomes increasingly important during missions requiring extended swims. The energy that a diver will expend during his mission will be directly influenced by this drag. Since the power requirements are proportional to the velocity cubed; i.e.

$$Power = f\left(V^3 \right) \tag{10-11}$$

hydrodynamic drag also becomes increasingly important when the diver is traveling at higher speeds such as when diver propulsion vehicles (DPV's) are being utilized.

Efforts have been made to characterize the hydrodynamic drag of various UBA configurations using experimental methods similar to those used for modern underwater ship hull form analyses (Holloway, 1987). A diver, wearing various garment/UBA combinations, was towed in a 380 foot-long towing tank facility at a speed range from 1.0 to 2.5 feet per second (speeds at which an unassisted diver can reasonably expect to attain). During these towing experiments complete time histories of speed and diver drag were obtained. Drag coefficients, C_d, were then calculated for each combination of garment and breathing apparatus using the expression

$$C_d = \frac{F}{0.5 * \rho * V^2 * A} \tag{10-12}$$

where F is the measured drag on the diver as he was pulled through the water, lb; ρ is the density of the water through which the diver was towed (approximately 1.99 lb-sec^2/ft^4 at the conditions tested); V is the speed at which the diver was towed, ft/sec; and A is the wetted surface area of the diver, ft^2 (calculated using an approximation proposed by DuBois (1916))

$$A = 2.174 \; W^{0.425} \; H^{0.725} \tag{10-13}$$

where W is the diver weight in kilograms, and H is the diver height in meters.

As in the cases for hydrodynamic drag characterizations for ship hulls, these drag coefficients were plotted against the dimensionless Reynolds Number, Re_L, given by

$$Re_L = \frac{V * L}{\nu} \tag{10-14}$$

where L is the characteristic length, given as the diver height in feet (L, ft = H, m * 3.28 ft/m); and v is the kinematic viscosity of the water, ft^2/sec.

Drag coefficients ranging from 0.05 to 0.06 were recorded over the range of underwater velocities and suit/UBA combinations tested. Although the differences seen in drag coefficients when comparing combinations of suits/breathing devices were relatively small in these low speed tests, the highest drag was observed with the breathing apparatuses worn on the diver's chest. This was felt to be due to the increased frontal area that is presented to the flow with the chest packs. Conversely, the UBA's worn on the diver's back were observed to have lower drag due to the effect of the diver's head as a fairing for these apparatuses. Other testing (Staglin, 1993) has indicated that significant improvements in drag reduction (28% drag reduction) can be seen by improving this fairing of the backpack with the diver's head.

10.9 Summary and Closing Remarks

The design of an underwater breathing apparatus involves many concerns that are critical to the comfort and safety of the diver. By addressing these concerns adequately, the UBA designer can maximize the performance of the diver in an often harsh environment.

It is important to note, however, that tradeoffs between many of these concerns are frequently necessary when designing an underwater breathing apparatus. For instance, a closely packed, granular bed of lithium hydroxide may answer all of the diver's carbon dioxide absorption needs for a particular mission. However, the added absorption capability obtained by using this scrubber system must be weighed against the added flow resistance, resulting in increased respiratory effort, that such a packed bed may cause. Additionally, the excellent absorption capability gained from using this chemical during cold water missions must be weighed against the added risk of injuring the diver through an accidental exposure to the caustic slurries that are often generated in these absorbers.

It is also important to note that it is usually a wasted effort to adequately design one UBA component while neglecting the proper concerns for another component. For instance, it does the diver little service to have a scrubber with a useful service life of 2 hours if he only has enough gas supply for 30 minutes. A proper design balance, usually driven by wise tradeoffs between all the UBA components, is critical.

11

Hyperbaric and Dive System Design Considerations

Objectives

The objectives of this chapter are to:
- provide an overview of hyperbaric system design considerations.
- provide an approach for gas system design.
- present the basics of pressure vessel for human occupancy design.
- review atmosphere control and monitoring considerations.
- address habitability and human engineering considerations.
- list various certifying codes and authorities.

11.1 Introduction

In designing a hyperbaric or dive system we proceed from general mission or functional requirements through a series of steps leading to the design and construction of the system. Shipboard dive systems range from simple surface support air dive systems to complex saturation (SAT) dive systems. Hyperbaric systems may be basic air recompression chambers to hyperbaric research facilities such as the Ocean Simulation Facility (OSF) at the Navy's Experimental Diving Unit (EDU) located in Panama City, Florida.

This chapter will take us through a step-by-step approach to the design of a hyperbaric or dive system. Since each dive system is unique, the design engineer will have to adapt the approach for his particular mission requirements.

11.2 Gas System Design

The heart of our dive system is the gas system. We must establish the gas volume and flow requirements based on the overall mission and maximum expected operations. Once this is established, we can determine the functional layout, line sizes, gas storage and compressor requirements. The following is a six step design approach is based on a previously published work (Henkener and Adkins, 1972).

11.2.1 Ship or Hyperbaric System Mission

First, we must establish the overall mission requirements. This is usually a top level requirement which establishes how the system will ultimately be used. The system may be one of or a combination of the following:

11.2.1.1 Conventional Diving

A conventional diving system can be any number of air or mixed gas systems. Included are air, oxygen and mixed-gas SCUBA; and surface-supplied air, and mixed gas diving apparatus. Various gas storage containers and compressors are needed to support conventional diving operations.

11.2.1.2 Recompression Chamber

In conjunction with a conventional diving system, a recompression chamber may be required either for surface decompression or emergency treatment of divers. If diving operations are conducted in remote areas it is imperative that a chamber be available since there may not be sufficient time to transport an injured diver to a shore based treatment facility. Recompression chambers generally consist of a treatment chamber connected to a lock-in, lock-out chamber. Additionally, a small medical lock may be present for transferring medical supplies, food, and other small items.

The chamber atmosphere is maintained either by direct ventilation or by way of an atmosphere control system. With the ventilation approach, the chamber is pressurized with air to the treatment depth; then, based on a schedule, vent and pressurization valves are periodically opened while maintaining constant chamber pressure. This simultaneously adds make-up air while removing carbon dioxide. As you might imagine, this uses a considerable amount of air which must be available in storage flasks. An atmosphere control system, on the other hand, circulates the chamber gas through scrubbers and adds make-up oxygen as required similar to a closed-circuit SCUBA (see Chapter 10).

For emergency treatment, a built in breathing system (BIBS) may be incorporated into the chamber. BIBS is an independent gas breathing apparatus available to personnel in the chamber which may be used for oxygen decompression treatments, or as a backup gas supply in the event of chamber atmosphere contamination.

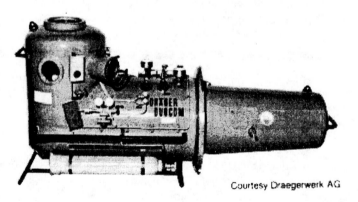

Courtesy Draegerwerk AG

Figure 11-1: Lightweight, one-person transportable chamber (Courtesy Draegerwerk AG)

Emergency transport under pressure of an injured diver may be done in a fly-away chamber. This is a small, one-man chamber which mates to a larger chamber. Because of its small size it can be easily transported from a remote site via aircraft, or other vehicle, to a treatment facility. On the down side, emergency medical treatment for other injuries can not be done. Recently, the Navy has approved a transportable two man chamber which circumvents this problem.

11.2.1.3 Saturation or Deep Dive Systems

Saturation systems are generally the largest and most complex of the hyperbaric systems. Saturation systems support deep dives which require divers to be under pressure for extended periods of time. The basic components of a typical saturation system include: one or more living/deck decompression chambers (DDC); a lock-in, lock-out chamber; personnel transfer capsule (PTC) for transporting divers to and from the work site under pressure; and medical locks for food and other supplies. While at the work site, divers wearing a helmet or full face mask are generally tethered to the PTC with a tended gas and communications umbilical.

11.2.1.4 Medical or Research Chambers

Land-based research chambers generally consist of one or more living chambers, lock-in, lock-out chambers, medical locks, and possibly a wet chamber for training or physiological testing. With the advent of hyperbaric oxygen treatment for a number of maladies, many hospitals have chambers for treatments of other than diving emergencies.

11.2.2   Diving Operations

After the overall mission is established, the next step is to determine the <u>maximum</u> diving operations. For each system the following interdependent factors must be addressed:

- Number of Divers
- Depth
- Time at depth
- Type and mixture of breathing gas
- Type of breathing apparatus

Both normal and emergency maximum diving operations need to be considered in designing the gas system. These factors are the basis for storage and flow calculations.

11.2.3   Storage Volume and Flow

The third step in designing a gas system is to determine the volume of gas needed and the gas flow rates based on the maximum diving operations. The storage volume of each gas (air, oxygen, and helium) determines the number and size of the storage flasks, compressors, and helium reclaim systems required. Gas flow rates are used to determine gas line sizes.

11.2.3.1 Storage Volume Factors

To determine the gas storage volume required, the following areas, as applicable, should be addressed:

<u>Equipment Volume</u>

The actual volumes of chambers, PTCs and locks are needed to calculate the volume of gas required for initial pressurization.

Decompression Schedule

In order to calculate the ventilation or physiological breathing gas requirements, the decompression schedule must be known. Depending on the certification authority, either commercial or Navy schedules may be used.

Below is a typical decompression schedule from the Navy Diving Manual for a saturation dive. This schedule is based on ascending 24 hours per day with no restrictions on diver sleep or activity.

Depth Range (FSW)	Rate of Ascent (ft/hr)
1000 to 200	4
200 to 50	2.5
50 to surface	2

Medical lock usage

Gas required for medical lock usage can be significant for long duration dives. The medical lock may be used ten to fifteen times a day for transferring food and supplies.

PTC/DDC Mating Schedule

Each time the PTC is decoupled from the DDC, gas is lost from the mating ring. The schedule is based on the working requirements, and is normally not more than twice a day.

Leakage

Estimated helium leakage from a saturation system needs to be included. In a complex system the following rates are reasonable:

Storage flasks and shipboard systems (assuming 500 leak points): 16.5 SCF per day
Deep-dive system chambers: volume equivalent to one foot drop in pressure per day

Reserve Gas

Sufficient gas should be in reserve to ventilate a DDC in the event of fire, smoke or other contamination.

Diver's Level of Work Activity

As discussed earlier in Chapter 3, the diver's respiratory minute volume (RMV) and oxygen consumption are directly related to the diver's exertion. For planning purposes the following consumption rates may be used.

	Oxygen Consumption	Respiratory Minute Volume
Moderate Work	1.5 slpm (3.4 SCFH)	40 liters/min (1.5 cfm)
Light Work	0.7 slpm (1.6 SCFH)	20 liters/min (0.75 cfm)

Breathing Apparatus

When diving outside of the PTC, the gas consumption for an open-circuit diving apparatus will be a function of the diver's RMV and the depth; with a closed-circuit system, the gas consumption will be based on the metabolic oxygen consumption alone.

Gas Temperature and Pressure

Gas charging temperatures should be considered. When rapidly charging the storage banks, the gas will be warm. If the banks are not topped-off, the pressure will decrease when the flasks cool down.

Minimum Bank Pressure

The minimum bank pressure is needed to determine the amount of storage gas available. For saturation diving operations to 1500 feet, the minimum bank pressure should be about 800 psia to assure 100 psi over bottom pressure. If a diaphragm booster compressor is used, all but one bank can be used to a minimum of 200 psia (the minimum compressor inlet pressure).

11.2.3.2 Storage Volume Calculations

For most calculations only three basic formulas are needed. For determining the mass of the gas required to pressurize a DDC, PTC, medical lock, etc., we simply multiply the volume times the change in gas density that will occur while pressurizing from the initial pressure to the working depth.

$$m_{gas} = V_{system} \Delta \rho_{gas} \qquad\qquad \textbf{(11-1)}$$

If we know the mass usage rate per diver, $\dot{m}_{diver}$, and the number of divers, we can determine mass of gas used for breathing apparatus or leakage for a given period t as follows:

$$m_{gas} = \dot{m}_{diver} N_{divers} t \qquad\qquad \textbf{(11-2)}$$

This mass of gas will be contained in a storage volume, V_{SCF} at standard temperature and pressure:

$$V_{SCF} = \frac{m_{gas}}{\rho_{STP}} \qquad\qquad \textbf{(11-3)}$$

11.2.3.3 Gas Flow Calculations

For gas flow calculations, the design engineer should be interested only in the maximum flow rates in order to properly size the distribution lines. Two areas need to be addressed for these flow calculations: chamber pressurization and gas flow to the diver.

<u>Chamber Pressurization</u>

To determine the maximum flows to a chamber, the designer needs to know the chamber volume and how quickly it must be pressurized or taken to depth. For normal treatment of decompression sickness, the rate of pressurization is 25 FSW per minute. For deep dive systems, a pressurization rate of 100 FSW per minute, or 50 lbf/in^2 per minute is reasonable. We can determine the volumetric flow rate, $\dot{V}_{SCFM}$ for a given pressurization rate and chamber volume as follows:

$$\dot{V}_{SCFM} = \frac{\Delta P/t}{P_{Ata}} \cdot V_{chamber} \qquad \qquad \textbf{(11-4)}$$

where ΔP is the change in pressure, Ata; t is the time for pressurization, Min: and $V_{chamber}$ is the volume of the chamber, ft^3.

11.2.4   Distribution System

The next step in our gas system design is to lay out the gas distribution system. The designer must decide on the best location for the gas supply components within a given set of constraints. The designer must determine the best routing for the piping including gages, valves, and pressure controls.

When designing the distribution system, the designer should design the system for easy cleaning in place. Drains and vents should be installed for removal of cleaning fluids. Low points and dead ends should be avoided. Adequate pipe supports should be provided.

Once the distribution system is laid out, we can determine the length of each pipe as well as flow resistances due to manifolds, valves, elbows, tees, etc.

11.2.5   Line Size and Pressure Drop

Our next step is to determine optimum pipe sizes. Using the approach discussed in Chapter 9, we can iteratively calculate the line size for a require flow rate, pressure drop, and effective line length. From Chapter 9, the total head loss in a hose or pipe in which an incompressible, viscous liquid is flowing (as well as compressible flow for small pressure drops) can be found by combining the hose loss with the minor losses to give

$$H_L = \left[f \cdot \frac{L}{D} + \sum K \right] \frac{V^2}{2g} \qquad \textbf{(11-5)}$$

and the mass flow rate through a pipe or hose can be found as

$$\dot{m} = \rho \dot{V} = \rho V A \qquad \textbf{(11-6)}$$

In sizing the pipes and unbilicals, it may be necessary to take an iterative approach based on initial assumptions for pressure and density, and assumed pipe diameter. Since the density of the gas changes as the pressure drops along the length of the pipe, the incremental head loss will decrease as the density increases. A general rule of thumb is that the maximum pressure drop, or head loss (H_L), in a pipe should be less than 20% of the difference between the source and use pressure. For example, if the gas is stored at 2500 psig and the pressure in the reducer is set for 500 psig, the pressure drop in the piping system should be less than 400 psi under maximum flow conditions.

Reasonable first order flow rate calculations can be obtained using the gas density based on the average pipe pressure. For the above example, we would calculate the density using the methods presented in Chapter 2 for a pressure of 2300 psig- the average of a maximum line pressure of 2500 psig and a minimum line pressure of 2100 psig. Alternatively, the density may be obtained from a gas properties table such as The Navy Diving-Gas Manual (1971). We repeat this procedure for determining pipe diameter for each of lines in our distribution system and tabulate our results.

11.2.6   Gas Storage and Compressors

The sixth and final step is: selecting storage flasks, compressors, gas mixers, reclaimers, filtration equipment and the like; and integrating them into our diving gas system. The design engineer must select components that supply high purity gas, are reliable and maintainable, and are designed with human factors in mind.

11.2.6.1 Storage Flasks

Storage flasks come in a variety of sizes and storage capacities. The gas may be stored in banks of standard gas cylinders used for transporting gas; submarine gas storage flasks; or cryogenically. Listed below are some typical volumes for various flasks and gasses.

Table 11-1: Gas Storage Flask Data

Gas	Container	Capacity (SCF)	Pressure (psig)	Diameter x Height (in.)	Internal Volume
Air	Cylinder	229	2,200	9 x 56	2,640 in³
Helium	Cylinder	286	2,640	9.25 x 60	3,000 in³
Nitrogen	Cylinder	224	2,200	9 x 56	2,640 in³
Oxygen	Cylinder	244	2,200	9 x 56	2,640 in³
Air	Storage Flask		4,600 max		26.9 ft³
Nitrogen	Storage Flask		4,600 max		26.9 ft³
Helium	Storage Flask		4,600 max		26.9 ft³
Oxygen	Storage Flask		3,000 max		26.9 ft³

Storage flasks are typically manifolded together in banks to permit pumping the gases back and forth between flasks containing the same gas. All flasks should be installed to permit removal and hydrostatic tests. Also the flasks should have vents, drains and pressure relief valves.

11.2.6.2 Compressors

Shipboard compressors provide air for air diving, and provide for charging Scuba cylinders. Oil lubricated air compressors for diving operations are of a special design to minimize the amount of oil reaching the cylinders which might contaminate the compressed air. **Under no circumstances should petroleum-based lubricants be used.**

In addition, diaphragm type gas booster compressors are used to transfer gas from shore stations, nearly depleted gas banks, or helium reclaimers. These compressors are normally low flow, motor or air driven, single or multistage.

11.2.6.3 Gas Mixers and Analyzers

For deep diving operations where a low percentage of oxygen is used, a gas mixer is essential to supply the large volume of gas required. For shallow mixed gas diving, gas can be manually pre-mixed using a time consuming mixing by pressure technique.

11.2.6.4 Reclaimers

Helium reclaimers are useful for back-to-back diving operations, particularly in remote areas where it may be logistically difficult to ship additional gas. However, reclaimers are big and bulky, and the cost of the helium reclaimed may not justify the reclaim system. A reclaim system typically consists of a reclaim bag and a booster compressor. During decompression, the DDC atmosphere is vented to the reclaim bag, and then transferred to the storage banks.

11.2.6.5 Coolers, Separators and Filtration Equipment

Coolers and separators remove water and cool air to a breathable temperature of 90° F or less. These components are particularly important for removing the bulk of the oil mists and vapors from air supplied from oil lubricated compressors. To meet breathing gas purity standards, special filtration equipment is especially necessary with oil lubricated compressors.

11.3 Pressure Vessels

In this section we are primarily interested in vessels subjected to internal pressure such as DDCs, PTCs, and recompression chambers. It is not meant to be an all inclusive guide to pressure vessel design, but rather a general approach for the first level of the design effort.

11.3.1   General Considerations

The shapes of greatest interest to us in designing the pressure vessels for a diving system are the cylinder and the sphere. Less frequently, other shapes, such as ellipsoidal dished heads and cones, may be used. These details will not be covered as their detail is beyond the scope of this book.

The materials used in the construction of pressure vessels are assumed to obey Hooke's Law; that is, they behave in an elastic manner with stress proportional to strain. These assumptions are generally valid in the skin or membrane area of the vessel, away from attachment points and discontinuities which lead to stress concentrations. Where stress concentrations do occur, local yield may occur thus relieving stress. The local yielding is called plastic deformation since it occurs in the plastic region of the stress/strain curve. Plastic deformation is very important in pressure vessel design, since it governs the low-cycle fatigue life for conditions of repetitive or cyclic loading. Materials with little or no plastic deformation such as glass and ultra-high strength steel are particularly susceptible to local stress raisers.

Pressure vessels are categorized as **thick-walled** or **thin-walled** based on the comparison of the wall thickness to the diameter. An extreme example of a thin-walled vessel is a balloon; while a gun barrel, having a wall thickness on the same order of magnitude as its diameter, is an example of a thick-walled vessel. We will be primarily interested in thin walled pressure vessels.

11.3.2   Stress

The thin-walled pressure vessels most commonly used in diving systems are cylinders closed by hemispherical or ellipsoidal dished ends, and spheres. For a pressurized cylinder, the average membrane stress is computed by equating the stresses to the forces generated by the internal pressure. While the stresses vary in the radial direction, for a thin-walled vessel we can use the average stress values.

For a cylinder with internal pressure p, diameter D, and wall thickness t we calculate the longitudinal stress σ_l as

$$\sigma_l = \frac{pD}{4t}$$

(11-7)

and the hoop stress as

$$\sigma_h = \frac{pD}{2t} \qquad\qquad (11\text{-}8)$$

For a sphere

$$\sigma_s = \frac{pD}{4t} \qquad\qquad (11\text{-}9)$$

the same as the longitudinal stress for a cylinder. We might note at this time that a sphere can contain the largest volume against a given pressure with the least shell area and thickness. Consequently, a sphere has the least shell volume and is thus the lightest pressure vessel shape. A detailed discussion of pressure vessel theory can be found in most strength of materials such as Timoshenko's *Strength of Materials*.

Rearranging the above equations, the wall thickness for a cylinder based on hoop stress is

$$t = \frac{pD}{2\sigma_h} \qquad\qquad (11\text{-}10)$$

and based on longitudinal stress and spherical stress is

$$t = \frac{pD}{4\sigma_l} \qquad\qquad (11\text{-}11)$$

From these two equations we can see that the hoop stress dictates the wall thickness of a cylinder. In actual practice, when using the appropriate certification code, the wall thickness will be greater than these theoretical values. Each code has its own empirical equations which take into consideration other factors such as joint efficiency values and include a safety factors. Applicable codes will be discussed later in this chapter.

11.3.3   Materials

When selecting materials for use in manned pressure vessels and their associated hatches, supporting structures, and viewports, we need to consider:

- Ultimate and yield strength under tensile, shear, compressive and combined loads.
- Ductility and notch resistance.
- Brittleness
- Fatigue resistance
- Density
- Weldability
- Compatibility with other materials
- Cost

Typically, hyperbaric chambers are fabricated from high strength steels such as HY-80 and HY-100 and aluminum. Table 11-2 lists some of the basic properties of these materials.

Table 11-2: Properties for Selected Materials

Material	HY-80 Steel	HY-100 Steel	Aluminum (7075-T6)
Density, lbm/in³ (gm/cm³)	0.28 (7.9)	0.28 (7.9)	0.10 (2.8)
Young's Modulus, Mpsi (GPa)	29 (200)	29 (200)	10.3 (71)
Compressive Strength, Kpsi (MPa)	80 (550)	100 (690)	73 (503)
Fracture toughness	Very good	Very good	Poor
Fatigue resistance	Good	Good	Fair
General corrosion resistance	Poor	Poor	Poor
Plate Cost	Low	Low	Medium

11.3.4 Corrosion and Fouling

For shipboard diving systems, corrosion and marine fouling can be a significant problem if not properly addressed. Marine fouling in the form of barnacles and other marine growth may add hydrodynamic drag or damage protective coatings. Corrosion, if not checked, may lead to the premature failure of the hyperbaric system.

Corrosion is an electrochemical reaction between the metal and the environment. There are four basic types of corrosion that the design engineer should take into account:

● General Corrosion occurs where a single base metal is exposed to sea water or sea spray in air. This form is characterized by relatively uniform corrosion over the exposed surface.
● Galvanic Corrosion occurs when two dissimilar metals in electrical contact form an electrochemical cell.
● Crevice Corrosion occurs where sea water penetrates a narrow, isolated area and a high concentration of metal ions and a low concentration of oxygen is present. Some metals, such as stainless steel are particularly susceptible to crevice corrosion.
● Stress Corrosion is observed on certain alloys when small flaws are subjected to tensile stresses in the presence of sea water.

A detailed treatment of corrosion, its measurement and control can be found in Uhlig's Corrosion Handbook (1948). General corrosion of carbon steels immersed in sea water is in the range of 0.002-0.007 in/year. These values double or triple in the splash zone. The effect of general corrosion can be addressed by increasing the thickness or the plate to allow for corrosion, or by special active and passive coatings. For relatively small or critical components, general corrosion can be minimized or greatly reduced by using the more noble metals such as nickel-chromium, nickel-copper, and type 316 and 304 stainless steel.

Galvanic corrosion can be minimized by keeping dissimilar metals which generate high electrical potentials apart from each other. The use of zinc or aluminum bars and plates can also be used as sacrificial anodes to provide cathodic protection to submerged structures.

11.4 Piping, Hoses and Umbilicals

As previously discussed, extensive piping is needed in the construction of a hyperbaric system. Pipes are needed to transport life support gasses, water, and sanitation. Hoses and umbilicals are used to supply gasses and liquids from the surface vessel to the PTC and from the PTC or vessel to the divers.

11.4.1 General

The design engineer should design the piping system to withstand service loadings such as:

- Weight of pipes, fittings, valves, and contained fluid.
- Internal or external pressure, both cyclic and static.
- Deflections and rotations of structures relative to the pipe attachment points.
- Restraint of hangers and supports.
- Thermal expansion and transients.
- Shock, vibration and water hammer.

High pressure piping used in man- rated systems should be protected against damage by suitable routing and shielding. Lines should be routed so they cannot be used as handholds. To the extent possible, lines should be made of one piece. Piping and tubing should be supported as close to bends as possible, and should not themselves be used to support components such as valves and filters. Joints should be kept to a minimum and should be easily accessible for inspection. All piping components should be designed to prevent incorrect assembly, and be clearly marked.

11.4.2 Connectors

The number of piping joints should be kept to a minimum. Welded joints should be used to the greatest extent possible. Lines which are required to be disconnected during normal operation, overhauls or inspection should use approved mechanical, bite-type, or threaded connectors. The use of flexible hoses for connectors should be considered only where flexibility of vibration dictates its use.

11.4.3 Umbilicals

Umbilicals include hoses and cables that tether a PTC or diver to a base. Umbilicals supply gas, liquids, electrical and hydraulic power, and communications. Individual hoses and cables may be bundled together on site, or may be encased in a pre-manufactured composite umbilical. Composite umbilicals are preferable due to their resistance to abrasion, damage, and deterioration. However, composite umbilicals are more difficult to repair, and are generally more expensive. Umbilicals should have adequate tensile strength for their design use, flexural strength for storage, and burst strength to withstand internal pressure.

11.5 Ancillary Components

11.5.1 Hatches and Closures

An opening is needed to get men and materials in and out of a pressure vessel with a pressure tight closure. The opening size must first be determined based on what must pass through it. It is important to keep the opening as small as possible since: a larger hatch means more weight with its associated handling problems; and the larger opening leads to additional reinforcement and fabrication problems. For the relatively modest pressures associated with diving chambers, flat hatch covers with an O-ring face seal are adequate.

Most hatches are round in saturation diving systems for reasons related to the ease of machining the sealing surfaces. When possible, a pressure-sealing hatch on the inside of the pressure vessel is desirable for reasons of safety and reliability. If this is not possible, a movable locking mechanism is required which will be strong enough to withstand shear forces generated by the pressure on the hatch surface. Breech-lock, radially expanding cylindrical plungers, and cammed clamp closures are examples of movable locking mechanisms. The outer hatch on the provision lock or medical lock, generally seals against pressure. An interlock, preventing opening of the lock until it is vented to atmosphere provides protection against accidental blowdown.

11.5.2   Viewports

Viewports must have adequate fatigue strength for the stresses imposed upon them during the service life. Where necessary, they should be protected against accidental blows or mechanical abuse. Typically, acrylic plastic viewports are used in man-rated systems.

11.5.3   Seals

Sealing materials and techniques must be adequate for the range of pressures, gas mixtures, temperatures, vibrations and atmospheric environments encountered. The effect of pressure cycling, stress concentrations, differential thermal expansion, differences in modulus of elasticity, and aging should be considered. Tolerances must be considered to prevent seal failures such as nibbling and extrusion.

11.5.4   Lighting

Lighting inside a hyperbaric chamber should be protected against accidental blows, and be able to withstand the pressurized environment. External light pipes are often used to illuminate chambers and have the advantage of having no internal fixtures and elements. An alternative emergency power source or emergency lamps should be available.

11.6   Control and Electrical Power

11.6.1   Control Systems

Control systems accomplish functions such as maintaining pressure, temperature and humidity within the pressure vessel. These generally consist of three parts: power supply, instrumentation, and control actuators. The control power supply may be manual, mechanical, pneumatic, hydraulic, or electrical. All critical controls should have two sources of power. Generally instrumentation includes sensors, warning devices, and displays. They include: carbon-dioxide sensors, oxygen sensors, gas-flow sensors, electrical-defect sensors, environmental sensors, interlock monitors, and video monitors. Control actuators need to be reliable and designed to fail safe. Individual actuators should be capable of being isolated from other actuators where a common power supply is used, and should allow for manual operator control.

11.6.2   Electrical Power

The environment for electrical systems used in hyperbaric and deep dive systems may differ markedly from normal shipboard conditions. The components may be oil immersed, subject to full sea pressure, operate at low temperatures, or be subject to high vibration and humidity. All electrical powered equipment or enclosures should be adequately grounded to prevent shock hazards to personnel.

11.6.2.1 Cabling

Cables subjected to pressure should either be pressure compensated or have a solid core construction. Cables should be protected against damage by accidental contact, crushing, or being used as a handhold. Connectors exposed to water pressure should be sealed against water intrusion, and should be capable of being disconnected with no risk of shock. Connectors should be designed to prevent incorrect connection.

11.6.2.2 Penetrators and Connectors

Pressure vessel penetrators for electrical cables must provide an effective barrier to gas leakage or water penetration. Stuffing tube penetrations are generally not acceptable. Pin type connections for cable entrances into pressure compensated enclosures are acceptable. Since the electrical hull penetrator is part of the primary pressure boundary, care must be taken in its design and installation.

11.7 Atmospheric Control and Monitoring

As previously discussed, the gas system needs to be designed to provide sufficient gas for the longest expected mission. Sufficient gas should also be available for emergency situations. Partial pressures of oxygen and diluent gases must be carefully monitored and controlled to be within acceptable limits (See Chapter 3). As oxygen is consumed, make-up oxygen must be added and carbon dioxide removed with scrubbers as described in Chapter 5.

Diving gas must be free from unacceptable levels of impurities or contaminants in accordance with military or commercial standards. Gases which may be safe to breathe on the surface at standard atmospheric pressure may be toxic at elevated partial pressures. Contaminants may be removed with appropriate filters, scrubbers and traps.

Chapters 7 and 8 addressed temperature and humidity control of diving systems. Divers working at elevated pressures in a helium rich environment are more susceptible to the detrimental effects of hot or cold environmental conditions. Significant heat may be lost through the respiratory tract, as well as from the body's surface.

In the DDC or chamber, temperature and humidity are controlled with the heat exchangers and dehumidification chillers. Typically, the chamber gas circulates through a gas conditioning system which chills the gas to remove humidity, removes carbon dioxide with a scrubber, removes impurities, adds make-up oxygen, and then reheats the gas.

For total environmental control, the following eight subareas must be controlled (Reimers, 1972):

11.7.1   Total Pressure

As discussed earlier in this chapter, the hyperbaric chamber's basic function is to hold gas under pressure for the duration of the dive operation. Control of the total pressure should be maintained within an accuracy of +/- one foot of seawater. The instruments that read chamber pressure are normally calibrated in feet of seawater. Depth or pressure control is relatively easy to control by adding or venting gas. However, at deep depths, venting can be wasteful of gas.

As depth increases it is necessary to increase the proportion of diluent gas in order to maintain partial pressures of oxygen and carbon dioxide. Helium is generally used as the diluent for dives in excess of 200 FSW remove the nitrogen narcotic effect. Also, the low density of helium makes breathing relatively easy at depth. However, a primary problem with helium is that it readily permeates through materials, joints and seals.

11.7.2 Oxygen Partial Pressure

Oxygen partial pressure must be controlled within a partial pressure range (P_{O2}) of from 0.20 to 1.6 atmospheres absolute (Ata). To maintain this P_{O2} range at sea level, the percent of O_2 can be between 20-100%; whereas, at 1000 FSW the O_2 percent is confined to 0.7-5.3%. In larger chambers the designer should be aware of the potential for pocketing or incomplete mixing, and he must insure that the helium being added is uniformly mixed.

Occasionally higher P_{O2} (1.5-2.0 Ata) are required during decompression to decrease decompression time. Rather than adding the oxygen to the chamber, the divers would normally breathe oxygen enriched gas from the built-in-breathing-system (BIBS) mask. If the diver exhales into the chamber, the chamber P_{O2} will rise unless vented. High P_{O2} may create a fire hazard, as well as present the possibility of oxygen toxicity.

11.7.3 Carbon Dioxide Partial Pressure

Like oxygen, the physiological effect carbon dioxide is a function of its partial pressure (See Chapter 3). Percent surface equivalent (% SEV) Is the commonly used convention pro expressing the partial pressure of carbon dioxide. For prolonged exposures the desirable upper limit is 0.5% SEV or about 0.005 Ata. Divers may be exposed to levels of up to 2% SEV for short periods without serious problems. Carbon dioxide is removed from the system using one of the techniques covered in Chapter 5.

11.7.4 Fire Protection

A chamber fire can be particularly dangerous. Divers confined in the chamber are not able to leave the pressurized atmosphere until they have decompressed. A fire would rapidly contaminate the atmosphere if not brought immediately under control. Compressed air readily supports combustion as the chamber pressure increases. For a constant P_{O2} the risk of fire decreases as chamber pressure increases.

To reduce the risk of fire, removal of combustible materials from the chamber is essential. Divers' clothing and bedding constitute the main sources of such material. Pressurized water is used as the suppression medium because is less toxic than alternative choices. Water fog spray nozzles are strategically located throughout the chamber in case of fire. Sufficient volume and flow must be available to rapidly extinguish the pressurized chamber.

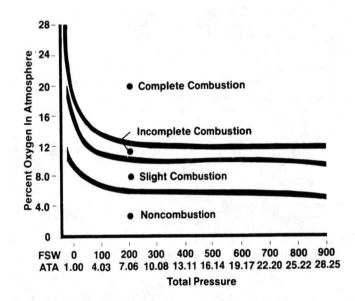

Figure 11-2: Hyperbaric Flammability Chart (Courtesy U. S. Navy)

11.7.5 Temperature and Humidity

Temperature and humidity are generally controlled to the same unit. Temperature control is normally required in the range of from 60-95°F with a tolerance of +/- 1°F. Loss of temperature control leads to divers' discomfort , but generally does not create a severe hazard. The comfort zone for air is relatively large (68-80°F); however, for a HeO$_2$ environment it is quite small (85-89°F). This is due to the high thermal conductivity of helium.

The respiratory system can tolerate a wide variation in the amount of water vapor in the breathing gas. Ideally the relative humidity should be maintained between 30- 40% for comfort and to minimize the potential for ear infection while providing sufficient moisture for good carbon dioxide scrubber efficiency.

11.7.6 Trace Contaminants

Trace contaminants in a breathing gas system include hydrocarbons, oxides of nitrogen, sulfur dioxide, halogen compounds such as carbon tetrachloride, and organic odors. Carbon monoxide may also be a major contaminant for compressor supplied systems. Generally trace contaminants are not a problem.

Toxicity of chemicals is generally related to their partial pressure, resulting in very low admissible concentrations at deep depths. Organic odors can be removed by granular type absorbents.

Table 11-3: Maximum Concentration for Some Contaminants in Saturation System Atmospheres. (Taken from U. S. Navy Diving and Manned Hyperbaric Systems Safety Certification Manual, 1987)

Contaminant	Limit (SEV)
Carbon Monoxide	10 ppm
Methane	1,000 ppm
Methanol	10 ppm
Total Hydrocarbons (less methane) as methane	10 ppm
Benzene	1 ppm
Halogenated hydrocarbons (methylchloride standard)	1 ppm
Oil mist	None detectable
Particulate matter	1 mg/cm^3

11.7.7 Bacteria

Bacteria pose a problem in wet chambers and dive systems. Severe ear infections are common on long dives. Water purification and filtration systems are essential for wet chambers to control bacteria. Chemical control may not be acceptable since the potential for chemical vapors may cause problems over prolonged periods.

11.7.8 Noise

Most pressurizing and venting systems create severe noise hazards. The high sonic velocities of the gases produce piercing, extremely high noise levels. Noise may be steady state or intermittent. Noise comes from sources such as machinery tools, compressors and gas expansion valves. Exposure to high background noise for extended periods can cause temporary as well as permanent hearing loss. Maximum allowable sound pressure levels (SPL) have been established by various certification authorities for steady-state background noise. The longer the exposure, the lower the allowable SPL. The U. S. Navy's Bureau of Medicine has established the following exposure limits for intermittent peak noise exposure instances not exceeding 15 minutes duration:

Daily Number of Exposures	Maximum Allowable SPL in decibels (dB)
1	105
4	100
8	95

11.8 Habitability and Human Engineering

Divers working at depth for extended periods need to be provided a comfortable, safe working and living environment. Human engineering factors need to be taken into account in the design of a dive system to enhance productivity and safety.

Provisions must be made for providing food and water to the divers. Normally food is provided via the medical or utility lock rather than prepared within the chamber. Additionally, water must be provided for drinking, bathing and sanitation.

Provisions must be made for disposal of waste products, including metabolic wastes, food, and wash water. Water and sanitary lines should be designed for the maximum pressure to be used in the hyperbaric chamber. Interlocks need to be included in the plumbing design to prevent inadvertent depressurization.

Communications devices may be necessary for divers to communicate with each other and with surface support personnel. When helium gas mixtures are being used, divers may need a helium speech unscrambler for their speech to be intelligible. For longer missions, in addition to reading materials, TV and radio may be piped into the chamber.

11.9 Codes and Certification

All life supporting hyperbaric systems must be designed and built to an appropriate military of commercial code or standard. Specific procedures are provided which must be followed during the design, operation, maintenance, and modification of diving systems. Certifying codes and authorities include (detailed callouts for these sources can be found in the references at the end of this book:

● " U. S. Navy Diving and Manned Hyperbaric Systems Safety Certification Manual" (1987)
● U. S. Navy "NAFAC DM 39, Hyperbaric Facilities" (1972)
● American bureau of Shipping "Rules for Building and Classing Underwater Systems and Vehicles" (1979)
● American Society of Mechanical Engineers (ASME) "Boiler and Pressure Vessel Code, Section VIII, Unfired Pressure Vessels"
● ASME PVHO-1, "Safety Standards for Pressure Vessels for Human Occupancy" (1993)
● Det Norske Veritas (Norwegian) "Rules for Certification of Diving Systems" (1982)

11.10   Closure

The forgoing chapters provide the student an overview of the considerations which must be addressed in the design and construction of a life supporting hyperbaric system. Clearly, hyperbaric system design involves a full spectrum of engineering disciplines and physiological considerations.

References

1. Boiler and Pressure Vessel Code, Section VIII, Unfired Pressure Vessels, American Society of Mechanical Engineers, New York (1993).

2. Boycott, A.W., G.C.C. Damant, and J.S. Haldane, "Prevention of Compressed Air Illness," J. Hygiene, 8:342-443 (1908).

3. Braithwaite, WR, "The Calculation of Minimum Inspired Gas Temperature Limits for Deep Diving," Naval Experimental Diving Unit Report 12-72, (1972).

4. Brown, G.M., Bird, G.S., Boag, T.J., Boag, L.M., Delahaye, J.D., Green, J.E., Hatcher, J.D., and Page, J., "The Circulation in Cold Acclimatization", Circulation, 9, pp813-822, (1954).

5. Clarke, J.R., "Elastance Standards for Underwater Breathing Apparatus," Proceedings of Underwater Intervention 1995, Houston, TX, pp139-140, (January 1995).

6. Crane Company, Flow of Fluids Through Valves, Fittings, and Pipe, Technical Paper No. 410, New York, (1980).

7. Design Manual, Hyperbaric Facilities, NAVFAC DM 39, U. S. Navy, (1972).

8. Dubois, E.F., and D. Dubois, "Formula To Estimate the Approximate Surface Area If Height and Weight Are Known," Arch. Intern. Med., 17, p863 (1916).

9. Gagge, A.P., A.C. Burton, and H.C. Bazett, "A Practical System of Units for the Description of the Heat Exchange of Man With His Environment," Science, 94, 2445, pp428-430 (1941).

10. Gagge, A.P., J.D. Hardy, G.M. Rapp, "Proposed Standard System of Symbols for Thermal Physiology," J. of Appl Physiol, 27: 439-446 (Sept 1969).

11. Gebhart, B., Heat Transfer, 2nd Ed, McGraw-Hill, New York (1971).

12. Guyton, AC, The Textbook of Medical Physiology, 5th Edition, W. B. Saunders Co, Philadelphia, (1976).

13. Hawley, J. G., Nuckols, M. L., Reader, G. T., Potter, I. J., Underwater Intervention Systems, Kendall/Hunt, Dubuque IA, (1996)

14. Henkener, J.A. and D. Adkins, "An Approach to the Design of Shipboard Breathing Gas Systems," The Working Diver 1972 Symposium Proceedings, Marine Technology Society, (1972).

15. Hoke, B, Jackson, DL, Alexander, J, Flynn, E, "Respiratory Heat Loss From Breathing Cold Gas At High Pressures," Summary of NMRI/NEDU Studies, Naval Medical Research Institute, Bethesda, MD, (1971).

16. Holloway, E.C., "Hydrodynamic Resistance Tests of a Diver," U.S. Naval Academy Engineering Report, (Jan 1987).

17. Jackson, D.C. and Schmidt-Neilsen, K.,"Countercurrent Heat Exchange in the Respiratory Tract", Proceedings Nat. Acad. of Sci.,51:1192-1197, (1964).

18. Jackson, DC, Schmidt-Neilsen, K, "Countercurrent Heat Exchange in the Respiratory Tract," Proc. Nat. Acad. Of Sci., 51:1192-1197, (1964).

19. Jacob, M., Heat Transfer, Vol 1, Wiley, New York (1949).

20. Butler, H.S., R. H. Payne, "Thermal Conductance of Diver Wet Suit Materials Under Hydrostatic Pressure," Naval Ship Research and Development Laboratory Report 2903, Panama City, FL (1972).

21. Johnson, CE, Linderoth, LS, Nuckols, ML, "An Analysis of Sensible Respiratory Heat Exchange During Inspiration Under Environmental Conditions of Deep Diving", J. of Biomechanical Engineering, Vol 99, Series K, pp45-53, (Feb 1977).

22. Johnson, CE, Nuckols, ML, (Editors), Hyperbaric Diving Systems and Thermal Protection, American Society of Mechanical Engineers Publication OED-6, New York, (1978).

23. Joye, D.D., J.R. Clarke, N.A. Carlson, and E.D. Thalmann, "Characterization and Measurement of Elastance With Application to Underwater Breathing Apparatus," Undersea and Hyperbaric Medicine, 21:53-65, (1994).

24. Kang, B.S., Song, S.H., Suh, C.S., and Hong, S.K., "Changes in Body Temperature and Basal Metabolic Rate of the Ama", J. Appl. Physiol., 18, 483-488, (1963).

25. Kang, BS et al, "Changes in Body Temperature and Basal Metabolic Rate of the Ama," J. Appl. Physiol., 18, pp483-488, (1963).

26. Keenan, J. H., et al, Steam Tables, John Wiley and Sons, New York, (1969).

27. Knafelc, M.E., "Unmanned and Manned Evaluation of a Prototype Closed-Circuit Underwater Breathing Apparatus, the EX-19," NEDU Report 5-88, U.S. Navy Experimental Diving Unit, Panama City, FL (1988).
28. Kreith, F., <u>Principles of Heat Transfer</u>, Intl. Textbook Co., Scranton, PA (1960).
29. Kuehn, L.A., and Ackles, K.N., "Thermal Exposure Limits for Divers," <u>Hyperbaric Diving Systems and Thermal Protection</u>, American Society of Mechanical Engineers OED-6, New York, pp39-51, (1978).
30. Lippitt, MW, Nuckols, ML, "Active Diver Thermal Protection Requirements for Cold Water Diving", <u>Aviation, Space, and Environmental Medicine</u>, Vol 54, No. 7, pp644-648, (July 1983).
31. Lippitt, MW, Nuckols, ML, "The Development of an Improved Suit System for Cold Water Diving", <u>Proceedings of the 13th Intersociety Conference on Environmental Systems</u>, San Francisco, CA, (Jul 11-13, 1983).
32. Mausteller, JW, "Review of Potassium Superoxide Characteristics and Applications," <u>The Characterization of Carbon Dioxide Absorbing Agents for Life Support Equipment</u>, American Society of Mechanical Engineers, OED-10, New York, (1982).
33. McAdams, W.H., <u>Heat Transmissions</u>, 3rd Ed, McGraw-Hill, New York (1942).
34. Middleton, JR, Thalmann, ED, "Standardized NEDU Unmanned UBA Test Procedures and Performance Goals", U. S. Navy Experimental Diving Unit Report No. 3-81, Panama City, FL, (July 1981).
35. Military Standard MIL-W-82400, "Wet Suits, Neoprene," (22 Oct 1965).
36. Moody, L.F., "Friction Factors for Pipe Flow," <u>Transactions of the American Society of Mechanical Engineers</u>, Vol 66, pp 671-678, (1944).
37. Mooney, D.A., <u>Mechanical Engineering Thermodynamics</u>, Chapter 25, Prentice Hall, Inc., (1953).
38. <u>NOAA Diving Manual: Diving for Science and Technology</u>, National Oceanic and Atmospheric Administration, U.S. Department of Commerce, (Oct 1991).
39. Nuckols, M L, ed, <u>The Characterization of Carbon Dioxide Absorbing Agents For Life Support Equipment</u>, American Society of Mechanical Engineers OED-10, New York, (1982).
40. Nuckols, ML, "Heat and Mass Transfer in the Human Respiratory Tract", <u>Proceedings of the 34th Annual Conference on Engineering in Medicine and Biology</u>, Houston, TX, (21-23 Sept 1981).
41. Nuckols, ML, "Life Support Maintenance for Deep-Sea Diving", <u>Transactions of 1987 American Nuclear Society Meeting</u>, Vol 4, pp29-30, (June 1987).
42. Nuckols, ML, "Thermal Considerations In The Design Of Divers' Suits", <u>Hyperbaric Diving Systems and Thermal Protection</u>, American Society of Mechanical Engineers OED-6, New York, pp83-99, (1978).
43. Nuckols, ML, Courson, BF, "Passive Methods Of Thermal Protection For Cold Water Diving", <u>Proceedings of Underwater Intervention '94</u>, Marine Technology Society Meeting, San Diego, CA, (7-10 Feb 94).
44. Nuckols, ML, "The Development of Thermal Protection Equipment for Divers", <u>Proceedings of the 24th Undersea Medical Society Workshop: Thermal Constraints in Diving</u>, Bethesda, MD, (3-4 Sept 1980).
45. Nuckols, ML, Zumrick, JL, Johnson, CE, "Heat and Water Vapor Transfer in the Human Upper Airways at Hyperbaric Conditions", <u>J. of Biomechanical Engineering</u>, Vol 105, No. 1, pp 24-30, (Feb 1983).
46. Nuckols, ML, Lippitt, MW, Dudinsky, J, "The Liquid-Filled Suit-Intersuit Concept: Passive Thermal Protection For Divers," <u>Undersea Biomedical Research</u>, Vol 18, No. 3, pp 168-172, (1992)
47. Nuckols, M.L. and P. Sexton, "Optimization of Small Gas Ejectors Used in Semi-Closed Circuit Breathing Apparatus," <u>Current Practices and New Technology in Ocean Engineering--1987</u>, Am. Soc of Mechanical Engineers, OED-12, New York, pp87-90, (1987).
48. Nuckols, ML, Courson, BF, "Heated Diver Decompression Shelter: The Womb Concept", <u>Ocean Engineering</u>, Vol 21, No. 5, pp 433-443, (Jul 1994).
49. Nuckols, M.L., Purer, A., and Deason, G.A., "Design Guidelines for Carbon Dioxide Scrubbers," Naval Coastal Systems Center Technical Manual 4110-1-83, Rev A, Panama City, FL (1983).
50. Penzias, W, Goodman, MW, <u>Man Beneath the Sea: A Review Of Underwater Ocean Engineering</u>, Wiley-Interscience, New York, (1973).
51. Perry, R.H., and Chilton, C.H., (Editors), <u>Chemical Engineers' Handbook</u>, 3rd Ed, McGraw-Hill, New York, (1973).
52. Piantadosi, CA, Nuckols, ML, "Integration of Physiological and Physical Factors in the Design of Passive Thermal Garments for Divers", <u>J. of Undersea Biomedical Research</u>, Vol 6 (Suppl): 28, (Mar 1979).

53. Post, D.B., "Elementary Design Guidelines for CO_2 Scrubbing with LiOH," Naval Coastal Systems Center Technical Manual 4110-2-85, Panama City, FL (1985).

54. Purer, A., G.A. Deason, M.L. Nuckols, "The Effects of Chemical Hydration Level on CO_2 Absorption by High Performance Sodasorb," Naval Coastal Systems Center Technical Memorandum TM 363-82, Panama City, FL (1982).

55. Riegel, P.S., and Caudy, D.W., "Air Flow and Pressure Drop in Hyperbaric Baralyme Beds," The Characterization of Carbon Dioxide Absorbing Agents for Life Support Equipment, American Society of Mechanical Engineers, OED-10, New York, (1982).

56. Rules for Certification of Diving Systems, Det Norske Veritas, Norway, (1982).

57. Rules for Building and classing Underwater Systems and Vehicles, American Bureau of Shipping, New York, (1979).

58. Safety Standards for Pressure Vessels for Human Occupancy, ASME PVHO-1, American Society of Mechanical Engineers, New York, (1993).

59. Sarich, AJ, "Permeable Membrane Removal of Carbon Dioxide From Diving Gas," The Characterization of Carbon Dioxide Absorbing Agents for Life Support Equipment, American Society of Mechanical Engineers, OED-10, New York, (1982).

60. Schenk, Hilbert, Introduction to Ocean Engineering, New York: McGraw-Hill, (1975).

61. Schenk, Hilbert, Class Notes, URI Dept. of Ocean Engineering, (1970).

62. Sexton, P, "Universal Humidity Chart", Naval Coastal Systems Laboratory Report #122-72, Panama City, FL, (June 1972).

63. Silverman, L. *et al*, "Air Flow Measurements on Human Subjects With and Without Respiratory Resistance at Several Work Rates," Am. Med. Assoc. Archives of Industrial Hygiene and Occupational Medicine, Vol 3, pp461-478, (1951).

64. Staglin, B. "A Quantitative Investigation of Possible Means to Reduce the Drag of Swimming Scuba Divers," Master's Thesis, Thayer School of Engineering, Dartmouth College, (December 1993).

65. Systems Certification Procedures and Criteria Manual for Deep Submergence Systems, NAVMAT P9290.

66. Taylor, N.A.S., and J.B. Morrison, "Lung Centroid Pressure in Immersed Man," Undersea Biomedical Research, Vol 16, pp3-19, (1989).

67. Timoshenko, S., Strength of Materials, Part II, 3rd ed., Van Nostrand, Princeton, NJ, 1956

68. U.S. Navy Unmanned Test Methods and Performance Goals for Underwater Breathing Apparatus, U. S. Navy Experimental Diving Unit Technical Manual 1-94, (June 1994)

69. U.S. Navy Diving and Manned Hyperbaric Systems Safety Certification Manual, Naval Sea Systems Command, NSN 0910-LP-312-4600, (Oct 1987).

70. U.S. Navy Diving-Gas Manual, 2nd Ed, Navships 0994-003-0710, U.S. Navy Supervisor of Diving, Naval Ship Systems Command, Washington, DC, (June 1971).

71. U.S. Navy Diving Manual, Vol 2, Rev 3, NAVSEA 0994-LP-001-9020, Naval Sea Systems Command, Washington, DC, (1991).

72. Uhlig, H. H., (Ed.), The Corrosion Handbook, Wiley, New York, (1948).

73. Wang, TC, "Carbon Dioxide Scrubbing Materials in Life Support Equipment, " The Characterization of Carbon Dioxide Absorbing Agents for Life Support Equipment, American Society of Mechanical Engineers, OED-10, New York, (1982).

74. Wattenbarger, JF, Breckenridge, JR, "Dry Suit Insulation Characteristics Under Hyperbaric Conditions," Hyperbaric Diving Systems and Thermal Protection, American Society of Mechanical Engineers OED-6, New York, pp83-99, (1978).

75. Webb, P., Beckman, E., Sexton, P., and Vaughan, W., "Proposed Thermal Limits for Divers," Office of Naval Research Contract N00014-72-C-0057 (1976).

76. Witherspoon, *et al*, "Heat Transfer Coefficients of Humans in Cold Water," Proceedings of the Symposium Internationale Thermal Regulation Comportementale, Lyon, France, (7-11 Sep 1970).

77. Workman, R.D., "Calculation of Decompression Schedules for Nitrogen-Oxygen and Helium-Oxygen Dives," U.S. Naval Experimental Diving Unit Research Report 6-65, Washington, DC, (May 1965).

78. Zemansky, M. W., Heat and Thermodynamics, 5th ed., Chapter 6, McGraw-Hill, (1968).

Nomenclature

ACF	Volume, expressed in actual cubic feet at condition of the surrounding temperature and pressure.
A_f	Wall effect factor
A_{CS}	Cross-sectional area
A_S	Surface area
Ata	Atmospheres of pressure, absolute
Atm	Atmospheres of pressure, gage
BHP	Brake horsepower
BTPS	Body temperature and pressure, saturated (37°C, ambient pressure, 47 mmHg water vapor pressure)
°C	Degrees Celsius
C_d	Drag coefficient
CB	Center-of-buoyancy
CG	Center-of-gravity
CLO	A unit of thermal protection inherit in an article of clothing.
c_{N2}, c_{He} , etc	Molar concentrations of nitrogen, helium, etc dissolved in a liquid
cmH_2O	Centimeters of water pressure
CNS	Central nervous system
CO_2	Carbon Dioxide
c_P	Specific heat of a gas a constant pressure.
D	Depth
DDC	Deck decompression chamber
e	Absolute roughness of a pipe surface
e_P	Average particle diameter of a chemical absorbent
ERV	Expiratory reserve volume
F	Mixing effectiveness factor
F_B	Force due to buoyancy
°F	Degrees Fahrenheit
f	Breathing frequency measured in breaths per minute.
f	friction factor
f_m	Modified friction factor
FSW	Feet of sea water
g	Acceleration due to gravity = 32.174 ft/sec² at sealevel
g_c	Dimensional constant = 32.174 lbm-ft/lbf-sec²
Gr	Grashof Number; dimensionless free convection coefficient
h	Convective heat transfer coefficient
h_{fg}	Latent heat of water as it evaporates from a liquid to a vapor.
H_L	Frictional head loss associated with the flow of viscous fluids
Hp	Horsepower
HPNS	High pressure nervous syndrome
IRV	Inspiratory reserve volume
J/L	Joules per liter (unit of breathing effort, equivalent to 1 kPa)
K	Thermal conductivity
K	Minor loss coefficient
°K	Degrees Kelvin, absolute temperature scale
k	Ratio of gas specific heats
k_H	Henry's solubility constant which characterizes the amount of gases dissolved in liquids at a given temperature.
kg·m/L	kilogram meters per liter of respired volume (old method for expressing breathing effort; aka,

	Work-of-Breathing, WOB)
kPa	kilopascal (unit of pressure or breathing effort = 1000 Pa)
L	Liters
lbf	pounds force
lbm	pounds mass
LPM	Liters per minute
M_1	Mach number for a gas at the inlet of a pipe
M_{10}	Maximum tissue pressure for an inert gas at the 10-foot decompression stop; this is the maximum safe inert gas pressure within a tissue prior to surfacing.
ΔM	The change in maximum tissue pressures at each 10-foot stop interval.
MBT	Maximum bottom time.
$\dot{m}$	Mass flow rate for a gas or liquid.
$\dot{M}$	Metabolic heat production rate
M_{O2}, M_{N2}, etc	Molecular weights of elements and mixtures
MSW	Meters of sea water
N_W	Index of refraction
NEDU	Navy Experimental Diving Unit
$\overline{Nu}$	Nusselt number; dimensionless convective heat transfer coefficient
P, P_T	Ambient pressure
Pa	Pascal = 1 newton/m²
P_{O2}, P_{N2}, etc	Oxygen partial pressure, nitrogen partial pressure, etc
P_{H2O}	Hydrostatic pressure
Pr	Prandtl number
psi	Pounds per square inch
psia	Pounds per square inch, absolute
psig	Pounds per square inch, gage
PTC	Personnel transfer capsule
P-v	Pressure - volume
ΔP	Pressure differential
$\overline{P}_v$	Pressure, volume-averaged (term used to replace the old Work-of-Breathing, WOB)
$\dot{q}$	Rate of heat gain or loss
R	Thermal resistance
°R	Degrees Rankine, absolute temperature scale
R_{O2}, R_{N2}, etc	Gas constants for oxygen, nitrogen, etc
Re	Reynolds number = $\rho VD/\mu$
R_u	Universal gas constant = 1544 ft-lbf/mol-°R = 0.0821 L-atm/mol-°K
Resistive Effort	Volume-averaged pressure ($\overline{P}_v$) taken from a characteristic breathing loop; historically called Work-of-Breathing, WOB.
RMV	Respiratory minute volume; defined as the volume of breathing mixture exhaled by the diver in one minute (measured in liters per minute (BTPS)).
RNT	Residual nitrogen time.
RQ	Respiratory quotient; defined as the ratio of carbon dioxide produced - to - oxygen consumed during metabolism.
$\dot{s}$	Rate at which heat is being stored or depleted from the diver's body.
SCUBA	Self-contained, underwater breathing apparatus
%SEV	Percent surface equivalent volume
SCF	Standard cubic feet; volume at 1 Ata, 70°F
SCFM	Standard cubic feet per minute; volumetric flow rate at 1 Ata, 70°F
SI	Surface interval; defined as the time interval spent at the surface between dives.
SL	Standard liters; volume at 1 Ata, 32°C
SLPM	Standard liters per minute; volumetric flow rate at 1 Ata, 32°C

STPD	Standard temperature and pressure, dry
Suprasternal Notch	An anatomical reference point for oral/nasal differential pressure.
TBL	Theoretical bedlife for carbon dioxide scrubber canisters.
TFS	Trial first stop.
TV	Tidal volume; volume of gas that is either inspired or expired by the diver during each breath (measured in liters).
ΔT	Temperature difference
U_i, U_o	Overall heat transfer coefficient based on inside, outside surface area, respectively.
UBA	Underwater breathing apparatus
V	Volume
VC	Vital capacity
$\dot{V}_{CO_2}$	Metabolic carbon dioxide production rate; measured in standard liters per minute, SLPM.
$\dot{V}_{O_2}$	Metabolic oxygen consumption rate; measured in standard liters per minute, SLPM.
$\dot{V}_{gas}$	Gas ventilation rate, SCFM
$\overline{V}_s$	Superficial gas velocity
W	Humidity ratio; ratio of the mass of water per mass of dry gas.
$\dot{W}$	Rate at which work is being performed
wk_P	Mechanical work done on a fluid by a pump
WHP	Water horsepower
WOB	Work-of-Breathing normalized for tidal volume. A measure of volume-averaged pressure, also referred to as Resistive Effort. Currently measured in kPa or joules/L (measured in kg·m/L in the past).
X_{O2}, X_{CO2}	Volume fraction of oxygen, carbon dioxide, etc as a component in a gas mixture.
η	Efficiency
ρ	Density; mass per unit volume
μ	Gas viscosity
ν	Specific volume; volume per unit mass (inverse of density)
γ	Specific weight; weight per unit volume
σ	Stefan-Boltzmann constant = 0.1714×10^{-8} Btu/hr-ft^2-°R^4
ϵ_S	Emissivity of a gray body surface
Θ_M	Log mean temperature difference
ϕ	Relative humidity

Glossary

ACF Volume, expressed in actual cubic feet at conditions of the surrounding temperature and pressure.

ACFM An abbreviation for actual cubic feet per minute.

Alveolus A small membranous sac in the lungs in which gas exchange takes place.

Anoxia The absence of oxygen (see Hypoxia).

Apnea A brief cessation of breathing.

Asphyxia Anoxia caused by the cessation of effective gas exchange in the lung.

Atmosphere Diving System A pressure-resistant one-man diving system that has articulated arms and sometimes legs.

Ata Atmospheres of pressure, absolute.

Atm Atmospheres of pressure, gage.

Barotrauma Mechanical damage to, or distortion of, tissues caused by unequal pressures.

Bends A colloquial term meaning any form of decompression sickness.

Blowup The uncontrolled ascent of a diver who is wearing a deep sea diving suit or a variable-volume drysuit.

BHP Brake horsepower.

BTPS Environmental conditions at body temperature and pressure, and saturated with water vapor (37°C, ambient pressure, 47 mmHg water vapor pressure)

Chokes An imprecise term for the pulmonary symptoms of decompression sickness.

CLO A unit of thermal protection inherit in an article of clothing.

Closed-Circuit Breathing Apparatus A life support system or breathing apparatus in which the breathing gas is recycled, carbon dioxide is removed, and oxygen is added to replenish the supply as necessary.

Dead Space The space in a diving system in which residual exhaled gas remains. The dead space in diving equipment adds to the amount of dead space that occurs naturally in the lungs.

Decompression Dive Any dive involving a depth deep enough, or a duration long enough, to require decompression stops during ascent.

Decompression Schedule A set of depth-time relationships and instructions for controlling an ascent following a dive.

Decompression Sickness An illness caused by the presence of bubbles in the joints or tissues.

Dyspnea Difficulty in breathing.

Embolism A bubble in the arterial system that occurs when gas or air passes into the pulmonary veins after rupture of alveoli in the lungs.

Emphysema A pulmonary condition characterized by loss of lung elasticity and restriction of air movement.

Half Time (Half-life) — The time required to reach 50 percent of a final state. In diving, a half time is the time required for a tissue to absorb or eliminate 50 percent of the equilibrium amount of inert gas.

Heliox — A breathing mixture of helium and oxygen that is used at greater depths because it can be inhaled without narcotic effect.

Hemoglobin — The coloring matter of the red corpuscles of the blood; hemoglobin combines with oxygen, carbon dioxide, and carbon monoxide.

HPNS — Neurological and physiological dysfunction caused by hyperbaric exposure, usually associated with deep helium dives. Signs and symptoms include tremors, sleep difficulties, visual disturbances, nausea, dizziness, and convulsions.

Hypercapnia — A condition characterized by excessive carbon dioxide in the blood and/or tissues.

Hyperthermia — Elevation of the body temperature to levels above normal.

Hyperventilation — Rapid, unusually deep breathing at a rate greater than is necessary for the level of activity.

Hypothalamus — The nerve center in the brain that influences certain bodily functions such as metabolism, temperature regulation, and sleep.

Hypothermia — Reduction of the body's core temperature below normal levels.

Hypoxia — A condition characterized by tissue oxygen pressures that are below normal.

Inert Gases — Gases that exhibit great stability and extremely low reaction rates; gases that are not biologically active.

Laminar Flow — Non-turbulent flow of a fluid.

Lockout Submersible — A submersible that has one compartment for the pilot and/or observer that is maintained at a pressure of one atmosphere and another compartment that can be pressurized to ambient pressure to allow a diver to enter and exit while under water.

LPM — An abbreviation for liters per minute.

Mediastinal Emphysema — Excessive gas in the tissues below the breastbone and near the heart, major blood vessels, and trachea; caused by gases being forced into this area from the lungs.

Metabolism — The phenomenon of transforming food into energy; accompanied by oxygen consumption, carbon dioxide production and heat.

Narcosis — A state of stupor or unconsciousness caused by breathing certain narcotic gases, such as nitrogen, at elevated pressures. Symptoms usually include light-headedness, loss of judgment, and euphoria.

Nitrox — A breathing mixture containing nitrogen and oxygen in varying proportions.

Partial Pressure — The proportion of the total pressure contributed to a mixture by a single gas in that mixture.

Pneumothorax	The presence of gas within the chest cavity but outside the lungs.
Psia	Abbreviation for pounds per square inch, absolute.
Psig	Abbreviation for pounds per square inch, gauge; a term used to express the difference between absolute pressure and the specific pressure being measured.
Rebreather	A semi-closed, or closed-circuit breathing apparatus that removes carbon dioxide exhaled by the diver and adds oxygen as necessary.
Refraction	The bending of light rays as they pass from one medium to another of different density.
Repetitive Dive	Any dive conducted after 10 minutes to 12 hours of a previous dive. Dives conducted within 10 minutes of a previous dive are considered a continuation of the previous dive.
Repetitive Group Designation	A letter that is used in decompression tables to designate the amount of nitrogen remaining in a diver's body for 12 hours after the completion of a dive.
Residual Volume	The amount of gas that remains in the lungs after a person voluntarily exhales fully.
Residual Nitrogen	A theoretical concept that describes the amount of excess nitrogen that remains in a diver's tissues after a hyperbaric exposure.
Residual Nitrogen Time	The time (minutes) that is added to the actual dive time when calculating the decompression schedule for a repetitive dive.
Resistive Effort	Volume-averaged pressure ($\overline{P_v}$) taken from a characteristic breathing loop; historically called Work-of-Breathing, WOB.
Respiration	The process by which gases, oxygen and carbon dioxide, are interchanged among the tissues of the body and the atmosphere.
Respiratory Minute Volume	The volume of breathing mixture exhaled by the diver in one minute (measured in liters per minute (BTPS)).
Respiratory Quotient	The ratio of carbon dioxide produced - to - oxygen consumed during metabolism.
Saturation	A term used in diving to denote a state in which the diver's tissues have absorbed all the inert gases they can hold at any particular pressure. Once this state is reached, no additional decompression obligations will be required if the diver spends additional time at that depth.
SCF	An abbreviation for standard cubic feet; at 1Ata, 70°F.
SCFM	An abbreviation for standard cubic feet per minute; commonly used to express the output volume of air compressors at 1 Ata, 70°F.
Scrubber	A component of an atmospheric control system (ECS) that removes carbon dioxide from the breathing gas; usually by absorbing it with a chemical absorbent.
SCUBA	An abbreviation for self-contained, underwater breathing apparatus.

SL	Standard liters; volume at 1 Ata, 32°C.
SLPM	Standard liters per minute; volumetric flow rate at 1 Ata, 32°C.
Squeeze	Deformation of tissue or some portion of the body caused by a difference in pressure.
Stage Decompression	A decompression procedure involving decompression stops of specific durations at given depths; usually at 10-foot intervals.
STPD	Standard temperature and pressure, dry
Subcutaneous Emphysema	A condition in which air enters the tissues beneath the skin of the neck and extends along the facial planes; caused by air escaping from the lungs through a rupture of the alveoli.
Suprasternal Notch	An anatomical reference point for oral/nasal differential pressure.
Surface Interval	The period elapsing between the time a diver surfaces from a dive and the time the diver leaves the surface to perform a repetitive dive.
Tidal Volume	Volume of gas that is either inspired or expired by the diver during each breath (measured in liters).
Total Bottom Time	The total amount of time between the time a diver leaves the surface and the time that the diver begins his ascent.
Turbulent Flow	A type of flow in which the fluid velocity a t a fixed point fluctuates with time in a nearly random way.
Tympanic Membrane	The thin membranous partition that separates the external ear from the middle ear (also called eardrum).
UBA	An abbreviation for underwater breathing apparatus.
Variable-Volume Drysuit	A type of drysuit that has both an inlet gas valve and an exhaust valve to allow the diver to change the gas volume within the drysuit during a dive.
Vital Capacity	The maximum volume that can be expired after maximum inspiration.
Work-of-Breathing	A measure of volume-averaged pressure that occurs at the mouth of a diver during a complete breathing cycle; also referred to as Resistive Effort. Currently measured in kPa or joules/L (measured in kg·m/L in the past).

Problems

1. A gas consists of 20% oxygen and 80% helium by volume. Fill in the table below:

Depth (FSW)	Pressure (ATA)	PO_2 ATA	mmHg	Phe ATA	mmHg
0					
33					
500					
1000					

2. Complete the table below:

Depth (FSW)	Pressure (psia)	Temperature °F	Volume ACF	SCF
0		70	8	
50		50		80
600		90	120	
500		32		2500

3. Determine the conversion factor to convert SCFM into SLPM.

4. A charged SCUBA bottle reads 2250 psig when read on the surface at 70° F using a bourdon tube pressure gage. What would the same gage read on the same bottle inside a PTC that is pressurized to 1500 FSW when the temperature is 45° F?

5. A gas mixture contains 0.5% CO_2 by volume. What is the CO_2 percent surface equivalent (%SEV) of this mixture when pressurized to 297 FSW?

6. A gas cylinder with an internal volume of 1 ACF is pressurized with air at 2250 psig. A cylindrical diving bell, accidently flooded with seawater while suspended at a depth of 66 FSW, will be evacuated with the air cylinder.

a) At what height will the water surface be displaced from the bell ceiling after emptying the gas cylinder? The diving bell dimensions are 6 ft diameter by 5 ft height (inside dimensions). Assume constant temperature.

b) How much ballast must be added to counteract the buoyancy of this trapped air?

7. A life jacket is being designed to provide 25 pounds of positive buoyancy to a diver at a depth of 130 fsw at a temperature of 40° F. Determine the air cartridge volume required to inflate the life jacket if the cartridge is pressurized to 600 psig at 70° F. (Don't ignore residual volume.)

8. What is the maximum depth that a 70% helium, 20% nitrogen, 10% oxygen mixture can be used if the partial pressure of the oxygen is not permitted to exceed 2 ATA and the partial pressure of the nitrogen is not permitted to exceed an equivalent seawater depth of 150 fsw?

9. A 1.5 ACF cylinder filled with air at 2250 psig is used to fill a lift bag. How much lift will be provided by the inflated bag at a depth of 80 fsw? Do not ignore the residual volume of the cylinder.

10. Calculate the molecular weight, density, specific heat, gas constant, and viscosity of a gas mixture containing 10% oxygen, 70% helium, and 20% nitrogen at a depth of 500 fsw and a temperature of 50° F.

11. A diver is swimming at 100 FSW where the temperature is 45° F. He is consuming 1.5 ft³/min (BTPS) air while swimming at this depth. How long will it take the diver to empty an air bottle rated at 80 standard cubic feet (SCF) at this depth if the actual volume of the bottle is 0.4 ft³ ? (Note: Don't ignore the residual volume in the tank.)

12. At the surface a diver inflates his life vest to an internal volume of 140 in³ to make himself neutrally buoyant in seawater.

a) Before inflating his vest how negatively buoyant was the diver?

b) What will be the internal volume of his vest after the diver reaches a depth of 150 FSW if no additional air is added to the vest? (Assume no temperature change.)

c) What change in buoyancy will the diver see, in comparison with surface buoyancy, after the diver reaches 150 FSW?

13. A lift bag is inflated underwater to a volume of 3 ft³ with air at 90° F. If this bag travels through a thermocline such that the surrounding water temperature dropped to 50° F, how would the lifting capability of the bag change? (Depth remains constant. Assume seawater.)

14. What is the maximum depth that air (79% nitrogen/21% oxygen) can be safely used if the partial pressure of oxygen is not to exceed 1.6 ATA and the partial pressure of nitrogen is not permitted to exceed 5.5 ATA?

15. A scuba bottle, charged to 2250 psig at 70° F, has a burst pressure of 4900 psig. At what temperature would it rupture if caught in a fire? (Assume atmospheric pressure is 15 psia.)

16. Write a computer program to calculate the physical and thermal gas properties for

a) a mixture containing 10% oxygen/90% helium
b) a mixture containing 50% oxygen/50% nitrogen
c) a mixture containing 16% oxygen/50% helium/34% nitrogen

 at depths of 0, 200, 500 FSW and temperatures of 40°, 70°, and 90°F.

17. A life jacket is designed to provide 10 pounds of positive buoyancy at 150 FSW where the temperature is 30°F.

a) What is the required volume of this jacket?

b) What gas cartridge volume rated at 500 psig and 80°F will be required to inflate this jacket? (Note: Do not ignore the unavailable gas volume.)

18. A diver completes a work dive to 130 FSW with a bottom time of 60 minutes.

a) What is his decompression schedule and repetitive group?

b) After a 1-hour surface interval the diver makes a 30-minute dive to 80 FSW. What schedule should be used for this dive?

c) Following a 3 hour surface interval after the second dive, what is the longest dive to 80 feet that the diver can make without decompression?

19. Two **Navy** divers (SCUBA) dive to 100 FSW for 15 minutes. After surfacing they are told that they need to make a second dive to 60 FSW for an estimated bottom time of 40 minutes.

a) What surface interval will be required to avoid decompression for the second dive?

b) What is their repetitive group following the second dive?

20. Show repetitive group indices, RNT's, SI's, and total bottom times for each:

a) Dive to 90' for 20 minutes followed 30 minutes later by a dive to 40' for 80 minutes.

b) Dive to 40' for 80 minutes followed 30 minutes later by a dive to 90' for 20 minutes.

21. Show repetitive group indices, RNT's, SI's, and total bottom times for each:

a) Dive to 60' for 60 minutes followed 1 hour later by a dive to 30' for 60 minutes.

b) Dive to 75' for 30 minutes followed 2 hours later by a dive to 50' for 60 minutes.

22. Show repetitive group indices, RNT's, SI's, and total bottom times for each:

a) Dive to 90' for 15 minutes followed 5 minutes later by a dive to 100' for 15 minutes.

b) Dive to 60' for 30 minutes followed 30 minutes later by a dive to 60' for 30 minutes.

23. Show repetitive group indices, RNT's, SI's, and total bottom times for each:

a) Dive to 60' for 40 minutes followed 1 hour later by a dive to 60' for the maximum time without decompression stops.

b) Dive to 100' for 25 minutes followed 1-1/2 hours later by a dive to 50' for the maximum time without decompression stops.

24 . Show repetitive group indices, RNT's, SI's, and total bottom times for each:

a) Dive to 100' for 15 minutes to be followed by a second dive to 100' for 15 minutes with the minimum surface interval for no decompression.

b) Dive to 110' for 20 minutes to be followed by a second dive to 80' for 20 minutes with the minimum surface interval for no decompression.

25. A diver descends to 70 FSW on air for a bottom time of 100 minutes. Calculate the decompression schedule for this dive based on tissue half-lives of 5, 10, 20, 40, 80, 120 minutes, and compare calculated schedule with that given in the Standard Navy Air Decompression Tables.

26. A diver leaves the surface where he was originally breathing air, and dives to 110 FSW for 70 minutes on air.

a) What will the tissue nitrogen pressures be at the end of this exposure for tissue half-times of 10, 20, 40, and 120 minutes?

b) At what depth will the diver make his first decompression stop when surfacing?

c) How long must the diver remain at the first stop?

27. Two researchers are trapped in a one atmosphere control sphere of an underwater vehicle which has been cut off from surface supplied gas and the CO_2 removal system. How long will it take for the researchers to become unconscious due to the CO_2 buildup or lack of oxygen? Clearly state all assumptions.

Volume of sphere: 100 ft^3
Initial Atmosphere: 0.21 ATA O_2, 0.79 ATA N_2
Assume an RQ of 1.1
Assume critical CO_2 limit is 6% SEV
Assume critical O_2 limit of 0.10 ATA
Assume an O_2 consumption rate of 0.5 slpm per man.

28. You, along with 20 other midshipmen (21 total) are trapped in classroom R224 taking the EN470 final exam when all outside ventilation to the room is cut off!

a) Will you have time to finish the exam before becoming unconscious due to carbon dioxide buildup in the room and/or lack of oxygen? You have a 3 hour exam. The average oxygen consumption rate per mid is 0.5 slpm. Volume of the room is 4000 ft^3. Initial Atmosphere: 0.21 ATA oxygen, 0.79 ATA nitrogen; Respiratory Quotient is 0.9. Assume critical CO_2 limit is 6% SEV; assume critical O_2 limit of 0.10 ATA. Surface air is 0.035% CO_2 by volume.

b) What ventilation rate would you recommend for this room?

29. A surface-supplied diver at 200 FSW is wearing a helmet with an internal volume of 8.0 liters. The diver is working moderately hard with an oxygen consumption level of 1.5 slpm.

a) What air flow rate, in ACFM, is required to keep a safe carbon dioxide level in the helmet during a long dive? Assume a RQ = 0.85. Surface air has 0.035% CO_2.

b) If the air flow is interrupted, how long does the diver have to get back to the surface before unconsciousness sets in?

30. The carbon dioxide scrubber in a closed-circuit breathing apparatus has the capability to absorb 495 standard liters of carbon dioxide in an underwater mission at 100 FSW, 40°F. What is the safe mission duration when using this apparatus if the diver has a respiratory minute volume of 45 liter/min and a respiratory quotient of 0.85?

31. A diver has a tidal volume of 2.5 liters and a breathing rate of 25 breaths per minute. He is producing carbon dioxide metabolically at the rate of 2.2 SLPM. Calculate

a) the diver's respiratory minute volume (RMV), BTPS

b) the diver's oxygen consumption rate, slpm

c) the diver's respiratory quotient (RQ)

32. LiOH absorbs carbon dioxide according to the following chemical reaction:

$$2\ LiOH + CO_2\ \text{---------}> Li_2CO_3 + H_2O$$

a) If a diver is producing 1.5 slpm of CO_2, what is the theoretical bedlife of a canister which contains 6.0 lbs of LiOH?

b) What will be the predicted canister breakthrough time (time until the exit CO_2 level reaches 0.5% SEV) if the canister efficiency is 78%?

c) What theoretical weight of calcium hydroxide, $Ca(OH)_2$, is required to give the same mission duration as that calculated in part a)? The reaction for calcium hydroxide is

$$Ca(OH)_2 + CO_2\ \text{----------}> CaCO_3 + H_2O$$

33. KO_2, potassium superoxide, has been suggested as a potential chemical for absorbing carbon dioxide, as well as, providing oxygen by the net reaction

$$2KO_2 + CO_2\ \text{---------}> K_2CO_3 + 1.5\ O_2$$

If used in a closed-circuit UBA, will a supplemental oxygen supply be necessary? Explain.

34. You have been asked to design a new CO_2 scrubber system for the submersible Atlantis. Sodium hydroxide, an alkali metal hydroxide from group 1A on the periodic table, is being considered for this design. The net reaction is

$$2\ NaOH + CO_2\ \text{---->}\ Na_2CO_3 + H_2O$$

The chemical has a bulk density of 25.6 lb/ft³. Atlantis will have a crew of twenty, each having an oxygen consumption level of 0.5 slpm and a respiratory quotient of 0.9. Its cabin has an internal volume of 1800 ft³, and the atmosphere is air (21% oxygen/79% nitrogen) maintained at 14.7 psia and 65°F.

a) What is the theoretical absorption capacity of this scrubber material, lbCO₂/lb?

b) At what rate is the Atlantis crew producing CO_2, lbCO₂/hr?

c) If the new canister has been found to have an efficiency of 75%, how much absorbent must the canister hold to give a breakthrough of 24 hours, lbm?

d) How much water will be produced by the absorption process during the 24 hour period, lbm?

35. Seawater is being supplied to a diver at 300 FSW at 50 psi over bottom pressure through a 0.6-inch diameter smooth hose that is 500 feet long. The water enters the hose at the surface at a pressure of 500 psig. Two 90 degree elbows, each with a minor loss coefficient of 0.5 and a check valve (k=8.0) are included in this hose circuit. What flow rate (ft³/min will be delivered to the diver? (Assume seawater properties: density=64 lbm/ft , viscosity=0.458 x 10-3 lbm/ft-sec)

36. A Bronco underwater cutting torch is being used at a depth of 30 FSW. A 150 foot long smooth hose with 3/8-inch ID delivers oxygen to the torch at 100 psi over bottom when the topside regulator setting is 130 psig. If the oxygen is being delivered from a high pressure storage bottle with a capacity of 200 SCF, how long can we operate the torch

before the bottle is emptied? Assume: a) All oxygen in the tank is available.
   b) Temperature is 70°F, gas constant is 48.29   ft-lbf/lbm-°R, k=cp/cv=1.4

37. A 1000-ft long umbilical supplies a heliox mixture containing 99% helium to a PTC at a depth of 850 FSW. The pressure at the umbilical inlet is 700 psig. Determine the pressure of the gas at the PTC inlet valve for a gas flow rate of 300 SCFM if the hose diameter (ID) is 0.5 inches and the gas temp is 50°F. k=1.67. Assume smooth pipe.

38. The wall of the space shuttle cabin consists of an inside finish of 1/2-inch thick polyethylene (k=0.15 Btu/hr-ft-°F), two layers of 2-inch thick corkboard (k=0.03 Btu/hr-ft-°F), an outside layer of 1/8-inch thick aluminum (k=118 Btu/ft-hr- °F) with a coating of 1/4-inch thick ceramic tile (k=10 Btu/ft-hr-°F). The internal and external convective heat transfer coefficients (film coefficients) at 1 atmosphere are 1.65 Btu/hr-ft-°F. The internal air temperature is 70°F and outside temperature at an altitude of 40,000 feet is -68°F. Calculate:

a) the overall heat transfer coefficient, U (assume flat plate)

b) the rate of heat transfer through the wall at 40,000 feet, Btu/hr. (wall consists of a 30 foot diameter cylinder, 25 feet long; assume flat ends.)

39. A well insulated breath heater is mounted to a diver's helmet to warm his inspired gases using a steady stream of hot water. The breathing gas flows through the heater at a rate of 6 acfm, with an inlet temperature of 40°F and an exit temperature of 90°F (gas density is 0.355 lbm/ft^3, gas specific heat is 0.68 Btu/lbm-°F). The hot water enters the heater at 110°F and exits
at 95°F (water density is 64 lbm/ft^3, specific heat for water is 0.94 Btu/lbm-°F). Calculate:

a) the log mean temperature difference across the breath heater if the flow of water is in opposite direction to the gas (ie, counterflow)

b) the total heat being transferred to the breathing gas

c) the overall heat transfer coefficient of the heater if its surface area is 9 ft^2.

40. Hot water is being supplied at 5 gpm to a surface supported diver through a 350 foot umbilical hose (0.5 inch ID by 0.92 inch OD). It is desired that the water temperature at the diver site be 100°F. If the diver and umbilical are surrounded by 35°F water, what temperature would you recommend that the water be heated at the surface? The film coefficients for the hose have been found to be: h_o=400 Btu/hr-ft^2-°F , h_i =100 Btu/hr-ft^2-°F
   The thermal conductivity of the hose is 0.12 Btu/hr-ft-°F.
   Thermal properties of the hot water are: density = 62 lbm/ft^3
   thermal conductivity = 0.364 Btu/hr-ft-°F
   specific heat = 1.0 Btu/lbm-°F

41. A spherical diving bell, with an outside diameter of 7 feet and a wall thickness of 1 inch, is lowered into 40°F water. A water current of 1 knot flows over the bell (1 kt=1.688 ft/sec).
Assume:
i) film coefficient on inside surface of bell is 1 Btu/hr-ft^2-°F
ii) for outside surface: $\overline{Nu_D} = 0.37\ Re_D^{0.6}$

iii) thermal conductivity of bell material, k=8 Btu/hr-ft-°F
iv) for water at 40°F, density = 62.4 lbm/ft^3
                    viscosity = 1.04 x 10^{-3} lbm/ft-sec
                    thermal cond, k=0.33 Btu/hr-ft-°F

a) What is the heat loss from the bell if the internal temperature is maintained at 90°F by an environmental control system?

b) What is the reduction in heat loss if 1-inch thick insulation is added to the inside of the diving bell (k_{ins}=0.06 Btu/hr-ft-°F)?

42. A diver is using a hot water suit (surface area of 18 ft^2) in 35°F water to surround his body with a thin layer of warm water. The suit is constructed of 3/16-inch thick foam neoprene (k=0.03 Btu/hr-ft-°F). If hot water is supplied at 110°F, what flow rate (ft^3/min) will be required to give an exhaust temperature from the suit of 95°F? Convective heat transfer coefficients have been found to be: h_i= 106 Btu/hr-ft^2-°F ; h_o= 84 Btu/hr-ft^2-°F

Water properties are as follows: density=62 lb/ft^3, specific heat= 1 Btu/lb-°F.
(Hint: Assume the suit is a flat plate.)

43. Air has a dry bulb temperature of 90°F and a wet bulb temperature of 70°F. For atmospheric pressures of 14.7 and 30 psia, find for each:

a) relative humidity
b) enthalpy of the gas mixture
c) humidity ratio

44. An environmental control system (ECS) dehumidifies and reheats 120 acfm of air (entrance conditions) at a depth of 191 fsw (100 psia). The gas enters the ECS at 70°F and 90% relative humidity and leaves at 80°F and 30% relative humidity. Determine:

a) dehumidification energy
b) reheat energy

45. For a 15% oxygen, 85% helium gas mixture, the wet-bulb temperature is 83°F, the dry-bulb temperature is 90°F, and the ambient pressure is 200 psia. Find:

a) relative humidity
b) humidity ratio
c) enthalpy of the mixture

46. An ECS is being designed for a deck decompression chamber with the following specifications: Depth=1100 FSW; Gas mixture: 2% oxygen/98 % helium; Gas flow rate= 150 acfm (entering conditions); Gas temperatures: entering=85°F, exiting=90°F; Relative humidity: entering=90%, exiting=40%.   For the proposed system determine:

a) Dehumidification coil temperature
b) Dehumidification energy
c) Reheat energy
d) Moisture removal rate

47. Air is stored in a scuba tank at 600 psia and 70°F.
a) What is the humidity ratio of this gas if it is saturated at 600 psia?

b) If we expand this air to 14.7 psia and 70°F, what will be the relative humidity after expansion?

c) If we breathe this air on the surface at 2.4 scfm, how much water must be added to the air to be fully saturated at body temperature (98.6°F), lb/hr?

d) How much heat is pulled from the lungs to humidify and heat the air to body temperature, Btu/hr?

48. Calculate the respiratory heat loss for a diver at 1100 FSW breathing a mixture of 98% He/2% O_2. Inspired gas temperature is 60°F and relative humidity is 10%. The exhaled gas is saturated at 89.8°F. The diver RMV is 1.5 ft³/min.

49. Seawater is being supplied to a diver at 300 FSW at a rate of 1.9 ft³/min. The water pump draws seawater from surface pressure and delivers it to the hose entrance at the surface at a pressure of 500 psig. What horsepower level must be supplied to the pump if the pump efficiency is 70%? (Seawater properties: density = 64 lbm/ft³, viscosity = 0.458 x 10⁻³ lbm/ft-sec)

50. A diesel engine is required to run an air compressor used on a dive to 300 FSW. The compressor exit pressure is set at 100 psi over bottom and inlet pressure is 14.7 psia. What size diesel (HP) is required to deliver 12 ACFM to the dive site at 300 FSW? Assume air inlet properties at 70°F; R = 53.3 ft-lbf/lbm-°R, k = 1.4, Isentropic efficiency of compressor = 0.65, mechanical efficiency = 0.7.

ANSWERS

1. 0 FSW: 1 ATA; 0.2 ATA, 152 mmHg, 2.94 psia;   0.8 ATA, 608 mmHg, 11.76 psia
2. 50 FSW: 36.97 psia; 30.6 ACF
3. 1 SCFM = 26.3 SLPM
4. 1475 psia
5. 5 %SEV
6. 1.78 ft; 3225.6 lbf
7. 96.5 in³
8. 627 FSW
9. ·4223.2 lbf
10. 11.6, 0.504 lb/ft³, 0.481 Btu/lb-°F, 133.1 ft-lbf/lbm-°R, 1.334 x 10⁻⁵ lbm/ft-sec
11. 12.3 min
12. 5.19 lbf, 25.2 in³, -4.25 lbf
13. -13.96 lbf
14. 196.7 FSW
15. 690 °F
16. EX: (10% O_2/90% He at 200 FSW, 70°F); DENSITY=0.124 lbm/ft³
     MOL WT=6.8, SPEC HT=0.76, GAS CONST=226.99, VISC=1.414 x 10⁻⁵
17. 0.156 ft³, 0.033 ft³
18. a) 30' for 9 min, 20' for 23 min, 10' for 52 min; Z

b) 20' for 11 min, 10' for 46 min

c) 12 min

19. a) SI=1:58   b) J

	RGI	RNT	SI	TBT
20.a)	F	61	30	141
b)	H	33	30	53(DECOMP)
21.a)	J	--	1:00	UNLIMITED
b)	G	29	2:00	89
22.a)	100' for 30 min (DECOMP)			
b)	F	30	30	60
23.a)	G	36	1:00	60 (24 min)
b)	H	47	1:30	100 (53 min)
24.a)	E	10	1:58	25 (15 min)
b)	G	18	2:00	38 (20 min)

25. 20' for 3 min, 10' for 29 min

26.   a) 113 fsw, 106 fsw, 88 fsw, 55 fsw

      b) 30 fsw

      c) 5 min

27. CO_2: 2.4 hrs; O_2: 4.8 hrs

28.   a) CO_2: 11.1 hrs; O_2: 18 hrs

      b) 77.3 SCFM

29.   a) 19.2 ACFM   b) CO_2: 0.32 min, O_2: 6.9 min

30. 310.6 min

31.   a) 62.5 LPM   b) 2.6 SLPM   c) 0.845

32.   a) 14.1 hrs   b) 11.0 hrs   c) 9.35 lb

33. No. SRQ=0.67 (over produces O_2)

34.   a) 0.55   b) 2.34   c) 136.2   d) 23.0

35. 2.25 CFM

36. 9.86 min

37. 575.3 psia

38.   a) 0.079   b) 41,099.6

39.   a) 34.6 °F   b) 72.4 Btu/min   c) 13.95

40. 111.1 oF

41. a) 7466 Btu/hr   b) 4234.7 Btu/hr reduction

42. 0.04 ft³/min

43.   14.7 PSIA: a) 36.7%   b) 34 Btu/lb   c) 0.0112 lbH_2O/lb

      30.0 PSIA: a) 20.8%   b) 25.1 Btu/lb

      c) 0.0031 lbH_2O/lb

44.   a) 440.6 Btu/min b) 520.2 Btu/min

45.   a) 28.6%   b) 0.0022 lbH_2O/lb   c) 60.6 BTU/lb

46.   a) 61°F   b) 1696 Btu/min   c) 1878 Btu/min d) 7.6 lbH_2O/lb

47.   a) 0.00037 b) 2.3%   c) 0.44   d) 560 Btu/hr

48.   sensible:1169 Btu/hr,   latent:206.5 Btu/hr,   total: 1375 Btu/hr

Appendix A: Conversion Tables

The following conversions use Sarich Notation© where $n^{\backslash m} = n \times 10^{m}$

LENGTH

	cm	in	ft	yd	m	fathom	km	miles	nautical mile
1 cm=	1	.3937	.03280	.01094	.01	$5.468^{\backslash-3}$	$1^{\backslash-5}$	$6.214^{\backslash-6}$	$5.396^{\backslash-6}$
1 in =	2.540	1	.08333	.02778	.0254	.01389	$2.54^{\backslash-5}$	$1.578^{\backslash-5}$	$1.371^{\backslash-5}$
1 ft =	30.48	12	1	.3333	.3048	.1667	$3.048^{\backslash-4}$	$1.894^{\backslash-4}$	$1.645^{\backslash-4}$
1 yd =	91.44	36	3	1	.9144	.5	$9.144^{\backslash-4}$	$5.682^{\backslash-4}$	$4.934^{\backslash-4}$
1 m =	100	39.37	3.281	1.094	1	.5468	.001	$6.214^{\backslash-4}$	$5.396^{\backslash-4}$
1 fath. =	182.9	72	6	2	1.829	1	$1.829^{\backslash-3}$	$1.136^{\backslash-3}$	$9.868^{\backslash-4}$
1 km =	$1^{\backslash5}$	$3.937^{\backslash4}$	3281	1094	1000	546.8	1	.6214	.5396
1 mile =	$1.609^{\backslash5}$	$6.336^{\backslash4}$	5280	1760	1609	880	1.609	1	.8684
1 Nmi =	$1.853^{\backslash5}$	$7.296^{\backslash4}$	6080	2027	1853	1013	1.853	1.152	1

AREA

	m²	cm²	in²	ft²	yd²	acres	miles²
1 m² =	1	$1^{\backslash4}$	1550	10.76	1.196	$2.471^{\backslash-4}$	$3.681^{\backslash-7}$
1 cm² =	$1^{\backslash-4}$	1	.155	$1.076^{\backslash-3}$	$1.196^{\backslash-4}$	$2.471^{\backslash-8}$	$3.861^{\backslash-11}$
1 in² =	$6.452^{\backslash-4}$	6.452	1	$6.944^{\backslash-3}$	$7.716^{\backslash-4}$	$1.594^{\backslash-7}$	$2.491^{\backslash-10}$
1 ft² =	.0929	929.0	144	1	.1111	$2.296^{\backslash-5}$	$3.578^{\backslash-8}$
1 yd² =	.8361	8361	1296	9	1	$2.066^{\backslash-4}$	$3.228^{\backslash-7}$
1 acre =	4047	$4.047^{\backslash7}$	$6.273^{\backslash6}$	$4.356^{\backslash4}$	4840	1	$1.563^{\backslash-3}$
1 mile² =	$2.59^{\backslash6}$	$2.59^{\backslash10}$	$4.015^{\backslash9}$	$2.788^{\backslash7}$	$3.098^{\backslash6}$	640	1

VOLUME

	cm³	in³	ft³	yd³	liters	pint	quart	gallon
1 cm³ =	1	.06102	$3.531^{\backslash\text{-}5}$	$1.310^{\backslash\text{-}6}$	$1^{\backslash\text{-}4}$	$2.113^{\backslash\text{-}3}$	$1.057^{\backslash\text{-}3}$	$2.642^{\backslash\text{-}4}$
1 in³ =	16.39	1	$5.787^{\backslash\text{-}4}$	$2.143^{\backslash\text{-}5}$	.01639	.03463	.01732	$4.329^{\backslash\text{-}3}$
1 ft³ =	$2.832^{\backslash4}$	1728	1	.03704	28.32	59.84	29.92	7.481
1 yd³ =	$7.646^{\backslash5}$	$4.666^{\backslash4}$	27	1	764.5	1616	807.9	202.0
1 liter =	1000	61.03	.03532	$1.308^{\backslash\text{-}3}$	1	2.113	1.057	.2642
1 pint =	473.2	28.88	.01671	$6.189^{\backslash\text{-}4}$	.4732	1	.5	.125
1 quart =	946.4	57.75	.03342	$1.238^{\backslash\text{-}3}$	.9463	2	1	.25
1 gallon =	3785	231	.1337	$4.951^{\backslash\text{-}3}$	3.785	8	4	1

MASS

	kg	gm	grains	ounces	lbm	tons (short)	tons (long)	tons (metric)
1 kg =	1	1000	15,432	35.27	2.205	$1.102^{\backslash\text{-}3}$	$9.842^{\backslash\text{-}4}$	0.001
1 gm =	0.001	1	15.43	$3.527^{\backslash\text{-}2}$	$2.205^{\backslash\text{-}3}$	$1.102^{\backslash\text{-}6}$	$9.842^{\backslash\text{-}7}$	$1^{\backslash\text{-}6}$
1 grain =	$6.480^{\backslash\text{-}5}$	$6.480^{\backslash\text{-}2}$	1	$2.286^{\backslash\text{-}3}$	$1.429^{\backslash\text{-}4}$	$7.143^{\backslash\text{-}8}$	$6.378^{\backslash\text{-}8}$	$6.480^{\backslash\text{-}8}$
1 ounce =	$2.835^{\backslash\text{-}2}$	28.35	437.5	1	0.0625	$3.125^{\backslash\text{-}5}$	$2.790^{\backslash\text{-}5}$	$2.835^{\backslash\text{-}5}$
1 lbm =	0.4536	453.6	7000	16	1	$5^{\backslash\text{-}4}$	$4.464^{\backslash\text{-}4}$	$4.536^{\backslash\text{-}4}$
1 shrt ton =	907.2	$9.072^{\backslash5}$	$1.4^{\backslash7}$	32,000	2000	1	0.8929	0.9072
1 long ton =	1016	$1.016^{\backslash6}$	$1.568^{\backslash7}$	35,840	2240	1.12	1	1.016
1 metric ton =	1000	$1^{\backslash6}$	$1.543^{\backslash7}$	35,274	2205	1.102	0.9842	1

VELOCITY

	ft/sec	km/hr	m/sec	miles/hr	cm/sec	knot
1 ft/sec =	1	1.097	0.3048	0.6818	30.48	0.5925
1 km/hr =	0.9113	1	0.2778	0.6214	27.78	0.5400
1 m/sec =	3.281	3.6	1	2.237	100	1.944
1 mile/hr =	1.467	1.609	0.4470	1	44.70	0.8689
1 cm/sec =	3.281^{-2}	3.6^{-2}	0.01	2.237^{-2}	1	1.944^{-2}
1 knot =	1.688	1.852	0.5144	1.151	51.44	1

FORCE

	dyne	NT	lb	gf	kgf
1 dyne =	1	1^{-5}	2.248^{-6}	1.020^{-3}	1.020^{-6}
1 NT =	1^{5}	1	0.2248	102.0	0.1020
1 pound =	4.448^{5}	4.448	1	453.6	0.4536
1 gram force =	980.7	9.807^{-3}	2.205^{-3}	1	0.001
1 kgf =	9.807^{5}	9.807	2.205	1000	1

ENERGY

	Btu	erg	ft-lb	hp-hr	joules	cal	kw-hr
1 Btu =	1	1.055^{10}	777.9	3.929^{-4}	1055	252.0	2.930^{-4}
1 erg =	9.481^{-11}	1	7.378^{-8}	3.725^{-14}	1^{-7}	2.389^{-8}	2.778^{-14}
1 ft-lb =	1.285^{-3}	1.356^{7}	1	5.051^{-7}	1.356	0.3239	3.766^{-7}
1 hp-hr	2545	2.685^{13}	1.980^{6}	1	2.685^{6}	6.414^{5}	0.7457
1 joule =	9.481^{-4}	1^{7}	0.7376	3.725^{-7}	1	0.2389	2.778^{-7}
1 calorie =	3.968^{-3}	4.186^{7}	3.087	1.559^{-6}	4.186	1	1.163^{-6}
1 kw-hr =	3413	3.6^{13}	2.655^{6}	1.341	3.6^{6}	8.601^{5}	1

Note: 1 erg = 1 gm-cm^2/sec^2
          1 kcal = 3.968 Btu

POWER

	hp	kw	joules/sec	ft-lb/sec	Btu/sec
1 horsepower =	1	0.7456	745.6	550	0.7068
1 kilowatt	1.341	1	1000	737.7	0.9480
1 joule/sec =	$1.341^{\backslash-3}$	0.001	1	0.7377	$9.480^{\backslash-4}$
1 ft-lb/sec =	$1.918^{\backslash-3}$	$1.356^{\backslash-3}$	1.356	1	$1.285^{\backslash-3}$
1 Btu/sec =	1.415	1.055	1055	778.2	1

PRESSURE

	atm	bars	dyne/cm^2	lb/in^2 (psia)	mm Hg	in Hg	in FW	ft FW	ft SW
atm =	1	1.013	$1.013^{\backslash6}$	14.7	760	29.92	407.0	33.91	33.07
bar =	0.9869	1	$1^{\backslash6}$	14.50	750.1	29.53	401.6	33.47	32.63
dyne/ cm^2	$9.869^{\backslash-7}$	$1^{\backslash-6}$	1	$1.45^{\backslash-5}$	$7.501^{\backslash-4}$	$2.953^{\backslash-5}$	$4.01^{\backslash-4}$	$3.347^{\backslash-5}$	$3.263^{\backslash-5}$
lb/in^2 =	$6.805^{\backslash-2}$	$6.895^{\backslash-2}$	$6.895^{\backslash4}$	1	51.71	2.036	27.69	2.308	2.25
mm Hg =	$1.316^{\backslash-3}$	$1.333^{\backslash-3}$	$1.333^{\backslash3}$	19.34	1	.03937	0.5355	0.04462	0.04351
in Hg =	0.03342	0.03386	$3.386^{\backslash4}$	0.4912	25.4	1	13.60	1.133	1.105
m FW =	0.0967	0.0980	$9.8^{\backslash4}$	1.422	73.52	2.895	39.37	3.281	3.199
in FW =	$2.456^{\backslash-3}$	$2.489^{\backslash-3}$	$2.489^{\backslash3}$	0.03609	1.867	0.07352	1	0.08333	0.08125
ft FW =	0.02949	0.02988	$2.988^{\backslash4}$	0.4333	22.41	0.8823	12	1	0.975
ft SW =	0.03024	0.03064	$3.064^{\backslash4}$	0.4444	22.98	0.9049	12.31	1.026	1

Note: 1. Column of Mercury (Hg) at 0° C.
2. Fresh water (FW) = 62.4 lbs/ft^3;   salt water (SW) = 64.0 lbs/ft^3 at 15° C.

MISCELLANEOUS

Specific Heat:	1 cal/g-°C = 1 Btu/lbm-°F
Thermal Conductivity:	1 cal/sec-cm-°C = 241.9 Btu/hr-ft-°F
	1 watt/cm-°C = 57.79 Btu/hr-ft-°F
Heat flux:	1 watt/cm^2 = 3171 Btu/hr-ft^2
	1 cal/hr-cm^2 = 3.687 Btu/hr-ft^2

Appendix B: Selected Properties of Water

Fresh Water

Temperature °F	Density lbm/ft³	Specific Heat Btu/lbm-°F	Thermal Conductivity Btu/ft-hr-°F	Viscosity lbm/ft-sec	Pr
32	62.4	1.01	0.319	1.20×10^{-3}	13.7
40	62.4	1.00	0.325	1.04×10^{-3}	11.6
50	62.4	1.00	0.332	0.88×10^{-3}	9.55
60	62.3	0.999	0.340	0.76×10^{-3}	8.03
70	62.3	0.998	0.347	0.658×10^{-3}	6.82
80	62.2	0.998	0.353	0.578×10^{-3}	5.89
90	62.1	0.997	0.359	0.514×10^{-3}	5.13
100	62.0	0.998	0.364	0.458×10^{-3}	4.52
150	61.2	1.00	0.384	0.292×10^{-3}	2.74
200	60.1	1.00	0.394	0.205×10^{-3}	1.88

Sea Water (Salinity of sea water 3.5%)

Temperature °F	Density lbm/ft³	Specific Heat Btu/lbm-°F	Thermal Conductivity Btu/ft-hr-°F	Viscosity lbm/ft-sec	Pr
32	64.2			1.26×10^{-3}	
40	64.2			1.10×10^{-3}	
50	64.1			0.93×10^{-3}	
60	64.0			0.81×10^{-3}	
70	63.9			0.71×10^{-3}	
80	63.8			0.62×10^{-3}	
90	63.7			0.55×10^{-3}	

Appendix C: Selected Navy Dive Tables

NO-DECOMPRESSION LIMITS AND REPETITIVE GROUP DESIGNATION TABLE FOR NO-DECOMPRESSION AIR DIVES

Depth (feet)	No-decompression limits (min)	A	B	C	D	E	F	G	H	I	J	K	L	M	N	O
10		60	120	210	300											
15		35	70	110	160	225	350									
20		25	50	75	100	135	180	240	325							
25		20	35	55	75	100	125	160	195	245	315					
30		15	30	45	60	75	95	120	145	170	205	250	310			
35	310	5	15	25	40	50	60	80	100	120	140	160	190	220	270	310
40	200	5	15	25	30	40	50	70	80	100	110	130	150	170	200	
50	100		10	15	25	30	40	50	60	70	80	90	100			
60	60		10	15	20	25	30	40	50	55	60					
70	50		5	10	15	20	30	35	40	45	50					
80	40		5	10	15	20	25	30	35	40						
90	30		5	10	12	15	20	25	30							
100	25		5	7	10	15	20	22	25							
110	20			5	10	13	15	20								
120	15			5	10	12	15									
130	10			5	8	10										
140	10			5	7	10										
150	5			5												
160	5				5											
170	5				5											
180	5				5											
190	5				5											

RESIDUAL NITROGEN TIMETABLE FOR REPETITIVE AIR DIVES

*Dives following surface intervals of more than 12 hours are not repetitive dives. Use actual bottom times in the Standard Air Decompression Tables to compute decompression for such dives.

Repetitive group at the beginning of the surface interval

Start	Z	O	N	M	L	K	J	I	H	G	F	E	D	C	B	A
A																0:10 / 12:00*
B															0:10 / 2:10	2:11 / 12:00*
C														0:10 / 1:39	1:40 / 2:49	2:50 / 12:00*
D													0:10 / 1:09	1:10 / 2:38	2:39 / 5:48	5:49 / 12:00*
E												0:10 / 0:54	0:55 / 1:57	1:58 / 3:22	3:23 / 6:32	6:33 / 12:00*
F											0:10 / 0:45	0:46 / 1:29	1:30 / 2:28	2:29 / 3:57	3:58 / 7:05	7:06 / 12:00*
G										0:10 / 0:40	0:41 / 1:15	1:16 / 1:59	2:00 / 2:58	2:59 / 4:25	4:26 / 7:35	7:36 / 12:00*
H									0:10 / 0:36	0:37 / 1:06	1:07 / 1:41	1:42 / 2:23	2:24 / 3:20	3:21 / 4:49	4:50 / 7:59	8:00 / 12:00*
I								0:10 / 0:33	0:34 / 0:59	1:00 / 1:29	1:30 / 2:02	2:03 / 2:44	2:45 / 3:43	3:44 / 5:12	5:13 / 8:21	8:22 / 12:00*
J							0:10 / 0:31	0:32 / 0:54	0:55 / 1:19	1:20 / 1:47	1:48 / 2:20	2:21 / 3:04	3:05 / 4:02	4:03 / 5:40	5:41 / 8:40	8:41 / 12:00*
K						0:10 / 0:28	0:29 / 0:49	0:50 / 1:11	1:12 / 1:35	1:36 / 2:03	2:04 / 2:38	2:39 / 3:21	3:22 / 4:19	4:20 / 5:48	5:49 / 8:58	8:59 / 12:00*
L					0:10 / 0:26	0:27 / 0:45	0:46 / 1:04	1:05 / 1:25	1:26 / 1:49	1:50 / 2:19	2:20 / 2:53	2:54 / 3:36	3:37 / 4:35	4:36 / 6:02	6:03 / 9:12	9:13 / 12:00*
M				0:10 / 0:25	0:26 / 0:42	0:43 / 0:59	1:00 / 1:18	1:19 / 1:39	1:40 / 2:05	2:06 / 2:34	2:35 / 3:08	3:09 / 3:52	3:53 / 4:49	4:50 / 6:18	6:19 / 9:28	9:29 / 12:00*
N			0:10 / 0:24	0:25 / 0:39	0:40 / 0:54	0:55 / 1:11	1:12 / 1:30	1:31 / 1:53	1:54 / 2:18	2:19 / 2:47	2:48 / 3:22	3:23 / 4:04	4:05 / 5:03	5:04 / 6:32	6:33 / 9:43	9:44 / 12:00*
O		0:10 / 0:23	0:24 / 0:36	0:37 / 0:51	0:52 / 1:07	1:08 / 1:24	1:25 / 1:43	1:44 / 2:04	2:05 / 2:29	2:30 / 2:59	3:00 / 3:33	3:34 / 4:17	4:18 / 5:16	5:17 / 6:44	6:45 / 9:54	9:55 / 12:00*
Z	0:10 / 0:22	0:23 / 0:34	0:35 / 0:48	0:49 / 1:02	1:03 / 1:18	1:19 / 1:36	1:37 / 1:55	1:56 / 2:17	2:18 / 2:42	2:43 / 3:10	3:11 / 3:45	3:46 / 4:29	4:30 / 5:27	5:28 / 6:56	6:57 / 10:05	10:06 / 12:00*

NEW → GROUP DESIGNATION: Z O N M L K J I H G F E D C B A

REPETITIVE DIVE DEPTH	Z	O	N	M	L	K	J	I	H	G	F	E	D	C	B	A
40	257	241	213	187	161	138	116	101	87	73	61	49	37	25	17	7
50	169	160	142	124	111	99	87	76	66	56	47	38	29	21	13	6
60	122	117	107	97	88	79	70	61	52	44	36	30	24	17	11	5
70	100	96	87	80	72	64	57	50	43	37	31	26	20	15	9	4
80	84	80	73	68	61	54	48	43	38	32	28	23	18	13	8	4
90	73	70	64	58	53	47	43	38	33	29	24	20	16	11	7	3
100	64	62	57	52	48	43	38	34	30	26	22	18	14	10	7	3
110	57	55	51	47	42	38	34	31	27	24	20	16	13	10	6	3
120	52	50	46	43	39	35	32	28	25	21	18	15	12	9	6	3
130	46	44	40	38	35	31	28	25	22	19	16	13	11	8	6	3
140	42	40	38	35	32	29	26	23	20	18	15	12	10	7	5	2
150	40	38	35	32	30	27	24	22	19	17	14	12	9	7	5	2
160	37	36	33	31	28	26	23	20	18	16	13	11	9	6	4	2
170	35	34	31	29	26	24	22	19	17	15	13	10	8	6	4	2
180	32	31	29	27	25	22	20	18	16	14	12	10	8	6	4	2
190	31	30	28	26	24	21	19	17	15	13	11	10	8	6	4	2

RESIDUAL NITROGEN TIMES (MINUTES)

U. S· NAVY STANDARD AIR DECOMPRESSION TABLE

Depth (feet)	Bottom time (min)	Time first stop (min:sec)	Decompression stops (feet) 50	40	30	20	10	Total ascent (min:sec)	Repetitive group
40	200						0	0:40	*
	210	0:30					2	2:40	N
	230	0:30					7	7:40	N
	250	0:30					11	11:40	O
	270	0:30					15	15:40	O
	300	0:30					19	19:40	Z
	360	0:30					23	23:40	**
	480	0:30					41	41:40	**
	720	0:30					69	69:40	**
50	100						0	0:50	*
	110	0:40					3	3:50	L
	120	0:40					5	5:50	M
	140	0:40					10	10:50	M
	160	0:40					21	21:50	N
	180	0:40					29	29:50	O
	200	0:40					35	35:50	O
	220	0:40					40	40:50	Z
	240	0:40					47	47:50	Z
60	60						0	1:00	*
	70	0:50					2	3:00	K
	80	0:50					7	8:00	L
	100	0:50					14	15:00	M
	120	0:50					26	27:00	N
	140	0:50					39	40:00	O
	160	0:50					48	49:00	Z
	180	0:50					56	57:00	Z
	200	0:40				1	69	71:00	Z
	240	0:40				2	79	82:00	**
	360	0:40				20	119	140:00	**
	480	0:40				44	148	193:00	**
	720	0:40				78	187	266:00	**
70	50						0	1:10	*
	60	1:00					8	9:10	K
	70	1:00					14	15:10	L
	80	1:00					18	19:10	M
	90	1:00					23	24:10	N
	100	1:00					33	34:10	N
	110	0:50				2	41	44:10	O
	120	0:50				4	47	52:10	O
	130	0:50				6	52	59:10	O
	140	0:50				8	56	65:10	Z
	150	0:50				8	61	71:10	Z
	160	0:50				13	72	86:10	Z
	170	0:50				19	79	99:10	Z

* See No Decompression Table for repetitive groups
**Repetitive dives may not follow exceptional exposure dives

U. S· NAVY STANDARD AIR DECOMPRESSION TABLE

Depth (feet)	Bottom time (min)	Time first stop (min:sec)	Decompression stops (feet)					Total ascent (min:sec)	Repetitive group
			50	40	30	20	10		
80	40						0	1:20	*
	50	1:10					10	11:20	K
	60	1:10					17	18:20	L
	70	1:10					23	24:20	M
	80	1:00				2	31	34:20	N
	90	1:00				7	39	47:20	N
	100	1:00				11	46	58:20	O
	110	1:00				13	53	67:20	O
	120	1:00				17	56	74:20	Z
	130	1:00				19	63	83:20	Z
	140	1:00				26	69	96:20	Z
	150	1:00				32	77	110:20	Z
	180	1:00				35	85	121:20	**
	240	0:50			6	52	120	179:20	**
	360	0:50			29	90	160	280:20	**
	480	0:50			59	107	187	354:20	**
	720	0:40		17	108	142	187	455:20	**
90	30						0	1:30	*
	40	1:20					7	8:30	J
	50	1:20					18	19:30	L
	60	1:20					25	26:30	M
	70	1:10				7	30	38:30	N
	80	1:10				13	40	54:30	N
	90	1:10				18	48	67:30	O
	100	1:10				21	54	76:30	Z
	110	1:10				24	61	86:30	Z
	120	1:10				32	68	101:30	Z
	130	1:00			5	36	74	116:30	Z
100	25						0	1:40	*
	30	1:30					3	4:40	I
	40	1:30					15	16:40	K
	50	1:20				2	24	27:40	L
	60	1:20				9	28	38:40	N
	70	1:20				17	39	57:40	O
	80	1:20				23	48	72:40	O
	90	1:10			3	23	57	84:40	Z
	100	1:10			7	23	66	97:40	Z
	110	1:10			10	34	72	117:40	Z
	120	1:10			12	41	78	132:40	Z
	180	1:00		1	29	53	118	202:40	**
	240	1:00		14	42	84	142	283:40	**
	360	0:50	2	42	73	111	187	416:40	**
	480	0:50	21	61	91	142	187	503:40	**
	720	0:50	55	106	122	142	187	613:40	**
110	20						0	1:50	*
	25	1:40					3	4:50	H
	30	1:40					7	8:50	J
	40	1:30				2	21	24:50	L
	50	1:30				8	26	35:50	M
	60	1:30				18	36	55:50	N
	70	1:20			1	23	48	73:50	O
	80	1:20			7	23	57	88:50	Z
	90	1:20			12	30	64	107:50	Z
	100	1:20			15	37	72	125:50	Z

* **See No Decompression Table for repetitive groups**
** **Repetitive dives may not follow exceptional exposure dives**

U. S. NAVY STANDARD AIR DECOMPRESSION TABLE

Depth (feet)	Bottom time (min)	Time to first stop (min:sec)	Decompression stops (feet)							Total ascent (min:sec)	Repetitive group
			70	60	50	40	30	20	10		
120	15								0	2:00	*
	20	1:50							2	4:00	H
	25	1:50							6	8:00	I
	30	1:50							14	16:00	J
	40	1:40						5	25	32:00	L
	50	1:40						15	31	48:00	N
	60	1:30					2	22	45	71:00	O
	70	1:30					9	23	55	89:00	O
	80	1:30					15	27	63	107:00	Z
	90	1:30					19	37	74	132:00	Z
	100	1:30					23	45	80	150:00	Z
	120	1:20				10	19	47	98	176:00	**
	180	1:10			5	27	37	76	137	284:00	**
	240	1:10			23	35	60	97	179	396:00	**
	360	1:00		18	45	64	93	142	187	551:00	**
	480	0:50	3	41	64	93	122	142	187	654:00	**
	720	0:50	32	74	100	114	122	142	187	773:00	**
130	10								0	2:10	*
	15	2:00							1	3:10	F
	20	2:00							4	6:10	H
	25	2:00							10	12:10	J
	30	1:50						3	18	23:10	M
	40	1:50						10	25	37:10	N
	50	1:40					3	21	37	63:10	O
	60	1:40					9	23	52	86:10	Z
	70	1:40					16	24	61	103:10	Z
	80	1:30				3	19	35	72	131:10	Z
	90	1:30				8	19	45	80	154:10	Z

Depth (feet)	Bottom time (min)	Time to first stop (min:sec)	Decompression stops (feet)									Total ascent (min:sec)	Repetitive group
			90	80	70	60	50	40	30	20	10		
140	10										0	2:20	*
	15	2:10									2	4:20	G
	20	2:10									6	8:20	I
	25	2:00								2	14	18:20	J
	30	2:00								5	21	28:20	K
	40	1:50							2	16	26	46:20	N
	50	1:50							6	24	44	76:20	O
	60	1:50							16	23	56	97:20	Z
	70	1:40						4	19	32	68	125:20	Z
	80	1:40						10	23	41	79	155:20	Z
	90	1:30					2	14	18	42	88	166:20	**
	120	1:30					12	14	36	56	120	240:20	**
	180	1:20				10	26	32	54	94	168	366:20	**
	240	1:10			8	28	34	50	78	124	187	511:20	**
	360	1:00		9	32	42	64	84	122	142	187	684:20	**
	480	1:00		31	44	59	100	114	122	142	187	801:20	**
	720	0:50	16	56	88	97	100	114	122	142	187	924:20	**

* See No Decompression Table for repetitive groups
**Repetitive dives may not follow exceptional exposure dives

U.S. NAVY STANDARD AIR DECOMPRESSION TABLE

150 / 160

Depth (feet)	Bottom time (min)	Time to first stop (min:sec)	90	80	70	60	50	40	30	20	10	Total ascent (min:sec)	Repetitive group
						Decompression stops (feet)							
150	5										0	2:30	C
	10	2:20									1	3:30	E
	15	2:20									3	5:30	G
	20	2:10								2	7	11:30	H
	25	2:10								4	17	23:30	K
	30	2:10								8	24	34:30	L
	40	2:00							5	19	33	59:30	N
	50	2:00							12	23	51	88:30	O
	60	1:50						3	19	26	62	112:30	Z
	70	1:50						11	19	39	75	146:30	Z
	80	1:40					1	17	19	50	84	173:30	Z
160	5										0	2:40	D
	10	2:30									1	3:40	F
	15	2:20								1	4	7:40	H
	20	2:20								3	11	16:40	J
	25	2:20								7	20	29:40	K
	30	2:10							2	11	25	40:40	M
	40	2:10							7	23	39	71:40	N
	50	2:00						2	16	23	55	98:40	Z
	60	2:00						9	19	33	69	132:40	Z
	70	1:50					1	17	22	44	80	166:40	Z

170 / 180

Depth (feet)	Bottom time (min)	Time to first stop (min:sec)	110	100	90	80	70	60	50	40	30	20	10	Total ascent (min:sec)	Repetitive group
								Decompression stops (feet)								
170	5												0	2:50	D
	10	2:40											2	4:50	F
	15	2:30										2	5	9:50	H
	20	2:30										4	15	21:50	J
	25	2:20									2	7	23	34:50	L
	30	2:20									4	13	26	45:50	M
	40	2:10								1	10	23	45	81:50	O
	50	2:10								5	18	23	61	109:50	Z
	60	2:00							2	15	22	37	74	152:50	Z
	70	2:00							8	17	19	51	86	183:50	Z
	90	1:50						12	12	14	34	52	120	246:50	**
	120	1:30				2	10	12	18	32	42	82	156	356:50	**
	180	1:20			4	10	22	28	34	50	78	120	187	535:50	**
	240	1:20			18	24	30	42	50	70	116	142	187	681:50	**
	360	1:10		22	34	40	52	60	98	114	122	142	187	873:50	**
	480	1:00	14	40	42	56	91	97	100	114	122	142	187	1007:50	**
180	5												0	3:00	D
	10	2:50											3	6:00	F
	15	2:40										3	6	12:00	I
	20	2:30									1	5	17	26:00	K
	25	2:30									3	10	24	40:00	L
	30	2:30									6	17	27	53:00	N
	40	2:20								3	14	23	50	93:00	O
	50	2:10							2	9	19	30	65	128:00	Z
	60	2:10							5	16	19	44	81	168:00	Z

* See No Decompression Table for repetitive groups
**Repetitive dives may not follow exceptional exposure dives

U.S. NAVY STANDARD AIR DECOMPRESSION TABLE

Depth 190 (feet)

Bottom time (min)	Time to first stop (min:sec)	110	100	90	80	70	60	50	40	30	20	10	Total ascent (min:sec)	Repetitive group
5												0	3:10	D
10	2:50										1	3	7:10	G
15	2:50										4	7	14:10	I
20	2:40									2	6	20	31:10	K
25	2:40									5	11	25	44:10	M
30	2:30								1	8	19	32	63:10	N
40	2:30								8	14	23	55	103:10	O
50	2:20							4	13	22	33	72	147:10	Z
60	2:20							10	17	19	50	84	183:10	Z

Depth 200 (feet)

Bottom time (min)	Time to first stop (min:sec)	130	120	110	100	90	80	70	60	50	40	30	20	10	Total ascent (min:sec)
5	3:10													1	4:20
10	3:00												1	4	8:20
15	2:50											1	4	10	18:20
20	2:50											3	7	27	40:20
25	2:50											7	14	25	49:20
30	2:40										2	9	22	37	73:20
40	2:30									2	8	17	23	59	112:20
50	2:30									6	16	22	39	75	161:20
60	2:20								2	13	17	24	51	89	199:20
90	1:50					1	10	10	12	12	30	38	74	134	324:20
120	1:40				6	10	10	10	24	28	40	64	98	180	473:20
180	1:20		1	10	10	18	24	24	42	48	70	106	142	187	685:20
240	1:20		6	20	24	24	36	42	54	68	114	122	142	187	842:20
360	1:10	12	22	36	40	44	56	82	98	100	114	122	142	187	1058:20

Depth 210 (feet)

Bottom time (min)	Time to first stop (min:sec)	130	120	110	100	90	80	70	60	50	40	30	20	10	Total ascent (min:sec)
5	3:20													1	4:30
10	3:10												2	4	9:30
15	3:00											1	5	13	22:30
20	3:00											4	10	23	40:30
25	2:50										2	7	17	27	56:30
30	2:50										4	9	24	41	81:30
40	2:40									4	9	19	26	63	124:30
50	2:30								1	9	17	19	45	80	174:30

Depth 220 (feet)

Bottom time (min)	Time to first stop (min:sec)	130	120	110	100	90	80	70	60	50	40	30	20	10	Total ascent (min:sec)
5	3:30													2	5:40
10	3:20												2	5	10:40
15	3:10											2	5	16	26:40
20	3:00										1	3	11	24	42:40
25	3:00										3	8	19	33	66:40
30	2:50									1	7	10	23	47	91:40
40	2:50									6	12	22	29	68	140:40
50	2:40								3	12	17	18	51	86	190:40

U. S. NAVY STANDARD AIR DECOMPRESSION TABLE

Depth (feet)	Bottom time (min)	Time to first stop (min:sec)	130	120	110	100	90	80	70	60	50	40	30	20	10	Total ascent time (min:sec)
230	5	3:40													2	5:50
	10	3:20											1	2	6	12:50
	15	3:20											3	6	18	30:50
	20	3:10										2	5	12	26	48:50
	25	3:10										4	8	22	37	74:50
	30	3:00									2	8	12	23	51	99:50
	40	2:50								1	7	15	22	34	74	156:50
	50	2:50								5	14	16	24	51	89	202:50
240	5	3:50													2	6:00
	10	3:30											1	3	6	14:00
	15	3:30											4	6	21	35:00
	20	3:20										3	6	15	25	53:00
	25	3:10									1	4	9	24	40	82:00
	30	3:10									4	8	15	22	56	109:00
	40	3:00								3	7	17	22	39	75	167:00
	50	2:50							1	8	15	16	29	51	94	218:00
250	5	3:50												1	2	7:10
	10	3:40											1	4	7	16:10
	15	3:30										1	4	7	22	38:10
	20	3:30										4	7	17	27	59:10
	25	3:20									2	7	10	24	45	92:10
	30	3:20									6	7	17	23	59	116:10
	40	3:10								5	9	17	19	45	79	178:10
	60	2:40					4	10	10	10	12	22	36	64	126	298:10
	90	2:10		8	10	10	10	10	10	28	28	44	68	98	186	514:10
260	5	4:00												1	2	7:20
	10	3:50											2	4	9	19:20
	15	3:40										2	4	10	22	42:20
	20	3:30								1	4	7	20	31		67:20
	25	3:30									3	8	11	23	50	99:20
	30	3:20								2	6	8	19	26	61	126:20
	40	3:10							1	6	11	16	19	49	84	190:20
270	5	4:10												1	3	8:30
	10	4:00											2	5	11	22:30
	15	3:50										3	4	11	24	46:30
	20	3:40									2	3	9	21	35	74:30
	25	3:30								2	3	8	13	23	53	106:30
	30	3:30								3	6	12	22	27	64	138:30
	40	3:20							5	6	11	17	22	51	88	204:30

U. S. NAVY STANDARD AIR DECOMPRESSION TABLE

Depth (feet)	Bottom time (min)	Time to first stop (min:sec)	130	120	110	100	90	80	70	60	50	40	30	20	10	Total ascent time (min:sec)
280	5	4:20												2	2	8:40
	10	4:00									1	2		5	13	25:40
	15	3:50									1	3	4	11	26	49:40
	20	3:50									3	4	8	23	39	81:40
	25	3:40								2	5	7	16	23	56	113:40
	30	3:30							1	3	7	13	22	30	70	150:40
	40	3:20						1	6	6	13	17	27	51	93	218:40
290	5	4:30												2	3	9:50
	10	4:10									1	3	5	16		29:50
	15	4:00									1	3	6	12	26	52:50
	20	4:00									3	7	9	23	43	89:50
	25	3:50								3	5	8	17	23	60	120:50
	30	3:40							1	5	6	16	22	36	72	162:50
	40	3:30						3	5	7	15	16	32	51	95	228:50
300	5	4:40												3	3	11:00
	10	4:20										1	3	6	17	32:00
	15	4:10									2	3	6	15	26	57:00
	20	4:00								2	3	7	10	23	47	97:00
	25	3:50							1	3	6	8	19	26	61	129:00
	30	3:50							2	5	7	17	22	39	75	172:00
	40	3:40						4	6	9	15	17	34	51	90	231:00
	60	3:00		4	10	10	10	10	10	14	28	32	50	90	187	460:00

Extreme exposures—250 and 300 ft

Depth (ft)	Bottom time (min)	Time to first stop (min:sec)	200	190	180	170	160	150	140	130	120	110	100	90	80	70	60	50	40	30	20	10	Total ascent time (min:sec)
250	120	1:50							5	10	10	10	10	16	24	24	36	48	64	94	142	187	684:10
	180	1:30					4	8	8	10	22	24	24	32	42	44	60	84	114	122	142	187	931:10
	240	1:30					9	14	21	22	22	40	40	42	56	76	98	100	114	122	142	187	1109:10
300	90	2:20					3	8	8	10	10	10	10	16	24	24	34	48	64	90	142	187	693:00
	120	2:00			4	8	8	8	8	10	14	24	24	24	34	42	58	66	102	122	142	187	890:00
	180	1:40	6	8	8	8	14	20	21	21	28	40	40	48	56	82	98	100	114	122	142	187	1168:00

SURFACE DECOMPRESSION TABLE USING AIR

Depth (ft)	Bottom time (min)	Time to first stop (min:sec)	Time at water stops (min)			Surface Interval	Chamber stops (air) (min)		Total ascent time (min:sec)
			30	20	10		20	10	
40	230	0:30			3			7	14:30
	250	:30			3			11	18:30
	270	:30			3			15	22:30
	300	:30			3			19	26:30
50	120	:40			3			5	12:40
	140	:40			3			10	17:40
	160	:40			3			21	28:40
	180	:40			3			29	36:40
	200	:40			3			35	42:40
	220	:40			3			40	47:40
	240	:40			3			47	54:40
60	80	:50			3			7	14:50
	100	:50			3			14	21:50
	120	:50			3			26	33:50
	140	:50			3			39	46:50
	160	:50			3			48	55:50
	180	:50			3			56	63:50
	200	:40		3			3	69	80:10
70	60	1:00			3			8	16:00
	70	1:00			3			14	22:00
	80	1:00			3			18	26:00
	90	1:00			3			23	31:00
	100	1:00			3			33	41:00
	110	:50		3			3	41	52:20
	120	:50		3			4	47	59:20
	130	:50		3			6	52	66:20
	140	:50		3			8	56	72:20
	150	:50		3			9	61	78:20
	160	:50		3			13	72	93:20
	170	:50		3			19	79	106:20
80	50	1:10			3			10	18:10
	60	1:10			3			17	25:10
	70	1:10			3			23	31:10
	80	1:00		3			3	31	42:30
	90	1:00		3			7	39	54:30
	100	1:00		3			11	46	65:30
	110	1:00		3			13	53	74:30
	120	1:00		3			17	56	81:30
	130	1:00		3			19	63	90:30
	140	1:00		26			26	69	126:30
	150	1:00		32			32	77	146:30
90	40	1:20			3			7	15:20
	50	1:20			3			18	26:20
	60	1:20			3			25	33:20
	70	1:10		3			7	30	45:40
	80	1:10		13			13	40	71:40
	90	1:10		18			18	48	89:40
	100	1:10		21			21	54	101:40
	110	1:10		24			24	61	114:40
	120	1:10		32			32	68	137:40
	130	1:00	5	36			36	74	156:40

Surface Interval column (vertical text): NOT TO EXCEED 5 MINUTES — TOTAL TIME FROM LAST WATER STOP TO FIRST CHAMBER STOP

SURFACE DECOMPRESSION TABLE USING AIR

Depth (ft)	Bottom time (min)	Time to first stop (min:sec)	Time at water stops (min)					Surface Interval	Chamber stops (air) (min)		Total ascent time (min:sec)
			50	40	30	20	10		20	10	
100	40	1:30					3			15	23:30
	50	1:20				3			3	24	35:50
	60	1:20				3			9	28	45:50
	70	1:20				3			17	39	64:50
	80	1:20				23			23	48	99:50
	90	1:10			3	23			23	57	111:50
	100	1:10			7	23			23	66	124:50
	110	1:10			10	34			34	72	155:50
	120	1:10			12	41			41	78	177:50
110	30	1:40					3			7	15:40
	40	1:30				3			3	21	33:00
	50	1:30				3			8	26	43:00
	60	1:30				18			18	36	78:00
	70	1:20			1	23			23	48	101:00
	80	1:20			7	23			23	57	116:00
	90	1:20			12	30			30	64	142:00
	100	1:20			15	37			37	72	167:00
120	25	1:50					3			6	14:50
	30	1:50					3			14	22:50
	40	1:40				3			5	25	39:10
	50	1:40				15			15	31	67:10
	60	1:30			2	22			22	45	97:10
	70	1:30			9	23			23	55	116:10
	80	1:30			15	27			27	63	138:10
	90	1:30			19	37			37	74	173:10
	100	1:30			23	45			45	80	189:10
130	25	2:00					3			10	19:00
	30	1:50				3			3	18	30:20
	40	1:50				10			10	25	51:20
	50	1:40			3	21			21	37	88:20
	60	1:40			9	23			23	52	113:20
	70	1:40			16	24			24	61	131:20
	80	1:30		3	19	35			35	72	170:20
	90	1:30		8	19	45			45	80	203:20
140	20	2:10					3			6	15:10
	25	2:00				3			3	14	26:30
	30	2:00				5			5	21	37:30
	40	1:50			2	16			16	26	66:30
	50	1:50			6	24			24	44	104:30
	60	1:50			16	23			23	56	124:30
	70	1:40		4	19	32			32	68	161:30
	80	1:40		10	23	41			41	79	200:30
150	20	2:10				3			3	7	19:40
	25	2:10				4			4	17	31:40
	30	2:10				8			8	24	46:40
	40	2:00			5	19			19	33	82:40
	50	2:00			12	23			23	51	115:40
	60	1:50		3	19	26			26	62	142:40
	70	1:50		11	19	39			39	75	189:40
	80	1:40	1	17	19	50			50	84	227:40

TOTAL TIME FROM LAST WATER STOP TO FIRST CHAMBER STOP NOT TO EXCEED 5 MINUTES

SURFACE DECOMPRESSION TABLE USING OXYGEN

Depth (feet)	Bottom time (min)	Time to first stop or surface (min:sec)	Time (min) breathing air at water stops (ft)				Surface interval	Time at 40-foot chamber stop (min) on oxygen	Surface	Total decompression time (min:sec)
			60	50	40	30				
70	52	2:48	0	0	0	0		0		2:48
	90	2:48	0	0	0	0		15		23:48
	120	2:48	0	0	0	0		23		31:48
	150	2:28	0	0	0	0		31		39:48
	180	2:48	0	0	0	0		39		47:48
80	40	3:12	0	0	0	0		0		3:12
	70	3:12	0	0	0	0		14		23:12
	85	3:12	0	0	0	0		20		29:12
	100	3:12	0	0	0	0		26		35:12
	115	3:12	0	0	0	0		31		40:12
	130	3:12	0	0	0	0		37		46:12
	150	3:12	0	0	0	0		44		53:12
90	32	3:36	0	0	0	0		0		3:36
	60	3:36	0	0	0	0		14		23:36
	70	3:36	0	0	0	0		20		29:36
	80	3:36	0	0	0	0		25		34:36
	90	3:36	0	0	0	0		30		39:36
	100	3:36	0	0	0	0		34		43:36
	110	3:36	0	0	0	0		39		48:36
	120	3:36	0	0	0	0		43		52:36
	130	3:36	0	0	0	0		48		57:36
100	26	4:00	0	0	0	0		0		4:00
	50	4:00	0	0	0	0		14		24:00
	60	4:00	0	0	0	0		20		30:00
	70	4:00	0	0	0	0		26		36:00
	80	4:00	0	0	0	0		32		42:00
	90	4:00	0	0	0	0		38		48:00
	100	4:00	0	0	0	0		44		54:00
	110	4:00	0	0	0	0		49		59:00
	120	2:48	0	0	0	3		53		65:48
110	22	4:24	0	0	0	0		0		4:24
	40	4:24	0	0	0	0		12		22:24
	50	4:24	0	0	0	0		19		29:24
	60	4:24	0	0	0	0		26		36:24
	70	4:24	0	0	0	0		33		43:24
	80	3:12	0	0	0	1		40		51:12
	90	3:12	0	0	0	2		46		58:12
	100	3:12	0	0	0	5		51		66:12
	110	3:12	0	0	0	12		54		76:12
120	18	4:48	0	0	0	0		0		4:48
	30	4:48	0	0	0	0		9		19:48
	40	4:48	0	0	0	0		16		26:48
	50	4:48	0	0	0	0		24		34:48
	60	3:36	0	0	0	2		32		44:36
	70	3:36	0	0	0	4		39		53:36
	80	3:36	0	0	0	5		46		61:36
	90	3:12	0	0	3	7		51		72:12
	100	3:12	0	0	6	15		54		86:12

Surface interval column: TOTAL TIME FROM LAST WATER STOP TO FIRST CHAMBER STOP NOT TO EXCEED 5 MINUTES

Surface column: 2-MINUTE ASCENT FROM 40 FEET IN CHAMBER TO SURFACE WHILE BREATHING OXYGEN

SURFACE DECOMPRESSION TABLE USING OXYGEN

Depth (feet)	Bottom time (min)	Time to first stop or surface (min:sec)	Time (min) breathing air at water stops (ft)				Surface interval	Time at 40-foot chamber stop (min) on oxygen	Surface	Total decompression time (min:sec)
			60	50	40	30				
130	15	5:12	0	0	0	0		0		5:12
	30	5:12	0	0	0	0		12		23:12
	40	5:12	0	0	0	0		21		32:12
	50	4:00	0	0	0	3		29		43:00
	60	4:00	0	0	0	5		37		53:00
	70	4:00	0	0	0	7		45		63:00
	80	3:36	0	0	6	7		51		75:36
	90	3:36	0	0	10	12		56		89:36
140	13	5:36	0	0	0	0		0		5:36
	25	5:36	0	0	0	0		11		22:36
	30	5:36	0	0	0	0		15		26:36
	35	5:36	0	0	0	0		20		31:36
	40	4:24	0	0	0	2		24		37:24
	45	4:24	0	0	0	4		29		44:24
	50	4:24	0	0	0	6		33		50:24
	55	4:24	0	0	0	7		38		56:24
	60	4:24	0	0	0	8		43		62:24
	65	4:00	0	0	3	7		48		70:00
	70	3:36	0	2	7	7		51		79:36
150	11	6:00	0	0	0	0		0		6:00
	25	6:00	0	0	0	0		13		25:00
	30	6:00	0	0	0	0		18		30:00
	35	4:48	0	0	0	4		23		38:48
	40	4:24	0	0	3	6		27		48:24
	45	4:24	0	0	5	7		33		57:24
	50	4:00	0	2	5	8		38		66:00
	55	3:36	2	5	9	4		44		77:36
160	9	6:24	0	0	0	0		0		6:24
	20	6:24	0	0	0	0		11		23:24
	25	6:24	0	0	0	0		16		28:24
	30	5:12	0	0	0	2		21		35:12
	35	4:48	0	0	4	6		26		48:48
	40	4:24	0	3	5	8		32		61:24
	45	4:00	3	4	8	6		38		73:00
170	7	6:48	0	0	0	0		0		6:48
	20	6:48	0	0	0	0		13		25:48
	25	6:48	0	0	0	0		19		31:48
	30	5:12	0	0	3	5		23		44:12
	35	4:48	0	4	4	7		29		57:48
	40	4:24	4	4	8	6		36		72:24

Surface interval column note: TOTAL TIME FROM LAST WATER STOP TO FIRST CHAMBER STOP NOT TO EXCEED 5 MINUTES

Surface column note: 2-MINUTE ASCENT FROM 40 FEET IN CHAMBER TO SURFACE WHILE BREATHING OXYGEN

Index